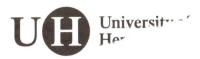

University of
He

College L

Lear

Research Practice

ii

Research Practice

Michael S. Lewis-Beck
editor

International Handbooks of Quantitative Applications
in the Social Sciences
Volume 6

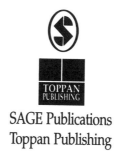

SAGE Publications
Toppan Publishing

For information address:

SAGE Publications Ltd.
6 Bonhill Street
London EC2A 4PU
United Kingdom

SAGE Publications, Inc.
2455 Teller Road
Thousand Oaks, California 91320
United States

SAGE Publications India Pvt. Ltd.
M-32 Market
Greater Kailash I
New Delhi 110 048 India

Printed in Singapore

British Library Cataloguing in Publication Data

Main entry under title:

Research Practice.—(International
Handbooks of Quantitative Applications in
the Social Sciences; Vol. 6)
   I. Lewis-Beck, Michael S. II. Series
   300.72
   ISBN 0-8039-5432-8

94 95 96 97 98 10 9 8 7 6 5 4 3 2 1

Sage Production Editor : Susan McElroy

CONTENTS

EDITOR'S INTRODUCTION

The methodological literature of the social sciences preoccupies itself with techniques of data analysis. Researchers fret over proper tests, indices, and estimations. While such concerns are of fundamental importance, they "put the cart before the horse." That is, before analysis can occur, the data must be gathered. Less has been written about this *sine qua non,* perhaps because it can appear something of an art. Fortunately, this volume shows that there is much of a systematic nature to be learned about research practice in the nonexperimental social sciences. (On experimental research, see our *International Handbook,* Volume 3.)

Quantitative work begins with empirical observation—an anthropologist records certain interactions in the village market, a sociologist conducts a public opinion survey, an economist gathers time series of macroeconomic indicators from government reports, an historian sorts through police reports of arrestees in a nineteenth century rebellion. Examples could be multiplied. In each, the investigator gathers data to answer research questions. How do they do it? More precisely, how do they do it in such a way that the data are of quality, offering the promise of answers?

In a rare paper, Bourque and Clark go "behind the scenes" of processing data to reveal the essential steps from collection to analysis. They illustrate the process by laying bear the decisions made in their own project, based on sample surveys of residents in two communities that had experienced earthquakes. The tasks of questionnaire development, interviewer training, computerized data entry, preliminary data preparation, and archiving are all helpfully described. The student gains a vital appreciation for the decision-making process that goes into any serious research effort. By way of summary, the authors provide a handy checklist for study documentation, a review of the care that must be exercised at each stage prior to analysis.

Converse and Presser, in the second paper, focus specifically on the construction of good survey questions. In an engaging manner, they write about the basic issues. How simple should an item be? How general? Is it better to have open-ended or closed-ended? What about a "no opinion" category? Are forced-choice items to be preferred over agree-disagree statements? What should the order of the questions be? How should a pretest be conducted? These, and many other, applied concerns are addressed by these leading scientists, drawing on their vast field experience and substantial experimental evidence.

In the beginning days of survey research, items were routinely administered by interviewers in face-to-face situations. Face-to-face interviews have been replaced to a large extent by telephone interviews, at least when virtually all the relevant survey population have telephones. Moreover, by the 1980s much of this was computer-assisted telephone interviewing (CATI), a technique clearly explicated in the third paper. Herein, Saris demonstrates how computer-assisted data collection (CADAC) in general can be used to replace pencil-and-paper questionnaires and even the interviewers themselves. Moreover, while Saris discusses potential advantages of CADAC, such as lowered per interview cost and increased data quality, he also notes possible disadvantages of this mode of data collection. His last sections, which offer guidelines on questionnaire design and computer programs for CADAC, seem especially valuable to would-be practitioners.

Responses to survey items, at least open-ended ones, lend themselves to content analysis, the data-gathering technique of the fourth paper, by Weber. The text of open-ended responses, say to an item such as °Discuss the most important problems facing the nation today" could be ordered into exhaustive categories, and the responses in each category counted. The analyst might then conclude, for example, that 43 percent of those surveyed mentioned "unemployment" as a "most important problem." Of course, content analysis—that is, the systematic classification of text—need not confine itself to open-ended survey responses. It can be applied as well to speeches, stories, documents, reports, indeed to any written material of research interest. To pursue the "unemployment" example further, suppose an American political scientist theorizes that the President's popularity goes down the more often the media reports on unemployment conditions. He or she might attempt a key-word-in-context (KWIC) computer-search of *New York Times* front-page stories, which could indicate the appearances of the key word "unemployment," along with the sentences around that key word (thus presenting the context of its mention). Such sophisticated procedures, and the computer software that makes them possible, are ably evaluated by Weber.

The last paper usefully reminds us of data sources (beyond surveys) that are published, and therefore available in libraries, archives, and public or private bureaus. Classic examples are census or economic data released by government. However, another large and growing source is data stored by individual researchers in member-accessible banks, such as the Inter-University Consortium for Political and Social Research (ICPSR) at the University of Michigan, or the European Consortium for Political Research (ECPR) at the University of Essex. In more and more nations, similar data banks are being established, and local investigators may find them well worth exploring.

Published, readily obtainable finished data are an invaluable resource, especially to researchers who chose not, or who are not able, to initiate an original data collection. However, published data may not be valid, perhaps due to poor sampling, changing definitions, improper standardization, clerical mistakes, or official corrections. Jacob sagely teaches us that, like survey data, these published data "are the consequence of one person asking questions of someone else." When considered in that light, it becomes obvious that it simply cannot be taken for granted that a published data-set is essentially error-free. Instead, following the tips of Jacob, we first establish its integrity. That done, we move with confidence to the challenges and rewards of the data-analysis stage.

—Michael S. Lewis-Beck
Series Editor

PROCESSING DATA   **PART I**
The Survey Example

LINDA B. BOURQUE

VIRGINIA A. CLARK

1. INTRODUCTION TO DATA PROCESSING

Data processing is like the backstage of a theater. It is rarely seen and frequently ignored, even by researchers. Few textbooks explain it, and instructors typically give it only passing comment. Yet, just as what goes on behind the scenes greatly contributes to the quality of a stage production, data processing critically affects an investigator's ability to carry out reliable, valid research.

In their haste to test hypotheses, researchers often do a slipshod or incomplete job of data processing. As a result, they may have to process data over and over again to put it into usable form. Such wasted effort eats up time and money budgeted for other things. In the worst cases, researchers may never get their data into a usable form such that their results can be trusted.

In this book, we will explain systematically how to perform data processing using today's technology. The term *data processing* commonly refers to converting verbal or written information into machine-readable data. Under this definition, data processing includes data coding, entering coded data into a computer, verifying data, and conducting range and consistency checks on data files. However, we prefer a broader definition. For us, data processing starts with selecting a data collection strategy and ends when data transformations are complete. This definition includes the following:

- developing response categories for precoded and open-ended questions, and incorporating the categories into the data collection instrument
- collecting the data
- creating data files that can be used by statistical packages such as the Statistical Package for the Social Sciences (SPSS), the Statistical Analysis System (SAS), or BMDP (a program developed for biomedical data)
- transforming data into variables useful for analysis
- documenting all aspects of the study, including the rationale and specifics of coding decisions and transformations

1

All these steps are not covered in equal detail in this volume. Readers who wish further information should refer to the pertinent references provided. This book can be used as a textbook for a course in data processing or as a reference by persons directing or performing data processing.

To set the stage for the chapters that follow: In the remainder of this chapter we briefly discuss what must be considered in choosing a data collection technique, and how this choice influences data processing. Chapter 2 describes the creation of response categories for both precoded and postcoded data. Chapter 3 discusses methods of ensuring accurate data collection. Chapter 4 outlines how data entry and management are combined to create a documented, computer-readable data file. Chapter 5 provides an overview of data transformations used to prepare data for analysis, and of ways to deal with missing data. Chapter 5 also includes a brief discussion of how to evaluate the adequacy of a scale. Chapter 6 discusses the documentation of data processing.

Overview of Data Collection Procedures

Data about people, their institutions, and their activities can be collected *directly*, using questionnaires, interviews, or direct observation, or *indirectly*, from written or electronic records and documents. The method selected is determined by the nature and content of questions that researchers wish to answer, available resources, and accessibility of potential subjects.

QUESTIONNAIRES

Questionnaires are used to collect data that are unavailable in written records or cannot be readily observed. This might include information about attitudes, opinions, and past, present, or anticipated behavior. The *major disadvantage* to the use of questionnaires is that the reliability and validity of data collected depend upon respondents' memories and forthrightness. (See Chapter 3 for a discussion of procedures that can be used to reduce bias and enhance the accuracy of data collection.) Questionnaires can be used only when respondents are available and willing to participate as research subjects. Questionnaires can be filled out by respondents or administered as part of face-to-face or telephone interviews.

In-Person and Telephone Interviews. There are *major advantages* to using interviews: Researchers can collect more information, and more complex information, from more subjects; based upon the requirements of the study, interviewers can select respondents and control the order in which data are obtained; and "skip patterns" can be set up (see Chapters 2, 4, and 5) to tailor questionnaires to respondents with different experiences, opinions, or attitudes. The cost of training, paying, and supervising interviewers is the *major disadvantage* of both in-person and telephone interviews. Telephone interviews are less costly than face-to-face interviews, but they restrict the pool of subjects to those who live in households with phones. Since interviews allow for longer and more complex data collection, *data processing* of interviews is likely to take longer and to cost more. The volume of data collected for each respondent may vary widely when skip patterns are used to allow for differences among respondents. This creates special challenges during data entry and processing. On the other hand, the use of interviewers can reduce the amount of unexplained missing data (see Chapter 5). The increased availability of computer-assisted telephone interviewing (CATI) and computer-assisted personal interviewing (CAPI) can greatly simplify data entry and the data processing that precedes analysis (see Aday, 1989).

Self-Administered Questionnaires. Self-administered questionnaires can be used with or without the researcher's presence. Mailed questionnaires are the most common example of interviews administered outside the presence of the researcher. Questionnaires distributed to classrooms of students are probably the most common example of researcher-supervised, self-administered questionnaires. Self-administered questionnaires are briefer, less complex, and more highly structured than interviewer-administered questionnaires. In general, questions in self-administered questionnaires should be "closed-ended," requiring, for example, yes, no, or multiple-choice responses, rather than "open-ended," requiring responses such as "fill in the blanks" or subjective narratives (see Chapter 2).

The *major advantage* of self-administered mail questionnaires is that there is no need to train and supervise interviewers who must then locate and interview subjects. This substantially reduces the time and money spent on data gathering. All study participants can be sent the questionnaire on the same day or given the instrument to fill out on a given day at a given location.

The *major disadvantage* of mailed questionnaires is the low and differential response rate. Uninterested persons fail to return questionnaires, illiterate respondents cannot participate, and out-of-date or inaccurate address lists prevent questionnaires from reaching targeted persons. Lack of control is also a problem. Although self-administered questionnaires usually are sent to a specific individual, once sent, there is no guarantee that the questionnaire will be completed by the designated person.

Data may be missing because respondents only partially complete what seem to them to be lengthy, repetitive, or incomprehensible questionnaires. When questionnaires are administered to groups of respondents, the respondents' perceptions of the researcher or the location (e.g., a clinic or a church) may cause them to change their answers to fit their perceptions of the responses desired. Researchers can reduce some of these problems by restricting the use of mail questionnaires to literate, highly motivated populations, by careful pilot testing, and by utilizing a variety of follow-up techniques to increase response rates (Dillman, 1978).

Special data processing is often needed because of the considerable amount of missing data (see Chapter 5), or because unsupervised respondents do not follow instructions on precoded questionnaires (see Chapter 4). On the other hand, the elimination of skips from self-administered questionnaires and the use of closed-ended questions simplify data entry and the creation of data files (see Chapter 4). In addition, respondents sometimes can be asked to record answers directly on scannable sheets, which greatly facilitates computer entry.

OBSERVATION

Observation can be either a direct or an indirect form of data collection. Subjects under observation may or may not be aware of being observed. Webb, Campbell, Schwartz, and Suchrest (1966) provide one of the best discussions available on the use of unobtrusive, indirect observational methods. Spradley (1980), Scrimshaw and Hurtado (1987), and Miles and Huberman (1984) discuss direct, overt observation in which the emphasis is on observing whether events occur, how they occur, with what timing, and in what order. Observations are frequently used to study interactions between people, and between people and their environment.

Videotapes, audiotapes, event recorders, or data collection forms can be used alone or in combination to collect observational data. When tapes are used, data must be transcribed and "content analyzed" prior to analysis (see Chapter 2). Data collection forms differ considerably depending on what is being observed and on the level of detail desired, but carefully structured, precoded forms can help the observer focus on what is to be observed, rather than on the mechanics of filling out the form.

The *major advantage* of direct observation is that the researcher directly observes events rather than relying on the respondent's memory or truthfulness in reporting. The *major disadvantages* are that observation is time-consuming and can be used only when the information desired is readily amenable to observation. As a result, samples of people or events frequently are small and unrepresentative. It is difficult to replicate direct observations and, like interviewers, observers must be carefully trained and monitored so that data are accurately and reliably recorded, both across observers and over time.

In many studies, more than one observer must be used. A preliminary study may be undertaken to determine if significant differences exist among the observers' ratings prior to beginning the main study. For a discussion of the design and analysis of such a study using continuous or equal interval data, see Fleiss (1986); for categorical data, see Fleiss (1981). (See Chapter 2 for our definition of interval data.) The results of the analyses can be used to determine whether it is best to retrain or drop one or more observers, stratify on observers in the analyses, use more than one observer for each observation, or proceed with the study. Often the problem can be avoided by having training sessions at which all the observers are present and differences in rating are discussed. As the study progresses, these analyses should be repeated at intervals to determine whether the observers are drifting out of agreement.

Special data processing requirements frequently include the need to manipulate large amounts of data for very few people. The length and content of data files often are not uniform and, when information is missing, it is difficult to know if a behavior did not occur or was not recorded. When the sample size is small or the behaviors observed simple, data processing may be performed more efficiently by hand than by computer.

RECORDS

Institutional records and other documents provide a major indirect source of data on people. Institutional records are developed by the government, educational institutions, corporations, the armed forces, and many other groups for a wide variety of reasons. Examples include the U.S. Census, work records, medical records, birth and death certificates, school records, and coroner's reports. Appointment and intake logs for medical or other facilities provide examples of less permanent records that may be used as a source of data.

The *major advantage* of records is their availability. When records are available in a centralized location, data collection is often cheaper and fewer cases may be missing. Records allow access to persons who are no longer available because of death or migration and allow the retrieval of information on events, such as immunizations, that a respondent may be unable to remember adequately or accurately. If it can be assumed that data were recorded uniformly across people, records provide an unbiased source of data.

From the researcher's point of view, the *major disadvantage* of records is that typically they are not collected for research purposes. This means that the data of interest may not exist or, if they do exist, they may be incomplete or not in readily usable form. Moreover, because data may have been collected by numerous people with differing levels of competence and interest, it may be difficult to establish the accuracy of the information. Finally, researchers may need to spend a great deal of time or may have difficulty gaining access to data they wish to use.

Data processing requirements vary widely when records are used as the source of information. Sometimes data must be collected by hand using forms similar to a questionnaire (see Chapter 2). However, if records are computerized, researchers may not have to do any data collection or data entry at all, which makes data processing quite simple. On the other hand, if very limited data are to be extracted from a large data file, large amounts of missing data or irregular files may add to the data processor's problems. In cases where information is to be collected from multiple computer files with different kinds of identifying information, and the researcher wishes to employ secondary data from several sources or to integrate secondary data with primary data, specialized computer expertise may be needed (see Brewer & Hunter, 1989; Hyman, 1972; Kiecolt & Nathan, 1985). Merging data sets is a common problem in such research.

Data Collection Techniques: Sources

Readers interested in more detailed information about data collection techniques may want to read some of the excellent publications on the subject. The following authors, among others, can provide a more in-depth understanding of the topic: Adams and Preiss (1960), Aday (1989), Alwin (1991), Boone and Wood (1992), Bradburn and Sudman (1979), Converse and Presser (1986), Dillman (1978), Fink and Kosecoff (1985), Hall (1966), Jobe and Loftus (1991), Miles and Huberman (1984), Patton (1990), Scrimshaw and Hurtado (1987), Sheatsley (1983), Spradley (1980), Stewart and Kamins (1993), Sudman and Bradburn (1982), and Webb et al. (1966).

Data Processing by Example: Earthquake Research

The remainder of this book will explain and describe data processing by example. Two surveys of community response to earthquakes that we have recently completed will serve as the primary source of our examples. Although our examples are drawn from studies of people, many of the data processing steps discussed are relevant to other kinds of data.

Both studies used similar questionnaires to collect data through telephone interviews lasting approximately 30 minutes each. All interviews were conducted by staff of the Institute for Social Science Research, University of California, Los Angeles.

The first study examined community behavior during and after the Whittier Narrows earthquake of October 1, 1987, which measured 5.9 on the Richter scale. Data were collected from 690 adult residents of Los Angeles County. The second study occurred approximately two years later in response to the Loma Prieta earthquake of October 17, 1989, of 7.1 magnitude. The slightly fewer (656) respondents in the second study were residents of five counties in the San Francisco Bay Area.

To reflect the normal progress and problems often associated with data processing during the course of conducting survey research, we discuss what worked, what did not work, and what could have been improved in our earthquake studies. We also indicate how our experiences during the Whittier Narrows study helped us modify and improve the Loma Prieta study.

2. DESIGNING FORMS FOR DATA COLLECTION

This chapter covers the design of data collection forms. First we describe types of data that can be collected, selection of variables, and how future analytical needs influence the format of a data collection form. Next we discuss how data collection forms used by other researchers can be adapted or adopted for use in current work, and differences between open- and closed-ended questions. We demonstrate how the format of a data collection form can facilitate computer entry, describe the development of response categories for closed-ended questions, and show how skip patterns and other characteristics of forms can influence data. In the final section we explain how to develop code frames for open-ended responses.

General Characteristics of Data Collection Forms

To gather accurate information to test theories or hypotheses, data collection forms must be reliable, systematic, and complete. To simplify the work of data collectors and ensure consistent and accurate use of forms, instruments must be self-explanatory, freestanding, and comprehensive. Persons who use them should not be expected to shuffle among several forms or be forced to refer to other documents while completing a form. A well-designed form will enable different data collectors to interview or observe in such a way that each will obtain identical information from a given respondent, record, or unit of analysis.

IDENTIFICATION NUMBER

Every respondent, case, or unit of analysis in your study must have a unique identification number. Names should not be used as identification because that would breach confidentiality. The simplest way is to assign ID numbers in sequence as data collection forms are returned to a central office, but often it is useful to embed information about the sample within the identification number.

TYPES OF DATA TO COLLECT

One of the worst things that can happen during the course of research is to arrive at the analysis stage and suddenly discover that you failed to collect an essential piece of information. To minimize chances of this happening, you should keep in mind the five types of information that may be collected: information about the respondent and information about his or her environment, behaviors, experiences or status, and thoughts or feelings. The first type is frequently referred to as *demographic data.* These data usually include gender, age, educational level, income, employment, marital status, ethnic or racial background, religion, and sometimes housing type. Novice researchers most often forget to collect information on one or more of these important demographic variables.

The other four types of data, alone or together, are usually the focus of research. Most commonly, studies are interested in two or more of these four types. For example, to assess the strength of opinions and attitudes, ordinarily it is also useful to know something about respondents' behavior and/or environment.

KEEPING YOUR ANALYSIS NEEDS IN MIND

It is important to keep analysis needs in mind while designing the data collection form. When there is uncertainty or when data can be collected in a variety of ways, it is best to collect them as interval data. By *interval data*, we mean continuous data that have equal intervals such that the difference between 1 and 2 always equals the difference between 2 and 3. From interval data, statistics such as the mean, standard deviation, and correlation can be interpreted.

Adopting, Adapting, or Developing a Data Collection Form

Researchers do one of three things when they develop a data collection form: *adopt* items developed by other researchers, *adapt* items developed by other researchers, or *develop* their own items. Obviously, it is most efficient to adapt or adopt pertinent sections of existing instruments. This also is essential when the objective of the research is to replicate another study or to use findings from another study as a standard.

ADOPTING INSTRUMENTS DEVELOPED BY OTHERS

Generally, there are five reasons that encourage researchers to adopt items from other studies. One is to replicate a study's findings on another population or at a later date. Another is when an investigator feels he or she cannot improve on another's instrument.

Adopting rather than adapting is also done when the desired instrument is under copyright, which assures the author that it cannot be used or changed without his or her permission. In the earthquake studies we used the Brief Symptom Inventory (BSI) to assess psychological well-being (Derogatis & Spencer, 1982) and the Mississippi Scale—Revised to assess levels of post-traumatic stress disorder (PTSD) (Keane, Caddell, & Taylor, 1988). Before we could use these instruments, however, we contacted the researchers who designed them, described what we intended to do, received permission, and paid fees to use the BSI. Even if a formal copyright does not exist, research ethics dictate that you document where you obtained the instrument and give credit to the original researcher.

A fourth reason a researcher may adopt items is to compare his or her study population with subjects used in other studies. The final motivation is to use instruments of known reliability and validity, to save the time and expense associated with constructing a new instrument.

In any case, when a researcher adopts items or sets of items from other researchers, no changes should be made in wording, answer categories, order or format of questions, or administrative procedures.

Selecting Items to Adopt. There are two major ways to go about finding items to include in a study. One is to be familiar with other research being conducted in the field, and the other is to consult one of the many books that contain lists of questions and summarize information on their prior use (e.g., Chun, Cobb, & French, 1975; George & Bearon, 1980; Kane & Kane, 1981; McDowell & Newell, 1987; Reeder, Ramacher, & Gorelnik, 1976; Robinson, Rusk, & Head, 1973; Robinson & Shaver, 1973; Robinson, Shaver, & Wrightsman, 1991; Shaw & Wright, 1967).

ADAPTING INSTRUMENTS DEVELOPED BY OTHERS

If any aspect of an instrument is changed, the instrument is considered adapted rather than adopted. Adaptation occurs for a variety of reasons: Some instruments are too long to be included in their entirety; a population other than the original population is being studied; instruments may need to be translated into other languages; or researchers may need to expand, reorder, or otherwise elaborate on items or change the procedure by which data are collected—for instance, an item written for an in-person interview may be modified for a mail questionnaire. If modifications are made in an instrument, pilot testing should be repeated and the instrument's reliability and validity must be reevaluated.

Adapting Turner, Nigg, and Heller Paz (1986). Questionnaires used in our earthquake research were adapted primarily from Turner et al. (1986). As part of their series of studies on earthquake predictions, Turner and his colleagues designed a questionnaire to be administered only when an earthquake of a certain size occurred. While they never used the instrument, our ability to adapt it saved us considerable time and expense. We could not adopt it in its entirety, however, because our research objectives were somewhat different from theirs, and we wanted to restrict our telephone interviews to 30 minutes each.

The major change we made was to create open-ended questions from closed-ended questions. Figure 2.1 shows a question as it was originally written, how we first modified it for the Whittier Narrows study, and then how we adapted it again for the Loma Prieta study.

Originally Turner had provided three answers for the question, "What kind of damage was this?" Each respondent who reported damage was asked whether

A. Question as Written by Turner et al. (1986)

16. Was the home you were living in damaged enough to need repairs?
     YES .... ASK A 1
     NO .... SKIP TO B 2
     A. What kind of damage was this? Was it:
        Major structural damage 1
        Some cracking, but not structural, or 2
        Very minor damage, such as objects
           moved around or damaged? 3

B. Question as Adapted for Whittier Narrows Study

12. Was the house you were living in damaged enough to need repairs?
     YES .... ASK A 1
     NO .... SKIP TO C 2
     A. What kind of damage was this?

     _____

     _____

C. Question as Revised for Loma Prieta Study

8. Was the home you were living in damaged enough to need repairs, or did you
   have any *other* personal property or belongings damaged during this earthquake?
     YES .... ASK A-K 1
     NO .... SKIP TO Q9 2
     A. What kind of damage was this?

     Damage to: CIRCLE ALL THAT APPLY
        PERSONAL PROPERTY BROKEN 01
        ENTIRE BUILDING DESTROYED 02
        FOUNDATION 03
        BUILDING OFF FOUNDATION 04
        HOUSE WALL(S) DAMAGED 05
        HOUSE WALL(S) COLLAPSED 06
        CHIMNEY COLLAPSED 07
        CEILING/ROOF DAMAGED 08
        CEILING/ROOF COLLAPSED 09
        WATER PIPES BROKEN 10
        WATER HEATER 11
        GAS LINES BROKEN 12
        FLOORS DAMAGED 13
        FLOORS COLLAPSED 14
        PATIO/PORCH DAMAGED 15
        FENCES/FENCE WALL DAMAGED 16
        DRIVEWAY DAMAGED/DESTROYED 17
        GARAGE DAMAGED/DESTROYED 18
        OTHER 19
           SPECIFY: _____

Figure 2.1. Comparison of Response Categories in Three Studies

he or she experienced "major structural damage," "some cracking, but not structural," or "very minor damage, such as objects moved around or damaged." Because we were not sure how consistent respondents would be in differentiating among these three levels, we deleted the alternative answers and had interviewers record whatever respondents said. These answers were then analyzed for content. As Figure 2.1 shows, the analysis of Whittier Narrows data yielded a rather long list of different kinds of damage. We then used this list as options for answers to the question in the Loma Prieta study.

TYPES OF QUESTIONS

Items in questionnaires can be either open-ended or closed-ended. Similarly, when data are collected by observation or from records, items included on the data collection form are either open-ended or closed-ended.

Open-Ended Questions. Open-ended questions have no lists of possible answers. Questions 1B, 2B, and 4B in Figure 2.2 are open-ended questions that generate brief answers, while Question 3 is an open-ended question that may generate a long and complex answer.

Questions 1B, 2B, and 4B are open-ended because it would be unreasonable to take up enough space to list all possible answers. In contrast, Question 3 is open-ended because the researcher was unsure what kind of answers respondents would give. While open-ended questions are much easier to write than closed-ended items, they generally are more difficult to answer, code, and analyze, because researchers must develop code frames or categories to organize and summarize the collected data. This process is sometimes referred to as *content analysis.*

Closed-Ended Questions. Closed-ended questions contain lists of possible answers from which the respondent selects the answer that best represents his or her view or situation. Questions 1, 1A, 2, 2A, 4, and 4A in Figure 2.2 are closed-ended questions.

When questionnaires are self-administered, respondents select answers to closed-ended questions by circling numbers or checking boxes or spaces. Interviewers administering questionnaires record respondents' answers similarly. Closed-ended questions are much more difficult to design but, if designed carefully and with sufficient pretesting, result in much more efficient data collection, processing, and analysis. Instead of having to write out an answer to the question, the interviewer or respondent selects the word, phrase, or statement from the list of answers that best matches the respondent's answer, the behavior observed if observations are the source of data, or the information available in a record if records are the source of data. When possible, answer categories should be alphabetized using key words.

1. As you probably know, there was an earthquake in Los Angeles on October 1st <u>last</u> <u>year</u>, that was 1987. Did you yourself feel the earthquake on October 1, 1987?

     YES .... SKIP TO Q2 1   V92
     NO .... ASK A 2

 A. Since you did not feel the earthquake, where were you when you found out it had occurred? Were you at:

                   <u>CIRCLE ONE ANSWER ONLY</u>

    a. Your own home? .... SKIP TO Q3 1
    b. Someone else's home? ..... ASK B 2
    c. Work? .... ASK B 3
    d. School? .... ASK B 4
    e. Traveling? .... ASK B 5   V93
    f. In a public place? .... ASK B 6
    g. Out of the area? ....SKIP TO C 7
    h. Or somewhere else? .... ASK B 8

 B. What area or city is that in?

   _____
   GEOGRAPHIC LOCATION   V94(2)

 C. When did you first become aware of or hear that this earthquake had occurred?

     SAME DAY 1
     NEXT DAY 2
     FEW DAYS LATER 3
     WEEK LATER 4   V95
     2-3 WEEKS LATER 5
     OTHER 6
      SPECIFY: _____
           V96

               | SKIP TO PAGE 6, Q8 |

2. When the earthquake struck, were you:

     Indoors, or 1   V97
     Outdoors? 2

 A. Where were you when the earthquake struck? Were you at:

                   <u>CIRCLE ONE ANSWER ONLY</u>

    a. Your own home? .... SKIP TO Q3 1
    b. Someone else's home? ..... ASK B 2
    c. Work? .... ASK B 3
    d. School? .... ASK B 4   V98
    e. Traveling on a road
      or freeway? .... ASK B 5
    f. In a public place like a
      building or store? .... ASK B 6
    g. Or somewhere else? .... ASK B 7

Figure 2.2. Creation of Precoded, Closed-Ended Questions

B. What area or city is that in?

_____
GEOGRAPHIC LOCATION   V99(2)

3. When you felt the earthquake, what was the very first thing you did?

_____
_____
                    V100(4)

4. When the earthquake struck, were you:

        Alone, or .... SKIP TO Q5 1   V101
        With others? .... ASK A 2

  A. Who were you with?

                                  CIRCLE ALL MENTIONS

        ADULTS IN MY HOUSEHOLD
          (OTHER THAN CHILDREN) 1   V102
        CHILDREN IN HOUSEHOLD 18 YRS
          AND OVER 1   V103
        CHILDREN IN HOUSEHOLD 17 YRS
          AND UNDER 1   V104
        OTHER RELATIVES NOT PART OF
          HOUSEHOLD 1   V105
        CO-WORKERS 1   V106
        FRIENDS/NEIGHBORS 1   V107
        OTHERS 1   V108
          SPECIFY: _____
                      V109(2)

  B. Not counting yourself, how many other people were you with?
     (RECORD AS GIVEN.)   _____
                        V110(4)

Figure 2.2. Continued

Facilitating Direct Computer Entry

Figure 2.2 presents a questionnaire that was set up to facilitate direct computer entry. Note that most questions are closed-ended, and many of the open-ended questions (e.g., 1B) require only brief answers. Moreover, all closed-ended questions have been precoded: A unique number has been assigned to each possible answer. The interviewer, data collector, or respondent simply circles the number corresponding to the answer selected. These codes are then used to enter data into the computer for analysis. Precoding simplifies answer selection and forces the researcher to decide in advance how data will be organized and coded for data entry and analysis. Computer-assisted telephone interviewing systems also facilitate direct entry of data into computers (Frey, 1989).

To reduce errors, answers in the questionnaire shown in Figure 2.2 are listed vertically, with dotted lines guiding the user to corresponding answer options. Researchers sometimes list answers horizontally in order to save space, but this significantly increases the chances for error. For instance, in the example below it would be easy for a respondent who wished to answer yes to check the line *after* rather than *before* the yes. His or her selection would then be incorrectly tallied as a no.

Did you yourself feel the earthquake on October 1, 1987?

_____ Yes _____ No

In the questionnaire represented in Figure 2.2, to mimic the way our eyes travel from left to right while reading English, codes are placed to the right of each alternative and lined up vertically on the right-hand side of the page. Because all answers are located on the right and answer categories are not mixed in with text, it is easy for data collectors or respondents to record answers; this layout also facilitates transfer of answers to a computerized data base.

Developing Response Categories
for Closed-Ended Questions

Listed below are rules that should be followed when designing answers for closed-ended or precoded questions and when devising data collection forms that contain those answers.

1. Answer categories should be exhaustive; that is, they should represent the full range of possible answers.
2. Answer categories should be mutually exclusive.
3. Answer categories should be designed to make it easy for data collectors, respondents, or coders to select appropriate options.
4. Answer categories should include a residual "other" option, with sufficient space for writing answers that were not anticipated.
5. Answer categories should anticipate analytical needs and enable the collection of data that are suitable for those analyses.
6. Open-ended questions should be used if they will provide interval data that closed-ended questions will not.
7. Consistent conventions should be used to record when data are unavailable and, when appropriate, to indicate the reasons data are missing.
8. Consistent codes for identical answers should be used throughout the instrument.

9. Codes that minimize transformations during analysis and correspond to everyday meanings of answers should be used throughout the instrument.

10. If the study will employ interviewers, it should be decided whether or not they will read aloud alternative answers to closed-ended questions.

11. It should be decided whether single or multiple answers are to be allowed, and consistent corresponding codes should be created.

12. Instructions on how to complete the form should be provided; whether and how skip patterns should be used should be carefully considered.

Due to ignorance, haste, or egocentrism, researchers frequently violate one or more of these rules. One of the most common mistakes is to assume that you know the range of possible responses and how to differentiate among them. Pilot studies and pretests will help you avoid these problems (see Frey, 1989).

In general, as solutions are created for one rule violation, at least a partial solution is provided for some others. As the following examples show, if answer categories really are exhaustive and mutually exclusive, they probably include a residual "other" category and are easy for respondents, interviewers, and coders to use.

EXHAUSTIVE RANGE OF RESPONSES

The following question from the Loma Prieta earthquake questionnaire failed to provide an exhaustive list, a residual "other," and, for some respondents, a mutually exclusive list.

5. Did you turn on or find a TV or radio to get more information about the earthquake?

    YES, REGULAR TV 1
    YES, BATTERY TV 2
    YES, REGULAR RADIO 3
    YES, BATTERY RADIO 4
    NO 5

We thought our list of answers was both exhaustive and mutually exclusive, so we did not include a residual "other" category in our list of answers. We discovered that we had failed to consider car radios. Many people reported that they were in cars at the time of the earthquake and turned on car radios to get information. We discovered our error during the pretest and were able to tell interviewers to add this answer to the list of possibilities. Including a residual "other," so that the interviewer could write down "car radio," would also have solved this problem.

Impact of Incomplete Lists on Data Quality. Generally, investigators end up with incomplete lists of categories because they have failed to examine questions developed by others or do not pretest instruments carefully enough. If a residual "other" category is included in an incomplete or poorly constructed list, a considerable number of respondents, interviewers, or coders will use it. This means investigators must later code what has essentially become an open-ended question. If no residual "other" category is provided, the respondent or interviewer may choose the single category that is closest to the desired response. This may result in lost information or in frequency distributions that "heap" or concentrate respondents in a single response category.

Heaping. An example of heaping occurred in the Whittier Narrows study when respondents were asked about their family income in 1987. Each respondent was asked to select the category that contained his or her family's income. We used prior Los Angeles County studies as our guide, and the top category we provided was "Over $40,000." However, the average family income in Los Angeles County increased rapidly during the 1980s, so when we started to analyze the data we found significant heaping of subjects in this highest category; 38% of our respondents reported family incomes over $40,000. As a result, we did not have a very clear idea of the distribution of family income in Los Angeles County.

Lost Data. The following question on marital status provides an example of an incomplete list that resulted in lost data.

47. What is your current marital status?
    NEVER MARRIED 1
    MARRIED 2
    DIVORCED 3
    SEPARATED 4
    WIDOWED 5

Although unmarried cohabitation is increasingly common throughout the United States, our question on marital status did not allow respondents to report cohabitation, so data about living arrangements were lost. Clearer specification of why we wanted information on marital status would have prevented this problem from occurring. If our objective was to obtain information about legal marital status, the question as written was sufficient. If, however, we also wished to find out about respondents' current living arrangements, additional questions should have been included.

MUTUALLY EXCLUSIVE ANSWERS AND EASILY USED CATEGORIES

The process of creating mutually exclusive answer categories overlaps with creating categories that are easy for the respondent, data collector, or coder to use. Figure 2.2 shows that Question 3 as posed in the Whittier Narrows study was open-ended. After analyzing the content of those data, we closed the question for the Loma Prieta study using categories of answers that resulted from the Whittier analysis:

```
GOT UNDER DOORWAY/TABLE/COVER  ............10
FROZE/STAYED WHERE WAS  ......................11
CAUGHT FALLING OBJECTS  ......................12
RAN OUTSIDE  .................................13
WENT TO CHILD ................................14
CALLED INSTRUCTIONS TO OTHERS IN AREA .......15
PULLED CAR OVER  .............................16
CONTINUED DRIVING  ...........................17
OTHER  .......................................18
     SPECIFY:_____
```

Our new list turned out to be exhaustive, but not always mutually exclusive. Many respondents reported doing several things, so interviewers had difficulty figuring out the *first* thing they did. Respondents might say they stayed where they were and called to others in the area, or that they grabbed a child and went to a door frame. In these instances, interviewers ignored the problem by acting as if the question were still open-ended and writing out everything respondents said.

INCLUDING A RESIDUAL "OTHER" CATEGORY

The lists of answers for Questions 1C and 4A in Figure 2.2 include a residual "other" category with space for the interviewer to write in responses not included on the answer list. We point this out to reiterate our belief that in general, researchers should always include a residual "other" category in the list of response alternatives to closed-ended questions.

ANTICIPATING ANALYTICAL NEEDS AND USING OPEN-ENDED QUESTIONS

We will consider rules 5 and 6 together. Researchers frequently create closed-ended questions when open-ended questions would provide better data and take up less space. For example, when he wanted information about injuries sustained, Turner asked:

> How many were injured? Would you say:
> A few people 1
> Some people, or 2
> Many people? 3

We adapted this question for the Loma Prieta study by making it open-ended:

> How many people *in all* do you know who were injured?
> NUMBER OF PEOPLE INJURED: _____

This change had three advantages. First, instead of creating an ordinal variable, we created discrete interval data (e.g., Bailey, 1987). This gave us much more flexibility when we analyzed our data. Second, it took up less space in the questionnaire, and third, it avoided the variable interpretation that results when "vague qualifiers" are used. While some respondents may consider three "a few," others may consider three "some."

Closed-ended questions often are used unnecessarily to collect data that are continuous in character. This error occurs most frequently in self-administered questionnaires. With the possible exception of questions about income, we have little reason to suspect that providing respondents with a list of answers rather than an open-ended question increases the validity of their answers. If the concern is that respondents will hesitate to answer because they don't think they remember the exact number, this can be avoided by instructing them to give their best estimate.

RECORDING MISSING INFORMATION

In the questionnaires shown in Figures 2.1 and 2.2 we have not provided an answer category or code for "don't know" or "no response." Researchers differ regarding the advisability of including such alternatives. Five interrelated issues are raised in discussions about "don't knows." The meaning or value of including a "don't know" category probably differs with the following factors: the researcher's objectives, how data are collected, whether factual or attitudinal information is being solicited, whether respondents are told that a "don't know" category is available, and the extent to which data collectors are trained and monitored. When the researcher's primary objective is to collect factual or behavioral information, we believe it is better not to include "don't know" answers in questionnaires because their existence in a list of alternatives encourages interviewers and respondents to use them when other answers are actually more appropriate. When collection of data on attitudes is the major objective of a study, we recommend that researchers consult the rapidly expanding literature on this topic before making a decision (e.g., Converse, 1970; Duncan & Stenbeck, 1988; Faulkenberry & Mason, 1978; Fieck, 1989; Frey, 1989; Poe, Seeman, McLaughlin, Mehl, & Dietz, 1988; Presser & Schuman, 1989; Sheatsley, 1983). Of course, when such answers are not included, the researcher must provide a way to signify that questions were left unanswered when data are entered into the computer (see Chapter 4).

In contrast, when records or observations are the source of data, we recommend *including* such alternatives in the data collection form. For example, coroner's records contain results from laboratory tests as well as notes recorded by the coroner. If test results are important to the study, then the data collection form should clearly *identify* which tests are to be examined, *specify* what data are to be recorded about each test, and include a way to indicate that a given person's file contains *no record* of that particular test.

Probably one of the biggest errors made in extracting data from records is failing to note that a recorder looked for a piece of information and did not find it. To correct this, instead of merely having a space in which to record results of, for instance, a hemoglobin test, the data form should include a way to indicate that the collector looked for the results but found no indication in the medical record that a hemoglobin test had been run. Without such a category, a blank space can indicate one of two things: Either no test result existed or the data collector missed it.

USING CONSISTENT CODES

Some categories of answers occur repeatedly throughout a data collection instrument, such as yes, no, refused, don't know, missing information, and inapplicable. Researchers can simplify data analysis by using consistent numeric codes throughout the data collection form for these common response options. Figure 2.3 shows the codes we used in the earthquake questionnaires. Yes was always coded 1, no was coded 2, and similarly consistent codes were designed to explain missing answers. For example, if someone was alone when the earthquake struck, obviously the interviewer did not ask the respondent who he or she was with (see Figure 2.2, Question 4A). In this case, the answer was coded 0, for "inapplicable." When respondents said they didn't remember who they were with, a code of 8, designating "don't know," was entered. Respondents who did not want to answer were coded 7 for "refused," and if an interviewer forgot to ask a question and we did not catch the error (see Chapter 3), the answer was coded 9, for "missing data." Depending on the research objectives, a researcher may want to combine or delete codes for missing data in later stages of analysis, but such distinctions should be included in the original data set.

Notice that, with the exception of zeros, the last digit in a field of numbers is used to distinguish among the various missing data codes. This is a convention

	Example Code		
Response	Single Digit	Double Digits	3+ Digits
Yes	1		
No	2		
Refused to answer	7	97	997
Don't know	8	98	998
Missing information	9	99	999
Not applicable	0	00	000

Figure 2.3. Examples of Consistent Codes

that has developed over time. If data were missing for a variable that normally is coded in a field of two or more digits, the "leading digits," all those to the left of the last digit, would be 9s. So, for example, if a respondent refused to give his or her age, age would be given a code of 97; if the question on age was not applicable, it would be coded 00; if it was not asked, it would be coded 99; and if a respondent did not remember (or claimed not to remember) his or her age, it would be coded 98. Of course, when a study is focused on an elderly population, the researcher might want to use three digits in coding age to ensure that the codes for respondents aged 90 and above are not confused with the codes used for missing data. In such a case, codes of 997 and 998 would be used for instances where respondents refused or did not know their age.

CODES THAT MINIMIZE TRANSFORMATIONS
DURING DATA ANALYSIS

Researchers frequently assign codes to answer categories arbitrarily, without thinking about how codes might facilitate later analysis of the data. For example, if one possible response to a question is "none," why not use zero as the code? In the earthquake questionnaires, respondents were asked whether their homes were damaged as a result of the earthquake. Respondents who reported damage were then asked to estimate the amount of damage in dollars. Consistent with our earlier suggestion to design open-ended questions when potential answers have a continuous range, we made this an open-ended question. This question was coded 0, connoting *inapplicable* for persons who experienced no damage. Codes for persons who reported damage were the dollar amounts entered as responses to the open-ended question. Thus when we analyzed the data we did not have to transform it; persons who reported no damage already were coded 0, and costs for those who did report damage were coded by the amount of damage reported.

ARE ALTERNATIVE ANSWERS TO BE READ TO RESPONDENTS?

When data are collected by interview, the researcher must decide whether or not the interviewer will read alternative answers to the respondent. In general, if the researcher wants a respondent to be aware of all the alternative answers or wants to maximize the accuracy of the respondent's recollections and the reporting of behaviors and attitudes, he or she will have the list read to the respondent. In face-to-face interviews, cards that list the possible alternatives are sometimes handed to the respondent. Lists of answers are *not* read to the respondent when doing so would be redundant with the question, or when the researcher does not want to "lead" the respondent by suggesting answers to him or her.

In Questions 1 and 2 in Figure 2.2, there was no reason for the interviewer to read "yes" and "no" or "indoors" and "outdoors" to the respondent because the answer alternatives essentially duplicate the substance of the question. In Questions 1A and 2A, however, the possible answers *were* read to the respondent and the respondent was asked to choose the single answer that best described where he or she was at the time of the earthquake.

In Question 3, we wanted respondents to tell us what they did during the earthquake without their obtaining any suggestions or "cues" from us regarding what we think they should have done. Thus the alternative answers reported earlier, which were created from the Whittier Narrows data for inclusion in the Loma Prieta questionnaire, were *not* read to respondents.

On our questionnaires, we differentiate between answers that are to be read to respondents and those that are not to be read: When answers are to be read to a respondent they are in lowercase type; when answers are only for the interviewer to use, they are in uppercase type.

WILL SINGLE OR MULTIPLE ANSWERS BE ALLOWED?

When creating closed-ended questions, it is important to decide whether respondents will be encouraged to give multiple answers to a question or be restricted to a single answer. In Question 4A in Figure 2.2, respondents were encouraged to report all the different kinds of people they were with at the time of the earthquake. In contrast, in Questions 1A, 2A, and 3, respondents were asked to provide a single answer.

When a list of alternative answers is included in a data collection form or questionnaire, the instructions must clarify whether single or multiple answers are desired. For example, in Questions 1A and 2A we state, "CIRCLE ONE ANSWER ONLY," while in Question 4A we state, "CIRCLE ALL MENTIONS." In concert with those instructions, the number of variables created from each answer shows whether single or multiple answers are intended; a single variable, V98, is assigned to Question 2A, while seven variables (one for each alternative response) are assigned to Question 4A.

12. Was the home you were living in damaged enough to need repairs?
      YES ....ASK A 1
      NO .... SKIP TO C 2

  A. What kind of damage was this?

      _____

      _____

  B. Was the damaged caused by: (CIRCLE ALL THAT APPLY)
      The earthquake itself on Oct. 1, or 1
      By aftershocks? 1
      OTHER 1
          SPECIFY: _____

  C. Did you have any other personal property or belongings damaged during this earthquake?
      YES ....ASK D 1
      NO .... SKIP TO Q13 2

  D. What is your estimate of the amount of damage to your home and property? (RECORD DOLLAR AMOUNT. PROBE FOR BEST ESTIMATE).

      DOLLAR AMOUNT: _____

  E. Have you applied for disaster assistance?
      YES ....ASK F 1
      NO .... SKIP TO Q13 2

  F. How much did you apply for?

      DOLLAR AMOUNT: _____

  G. Have you received disaster assistance?
      YES ....ASK H 1
      NO .... SKIP TO Q13 2

  H. How much assistance did you receive?

      DOLLAR AMOUNT: _____

Figure 2.4. Example of Skip Patterns

CREATING SKIP PATTERNS

The ability to create "skip patterns" is one of the most powerful features of data collection. These logical branches allow researchers to customize instruments for different kinds of respondents. We must point out, however, that creating good skip patterns is a difficult task. Even when well-designed skip patterns are used, it is still possible to gather incomplete data that will complicate the creation of variables useful for analysis.

In the Whittier Narrows study we asked respondents, "Was the home you were living in damaged enough to need repairs?" (see Question 12 in Figure 2.4).

Persons who answered yes were asked about the kind of damage suffered and its cause (see Questions 12A and 12B in Figure 2.4); persons who answered no were *not* asked these two questions and were "skipped" to Question 12C. *Both* groups of respondents were asked, "Did you have any *other* personal property or belongings damaged during this earthquake?" (see Question 12C in Figure 2.4). Persons who answered yes to this question were then asked to estimate the dollar amount of their damage and whether they applied for disaster assistance (see Questions 12D-12H); persons who answered no were skipped to the next section of the questionnaire.

When we designed the questionnaire, the logic of our skip pattern looked fine to us, but when we started analyzing our data we discovered a major logical flaw. A total of 85 people in this study reported damage to their homes, while 605 people reported no damage to their homes. In contrast, 120 people reported damage to personal property, while 534 people reported no damage to personal property. Our skip pattern assumed that *all respondents who reported damage to their homes would report damage to personal property!* In fact, 36 of the 85 people with damage to their homes reported no damage to personal property. Because our assumptions did not allow for this combination of responses, these 36 people were not asked to estimate the dollar amount of their damage or whether they sought disaster assistance. The problem caused by this particular sequence of skip patterns led to missing data for these 36 people that had to be estimated prior to analysis (see Chapter 5).

A simple flow diagram can help verify that the branching and skipping in a data collection instrument work as intended. Had we tested our design when we created the questions in Figure 2.4, we might have caught our error. Parts A and B of Figure 2.5 show how to develop a flow diagram using the material from questionnaire fragments included in Figures 2.2 and 2.4. They also document the structure of the data collection instrument.

In Figure 2.5, the questions for which responses are to be obtained are shown as rectangular boxes. Each major question is placed at the head of a column, with subsidiary questions below it. Changes in flow, based on the response to a question, are shown by diamond-shaped decision boxes directly below the question. Thus in part A of the figure a "yes" response to Question 1 results in transfer directly to Question 2, while a "no" response continues the flow through the subquestions of Question 1.

There is one basic difference between the two parts of Figure 2.5. The structure in part A (from Figure 2.2) is one of "branching," with a substantial series of subsequent questions on each subsequent branch. In contrast, the structure in part B (from Figure 2.4) is primarily one of "skipping" subordinate questions while continuing along one general track. Thinking about this distinction helps clarify how to structure a particular line of questioning. (Both of these structures are referred to as *networks*, in that they branch out and then rejoin, in contrast to a *tree*, where branches do not rejoin.)

A. Illustration of Skip "Branching" Pattern

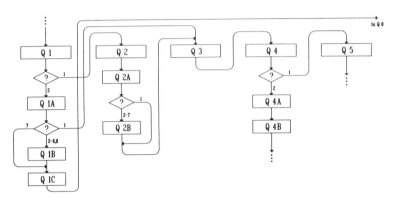

B. Illustration of Skip Pattern

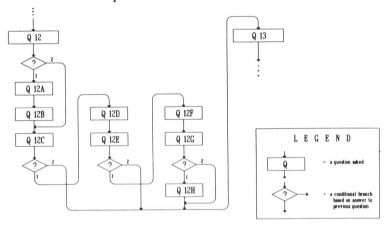

Figure 2.5. Flow Diagrams of Skip Patterns in the Questionnaire Fragments Presented in Figures 2.2 and 2.4

Developing Code Frames for Open-Ended Questions

When open-ended questions are used to collect data, verbal answers must be postcoded or content analyzed. During this process, text is transformed into numbers. This is similar to, but briefer than, what is done when newspapers and other publications are summarized for analysis (e.g., Weber, 1985).

SHORT OPEN-ENDED ANSWERS

Earlier we noted that questions may be left open to save space otherwise taken up by lengthy lists of options, because better-quality data are obtained, or because the researcher is unsure what the range and variety of answers should be. In the simplest example of the first case, coding involves creating a list of answers given, arbitrarily assigning number codes to the list, and recording codes for each respondent's answers. In the simplest example of the second case, coding involves recording a number that was given in response to a question asking, for example, the respondent's age.

Sometimes, however, seemingly simple open-ended questions of this sort require the researcher to develop more complicated answers; for example, Question 4B, "Not counting yourself, how many *other* people were you with?" While most respondents gave a single number, such as 1 or 5, respondents who were at work, in stores, or in other public places sometimes gave ranges, such as 20-25, or verbal answers, such as "a lot." In these cases, we decided to select the midpoint of the range given and round up to the nearest integer. The person who said 20-25 was given a code of 23. The answer "a lot" was arbitrarily given a code of 95. Regardless of *what* the decision is, once a decision is made, the researcher must carefully document the new "coding rule" and use it consistently throughout the remainder of the coding process. (For a thorough discussion of editing procedures and coding rules, see Sonquist & Dunkelberg, 1977.)

Coding Respondents' Occupations. Information on respondents' occupations frequently is collected using short-answer open-ended questions. In the earthquake studies, respondents were first asked about their current and past employment status. Those who had worked were then asked, "What kind of business, industry, or organization is that?"; "What do/did they make?"; "Is it wholesale, manufacturing, or what?"; "What is/was your main occupation?"; and "What do/did you actually do?" Interviewers did not code the answers. After questionnaires were returned to the central office, answers were coded using the *Alphabetical Index of Industries and Occupations* (U.S. Bureau of the Census, 1982). To maximize accurate coding, information about the industry and the occupation must be available (U.S. Bureau of the Census, 1970; Van Dusen & Zill, 1975). The coder then uses the *Index* to ascertain the appropriate code by assessing information provided about the type of work, the industry or business in which the respondent is employed, and whether or not he or she is self-employed.

Because the above process is relatively time-consuming, and therefore expensive, researchers frequently create less detailed closed-ended questions in which respondents are asked to report whether their jobs are professional, managerial, technical, sales, clerical, craftsman/foreman, service worker, operative, labor (not farm), farm manager, or farm worker.

CREATING A MULTIDIMENSIONAL CODE FRAME
FOR COMPLEX ANSWERS

The most important part of coding open-ended questions is creating a code frame. A code frame shows how verbal answers are converted to numbers. In the above examples and in other, short-answer questions, the creation of the code frame is straightforward and quite simple, but for most open-ended questions the process is more complex. This should come as no surprise, because open-ended questions themselves are designed to obtain information that cannot be summarized adequately in a closed-ended form. In essence, the objective of creating a code frame is to formulate a set of categories that accurately represents answers, and in which each category includes an appreciable number of responses.

The same rules specified earlier to create answer categories for closed-ended questions apply to creating code frames for open-ended questions. As with answer categories, code frames must have exhaustive, mutually exclusive categories that are easy to use. Codes must be meaningful and consistent, should maximize ease of transformation during data analysis, and should adopt the highest form of measurement possible. In addition to the earlier rules, six more must be followed when designing code frames for open-ended questions:

1. Specify the objectives for which the code frame is to be used.
2. Maintain a balance between too much detail and not enough detail.
3. Maximize the maintenance of information.
4. Create a sufficient range of codes, variables, or dimensions so that the coder need not force data into categories.
5. Allow for the systematic coding of missing data.
6. Group together related categories of information and use meaningful leading digits in multidigit codes.

Developing Code Frames: An Example. By analyzing the development of questions concerned with injury in the Whittier Narrows study, we can see how these rules help researchers develop code frames for open-ended questions. Beginning with Question 15, respondents were asked a series of questions about injuries.

ID Number	Answer
074	A headboard fell on a woman on the third floor. . . . She went unconscious.
106	Things fell on me in garage when I went out there.
125	The roof fell in on them and broke the table they were hiding under.
137	Threw me to ground—just had hysterectomy with stitches.
139	Friend's girl was killed when building fell on her at college in East L.A.
160	They sprained their feet as they were running to the doorway.
175	Got hit on head with falling object—Had bump for week.
270	My husband is a cardiologist and his patient had a heart attack—I know the patients slightly.
286	My husband jumped thru the window and suffered a laceration in the heel.
292	The chimney fell down.
327	Me—Mental injury—I came unglued. Dear friend had heart attack. . . . She has no history of heart trouble.

Figure 2.6. Answers to Open-Ended Questions About Injuries, Whittier Narrows Study

15. In this earthquake was anyone you know injured?

    YES . . . . ASK A 1
    NO . . . . SKIP TO Q16 2

    A. Can you tell me about that? Who exactly was this, and how were they injured?

In response to this question, 31 respondents said they knew someone who was injured. Figure 2.6 contains answers given by 11 of these 31 respondents. To include these responses in our study, we had to create a code frame to categorize and analyze these data.

We used all 31 responses to create our code frame. If, in contrast, 500 persons had reported an injury, we would have selected a sample of the 500 responses—possibly 100—to work with in developing our code frame. When creating a code frame, we find it helps to write each answer on an index card. The cards can then be sorted in different ways to determine how many categories are needed to include all responses. We also find it useful for two or more persons to work independently to develop a code frame, and then work together on the final code. This ensures maximum objectivity, validity, and reliability.

Objective of the Code Frame. Usually, answers to an open-ended question can be coded in several ways. For example, when looking at injuries caused by earthquakes, we might be interested in the number of injuries reported, the way an injury occurred, what parts of the body were injured, who (in relation to the respondent) suffered the injury, where it occurred, what the person was doing at the time, whether medical care was sought and obtained, and so on. The amount of detail included in a code

Code Category	Code Value	Number of Respondents
Hit by object	1	11
Cuts	2	3
Sprains, bruises, breaks	3	9
Heart attack	4	2
Don't know	5	1
Trapped	6	1
Other	95	2
Missing	99	2
Not Applicable	0	658
TOTAL		690

Figure 2.7. Simple Code of Injuries

frame is determined by the amount of information respondents give the researcher and what the researcher wants to do with that information. We developed two code schemes for the injury question in the Whittier Narrows study.

Maximizing Information and Encoding Ease. Figure 2.7 shows the first code frame that was developed at the time the data were entered into the computer. Only one variable was created, and each answer was coded into one of its nine categories. Unfortunately, this coding scheme confused how the person was injured (e.g., "hit by an object") with what happened as a result (e.g., "cuts"). Although some respondents gave both kinds of information (see Case 074), the coder was forced to decide which kind of information should be recorded in the machine-readable data set. Furthermore, this coding scheme did not allow us to retrieve information about whether anyone had died from these injuries (see Case 139 in Figure 2.6).

This first scheme is not a good code frame. Answer categories are neither exhaustive nor mutually exclusive, and coders will have difficulty deciding how to code many answers. For example, note that for Case 175, the coder must decide whether the answer is coded 1, for "hit by object," or 3, for "sprains, bruises, or breaks."

As we started analyzing the data, we discovered this single code was both inaccurate and incomplete. Fortunately, because our original answers were stored in a computer file, we were able to develop a new code frame (see Figure 2.8). Instead of coding each answer into one of several categories belonging to a single variable, this time we coded answers into four variables or dimensions. In the new code frame we recorded the *number* of people reported injured, the *identity* of people injured, the *cause* of the injury, and the *type* of injury. Moreover, to maximize information provided, we recorded information on injuries to two different people. "Maximizing information" does not mean the recording of data that do not exist, but it *does* include recording when a piece of information was sought but not found. For example, in this instance, it would

Q15B. You said (. . .) was injured in the earthquake. Can you tell me about that? Who exactly was this, and how were they injured?

Seven 2-digit fields, V512-V518, are set aside to code answers to Q15B. Record the number of injuries reported in Dimension 1 (V512). With the exception of persons who gave an inexact count of injured (e.g., some), the maximum number of injured reported was 2. Code dimensions 2-4 for up to two injured persons or groups. Information for the first injury reported is recorded in variables V513, V515 and V517; information for the second injury is coded in variables V514, V516 and V518.

DIMENSION 1: TOTAL NUMBER REPORTED INJURED   (V512: 2 digits)

       None, not applicable 00
       Code number given 01-89
       Some 90
       No information provided on number injured 99

DIMENSION 2: IDENTITY OF INJURED   (V513 & V514: 2 digits)

       Respondent 10
       Other household member, unspecified 20
           Spouse 21
           Parent 22
           Child 23
           Sibling 24
           Other relative (aunt, uncle, cousin) 25
           Roommate, friend 26
       Neighbor 30
       Relative, not in household, unspecified 40
           Spouse 41
           Parent 42
           Child 43
           Sibling 44
           Other relative (aunt, uncle, cousin) 45
       Co-worker 50
       Friend, acquaintance 60
       Other 70
       Person not identified 99
       Inapplicable, R knows no one injured 00

DIMENSION 3: CAUSE OF INJURY   (V515 & V516: 2 digits)

       Non-structural object(s) fell, unspecified 10
           Pictures 11
           Boxes 12
           Headboard 13
           Light fixture 14
           Broken glass (e.g., dishes, pictures) 15
           Shelves 16
       Parts of structure fell, unspecified 20
           Ceiling tiles 21
           Chimney 22

Figure 2.8. Complex Multidimensional Code for Injuries

Broken glass 23
Stairs collapsed 24
Roof collapsed 25
Building collapsed 30
Utilities, unspecified 40
Power outage resulted in darkness 41
Behavior of injured, unspecified 50
Injured person ran 51
Injured person attempted to take cover 52
Injured person jumped 53
Experience of being in earthquake, no detail 60
Earthquake caused fall 61
Trapped 70
Don't know how injury occurred 98
Cause of injury is not mentioned 99
Inapplicable, no injuries reported 00

DIMENSION 4: INJURY REPORTED (V517 & V518: 2 digits)

Death 10
Multiple severe injuries 20
Internal injuries 30
Broken bone(s), unspecified 40
Arm, wrist 41
Leg 42
Foot 43
Minor injuries, unspecified 50
Cuts 51
Bruises, sprains 52
Rug burn 53
Minor head injury 54
Aggravated prior surgery, injury 55
Concussion 60
Emotional, unspecified 70
Panic at time 71
Post-quake emotional 72
Heart attack 80
Unknown type of injury 98
Type of injury is not mentioned 99
Inapplicable; no injuries reported 00

Figure 2.8. Continued

mean that the coder sought information about a second injury but no information was provided.

Problems with the first code occurred for two reasons. First, we did not spend enough time discerning how the answers to open-ended questions related to objectives of the study. Second, we fell into the "single-dimension" trap, assuming that a single question can have only one answer. Researchers often assume this, even when multiple coding dimensions would more adequately represent the answers given.

Systematic Recording of Missing Data. In Figure 2.8, the first variable, V512, records the number of injuries reported by the respondent. When no injuries are reported, this variable is "not applicable" and a code of 0 is recorded. When an actual number of injuries is given or can be inferred, the actual number is coded. Respondents 125 and 160 gave general answers and received a code of 90 for "some." Finally, Case 292 gave no information about the number affected, so a 99 was recorded. Later, during analysis, that 99 told us that the coder looked for information about the number of people injured but no information was provided by Case 292. Recording the unavailability of information can be particularly informative when data are taken from records. The remaining three dimensions record information for up to two people reported injured by each respondent.

Grouping Related Categories and Using Meaningful Leading Digits. The second dimension or variable records information about who was injured. Here a two-digit code is used with a meaningful first digit. The codes for persons living in the same household all start with a 2, while codes for relatives outside the household start with a 4. This system enabled us to maintain detailed information in the code frame, while it also made it easy for us to combine categories during later analysis. This code also includes categories for respondents who said they "don't know who was injured," and for respondents who did not tell us who was injured (Case 292).

The third variable coded, V515 (and V516), records the cause of the injury, while the fourth variable, V517 (and V518), records data about the nature of the injury. Again, codes are grouped logically and in some instances include both general and more specific subcodes. We provided a code for persons who said they didn't know what caused the injury or what the injury consisted of as well as for those who did not mention the injury.

Leaving Sufficient Room in a Code Frame. As a rule, code frames are developed from a 20-50% sample of responses. While this gives the researcher a good selection of the total range of responses, some answers may not be represented. Unless properly instructed, coders will frequently try to force such answers into existing codes rather than add new categories. In the current example, we had no category for major burns that could have occurred if a water heater had broken or a gas line had caught fire. Clearly it would not be appropriate to code such burns under 53 for "rug burn," yet a coder might do just that if not instructed to do otherwise.

TIMING OF CODE FRAME CONSTRUCTION

Before data entry actually begins, researchers must decide how they will handle answers to open-ended questions. In the past, researchers had to code all open-ended responses at the time that machine-readable data files were created, or had to store the data collection instruments until they had time or needed to code open-ended responses. Microcomputers and data entry software changed all that. Now software programs allow researchers to store answers to open-ended questions in machine-readable files at the same time they convert other precoded data to machine-readable files for analysis. This is a valuable new resource, for, as we saw in our injury example, researchers are not always sure how the responses to open-ended questions should be coded until they have started analysis. Thus it is sometimes better to delay coding of open-ended responses until they are needed in analysis.

3. DATA COLLECTION AND QUALITY CONTROL

The data collection process itself influences the quality of data obtained. No matter how data are collected, the objective is to obtain accurate, complete data that are consistent across respondents, records, or other sources employed. When researchers conduct or supervise data collection, they must develop procedures to monitor its quality; when they hire someone else to do it, that individual or firm will handle most of the tasks discussed in this chapter. Nonetheless, researchers must understand the procedures used so that, where necessary, they can negotiate changes or additions, keeping in mind that such revisions will cost time and money. Careful data collection includes attention to pretesting and pilot studies, hiring and training data collectors, supervising data collectors, and logging and editing completed questionnaires or data collection forms.

Pretests and Pilot Studies

Before a data collection instrument is finalized, it should be pretested or used on a small subsample of the population in a pilot study. We refer to *pretesting* as testing parts of data collection instruments or procedures. This can be done in focus groups, in the laboratory, or out in the field. In a *pilot study* the entire instrument and its administrative procedures are tested in a miniature study. Pilot studies are particularly useful when data will be collected within the context of a larger ongoing activity such as admission to a hospital or attendance at a family planning clinic. In such situations, where investigators usually have received permission to gather data on-site, it is important to coordinate data collection with normal activities of the organization. This minimizes disruption and max-imizes cooperation between data collectors and organizational staff.

Many things can be evaluated in a pretest. Researchers may want to learn how well their questions and/or instructions on collection forms are understood, and in what sequence to order data collection. Pretests can reveal how comprehensive response categories are, how adequate a language translation is, how easily and reliably the data collection forms work, how well skip patterns work, and how best to identify, schedule, approach, and follow up on respondents or records. Pretesting can also help a researcher estimate how much the data collection will cost in time and money. We used pilot studies to test how much time it took to collect data from each respondent. Funding restrictions meant we could not allow interviewers to spend more than an average of 30 minutes per interview. After each set of pretests or pilot studies, we deleted unessential questions until we met that requirement.

The persons selected to conduct pretests or pilot studies vary according to the objectives. If the researcher intends to collect the final data personally, he or she should also do the pretesting and pilot work. Often pretests are used during the development of a data collection instrument. Here a pretest or pilot study provides firsthand information about the data collection situation and about problems that can be resolved more easily in this early stage. If other persons conduct pretests or pilot studies, the researcher must monitor or check their work.

In general, if the objective is to identify potential problems and suggest solutions, the best or most experienced data collector should conduct the pretest or pilot. In such cases, the researcher will get the most useful feedback from the pretester whom he or she has instructed to be particularly sensitive to things that do not work or that are being missed by the data collection instrument. When questionnaires are pretested by interview, the researcher may also ask respondents for feedback on how well they understood the instrument or on how easily they were able to complete it. This can be done informally by having the interviewer ask respondents for comments, or more formally by providing questions for the interviewer to ask about respondents' opinions.

It is unwise to use the most experienced interviewers or data collectors in pretests and pilots when the objective is to find out how much time and/or money it will cost to collect data. Obviously, the estimates of such interviewers will understate the difficulties and average time needed for the actual study, in which interviewers with varying levels of experience will be employed (see Aday, 1989; Weinberg, 1983).

Hiring Data Collectors

In general, data collectors must be able to read and write and should have at least a high school education. Advanced education or training may be necessary in some instances, for example, when collecting involves abstracting information from medical records. If data are to be collected by interview, the interviewers selected must have pleasant reading voices, use good diction, and be able to project well enough to be heard and understood easily. Both interviewers and observers must be interested in others, feel comfortable with the subject matter, and appreciate diversity. They also should feel confident about their ability to gather information, yet be able to interact with respondents in ways that do not influence the information they gather. Individuals who are easily shocked by others' attitudes or life-styles, or who try to convince others to accept their view of the world, will not be good interviewers.

Because data collectors often work in the field, away from the research office, they must be good at working alone with only occasional or minimal supervision. Moreover, they must have personalities and temperaments that enable them to get along with persons who control access to data sources and with potential respondents.

There are no restrictions on the age, gender, or race of persons who work with records, and the importance of such characteristics for interviewers is often overemphasized. The general conclusion that can be drawn from research is that the gender and ethnicity of interviewers become relevant only when sexual or ethnic attitudes or behaviors are the object of study (e.g., Anderson, Silver, & Abramson, 1988a, 1988b; Bradburn, 1983; Campbell, 1981; Cotter, Cohen, & Coulter, 1982; Frey, 1989; Reese, Danielson, Shoemaker, Chang, & Hsu, 1986; Schuman & Converse, 1989; Singer, Frankel, & Glassman, 1989; Weeks & Moore, 1981). When found, such effects seem to involve feelings of social deference on the part of the respondent that may more accurately reflect a desire to please the interviewer or differences in age or social class between the interviewer and respondent. Lack of interest in people, personal attitudes about the study's subject matter, and perceptions that information will be difficult to get probably interfere more with an interviewer's ability to conduct an interview than does his or her race, gender, or age.

The single greatest danger in data collection is that the data collector may "lead" the respondent or record data from an interview, record, or observation selectively. Although college students, former missionaries, salespersons, social workers, and nurses may all seem to have the types of experience necessary to be good interviewers, we have found that these persons frequently must unlearn old interpersonal styles before they can become effective interviewers. Giving data collectors thorough training and supervision is the best way to prevent them from leading respondents or gathering selective data. One method is to develop a completely scripted, carefully pretested questionnaire and to train interviewers to stick to it.

Training Data Collectors

Regardless of their past experience, *all* data collectors must be trained. Persons new to data collection need *general* training as well as the *specific* training that even experienced data collectors must receive.

TABLE 3.1
Agenda for Basic Training of Interviewers

1. Presentation of the nature, purpose and sponsorship of the survey
2. Discussion of the total survey process
3. Role of the professional survey interview (including a discussion of ethics of interviewing: confidentiality, anonymity, and bias issues)
4. Role of the respondent (helping respondent learn how to be a respondent)
5. Profile of the questionnaire (identification of types of questions and instructions, answer codes, precolumning numbers for data processing, etc.)
6. Importance and advantages of following instructions (examples of disadvantages to interviewer when instructions are not followed)
7. How to read questions (including correct pacing, reading exactly as printed and in order, conversation tone)
8. How to record answers (for each type of question)
9. How and when to probe (definition and uses of probes for each type of question)
10. Working in the field or on the phone (preparing materials, scheduling work, introduction at the door or on the phone, answering respondent's questions, setting the stage for the interview)
11. Sampling (overview of types of samples, detailed discussion of interviewer's responsibilities for implementation of last stage of sampling on specific survey)
12. Editing (reviewing completed interviews for legibility, missed questions, etc.)
13. Reporting to supervisor (frequency and types of reports required)

SOURCE: "Data Collection: Planning and Management" by E. Weinberg in P. H. Rossi, J. D. Wright, and A. B. Anderson (Eds.) *Handbook of Survey Research,* pp. 344-345. Copyright 1983 by Academic Press. Used with permission.

GENERAL TRAINING

Table 3.1 reproduces Eve Weinberg's (1983) list of items that should be covered when training inexperienced interviewers. Training resources and techniques include written materials, lectures by supervisors, group and individual role playing, practice interviews to be reviewed with the supervisor or in groups with other interviewers, and written exercises.

Most research organizations have training manuals that summarize their training procedures (e.g., Survey Research Center, 1976). We recommend that persons interested in carrying out research obtain copies of such documents and observe training sessions conducted by an experienced research organization. By writing to authors of studies in which data are gathered from records, interested readers may also be able to obtain copies of manuals outlining methods used to train record abstractors.

STUDY-SPECIFIC TRAINING

Specific training focuses on the unique needs of the study in question. The length of training varies with the complexity of the research and past experience of data collectors. If data are to be collected that reveal that subjects are vulnerable to harm from themselves (e.g., suicide) or others (e.g., sexual assault), or that they have harmed or may harm others (e.g., child abuse), data collectors must be taught how to handle such information. If topics are likely to be raised during interviews that may upset interviewers, specialized training and debriefing procedures may need to be developed that allow interviewers to discuss their feelings. When data collection and entry are subcontracted to a full-service survey organization, the researcher and the organization must agree on specifics of the training program.

In the case of the earthquake studies, which employed relatively experienced interviewers, half-day "briefings" were conducted. During training, the objectives of the study were explained and then interviewers were led through the questionnaire using a variety of role-playing techniques. Interviewers were encouraged to ask questions throughout the briefings.

Selecting Respondents. No matter what procedure is chosen to select respondents or records, the data collector must understand and follow it, because this procedure determines characteristics of the sample. If sample selection procedures are not followed exactly, the sample obtained will differ from what was intended.

Debriefing. After the briefing for the Loma Prieta study was completed, interviewers were sent home with lists of telephone numbers generated randomly by the computer. Each interviewer was to complete a minimum of two interviews within a 48-hour period. These were returned immediately to the Institute for Social Science Research for review, and the interviewers were "debriefed." The data collection supervisor discussed with each interviewer his or her experience while interviewing, corrected recording and procedural errors, and ensured that all instructions were followed. In studies employing inexperienced data collectors, researchers may want to arrange practice interviews to give interviewers more experience before their work is assessed by supervisors.

The objective throughout training is to ensure that all data collectors use the questionnaire or data collection instrument as intended. Upon occasion, one may discover that an experienced data collector who has done good work in the past is simply not suited to work on the current study, because of negative or strong attitudes or experiences concerning the topic, or for idiosyncratic situational or personal reasons. (For more information and sources on hiring and training of interviewers, see Aday, 1989; Bradburn, 1983; Weinberg, 1983.)

Supervision During Data Collection

Data collectors must be supervised most closely in the beginning of a study, when they are least experienced in using the instrument and in following study procedures. In this initial stage, the supervisor must verify or validate all completed questionnaires and data collection forms. To verify the accuracy of data collection, the field supervisor recontacts the subject and reconducts all or part of the face-to-face interview. When data are collected by telephone from a central location, supervisors on the premises can monitor actual interviews. When computer-assisted telephone interviewing (CATI) systems are used or data are entered into the computer immediately, the quality of interviewing can also be monitored by conducting analyses of responses to specific questions by the interviewer. If systematic differences are found, they may represent a problem with the quality of the data. (For more information on monitoring of data collectors, see Aday, 1989; Frey, 1989; Weinberg, 1983.)

Abstracted records are verified by supervisors or experienced abstractors who reabstract records. Unfortunately, the only way to verify observations is to have two observers collect data simultaneously. This increases expense, but it does allow the researcher to compare the data obtained across observers and to make empirical estimates of reliability (e.g., Fleiss, 1981, 1986).

Once a data collector is well trained, complete verification is conducted only on a small portion (usually 10%) of his or her interviews or record abstractions, or only when problems are identified as the data are edited or checked. At this stage, verification can involve a complete reinterview or simply the confirmation of demographic information or reported behavior.

Project coordinators or field supervisors are also responsible for monitoring the progress of all interviewers, and for keeping track of all data that have been collected. The "call record" is one way to assess an interviewer's performance.

USING CALL RECORDS TO CHECK INTERVIEWER PERFORMANCE

Interviewers keep a call record for each attempt they make to identify and contact a subject. Figure 3.1 shows a call record from the Loma Prieta study. In this instance the designated respondent was particularly difficult to reach. The first call to the household was made at 5:35 p.m. on May 1, 1990. The interviewer conducted the screening interview (referred to as the *screener*) with the adult resident who answered the phone. The purpose of the screener in the Loma Prieta study was to find out whether the telephone number dialed was a residence, to determine who lived there, and whether adults in the household had also lived there on October 17, 1989, the date of the earthquake. The data collector listed all adult residents over 18, and then, using a Kish (1965) table, randomly selected a respondent from among them. The two rows of numbers in the upper right-hand corner of Figure 3.1 are a Kish table. The interviewer has circled the 2 in the top row and the 1 beneath it in the second row to indicate that there are 2 adults over 18 in this household who lived there on October 17, 1989, and that the first person listed on the household roster is the designated respondent.

Because the interviewer was speaking with the other adult during the screener, she now had to arrange to interview the designated respondent. The interviewer

38

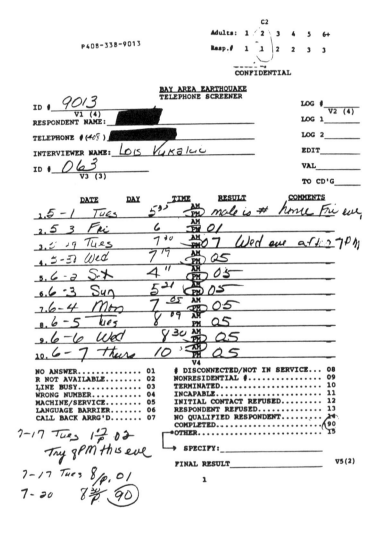

Figure 3.1. Using a Call Record to Monitor Interviewer Behavior

learned that the other adult was a male who would be home Friday evening. She called back on Friday evening, but there was no answer. On the following Tuesday evening she called again, and was told to call on Wednesday evening after 7:00 p.m. When she called on Wednesday, she got an answering machine. She then changed tactics and tried to contact the respondent on the weekend, but had no success. Periodically over the next week she made several more unsuccessful attempts to reach the targeted respondent. Then she gave up trying to reach him for a month, while she was busy interviewing others. Finally she reached and interviewed the respondent on Friday, July 20, at 8:30 p.m.

This call record documents the work of a conscientious interviewer. Notice how the interviewer persisted and called at different times of the day and on different days of the week. Obviously, attempts cannot go on forever. Usually, the number of callback attempts is determined by the research budget.

Call records provide a good one-page summary of an interviewer's work, particularly as it affects the makeup of the sample. While call records can be falsified, falsified records usually do not result in completed interviews. For example, in the Loma Prieta study, one new interviewer was given a list of 10 telephone numbers from the computer-generated list. A week later he returned 10 screeners to the office and reported that all 10 numbers did not exist, were disconnected, were businesses, or were for FAX machines. Because this was such an exceptionally low yield (generating zero out of a potential 10 interviews), the field supervisor called the numbers and found that the call records had been falsified. The interviewer was fired.

Call records are a valuable way to document and validate both personal interviews and off-site telephone interviews. When telephone interviews are conducted from a central location or computer-assisted telephone interviewing is used, there are more efficient ways to monitor data collectors' behavior and the status of the sample. CATI, for example, keeps track of whether a number was dialed and what the outcome was. Direct supervision can be used when calls are made from a central location.

Editing

Once data are collected, editing and data entry begin. Editing involves identifying and correcting errors that occur over the course of the study. Researchers must not forget to allow enough money for editing in their research budgets; the U.S. Office of Management and Budget (1990, p. 13) estimates that editing absorbs a minimum of 20% of the cost of most federal surveys.

Errors can occur in the design of data collection (see Chapter 2), because respondents intentionally or unintentionally make errors, because data collectors make errors, or during the creation of machine-readable files (see Chapter 4). Here we will describe how to identify and correct errors created by respondents and data collectors.

INTERVIEWER EDIT

The first stage of editing is done by the data collector or interviewer, who should carefully review each questionnaire as soon as possible after completion, while the interview is still fresh in mind. An *interviewer edit* ensures that handwriting is legible, no questions were missed, all skip instructions were followed, all information in boxes is coded, numbers corresponding to precoded answers have been circled, and all identifying information has been appropriately filled out.

When a questionnaire has open-ended questions or residual "other" categories for closed-ended questions, the interviewer must make sure that answers are filled out legibly and completely. During the interview, interviewers can reduce the likelihood of incomplete answers if they record *all* probes used to elicit responses and write down *everything* respondents say. Only when a subject says something like "I can't think of anything else" in response to the final probe: "What else can you tell me about [. . .]?" should the interviewer go on to the next question.

Sometimes the interviewer needs to clarify material so that supervisors or other office staff know data are correct. For example, if there is a discrepancy between the roster of persons living in the household and the number of persons reported as dependent upon household income, an interviewer needs to explain this or the supervisor might assume there is an error in the data. This situation occurred more than once in our earthquake studies. The "error" was explained by a note written by the interviewer stating that children were away at college or alimony was being paid to an ex-spouse.

If during this editing process an interviewer finds that answers to one or more questions are missing, he or she must call the respondent back immediately to obtain the missing data. Once the interviewer has completed the edit and made corrections, he or she returns the questionnaire or data form to the central office for logging-in and further editing.

LOGGING OR FIELD EDIT

The next edit is called the *logging* or *field edit*. Logging gives the researcher a quick assessment of how the data collectors are performing. Here supervisors make sure that the proper respondent was interviewed or the proper record was abstracted. They check the skip patterns to verify that they were followed correctly and review the call record sheet to ensure that it was completed properly. If errors are found, the questionnaire is returned to the interviewer for reinterview or correction. Similar checks are made if records are the source of data.

The field edit provides the major source of information about whether data collection is proceeding on schedule and whether the selected sample size is large enough to produce the necessary number of completed interviews. In every method of data collection, researchers must estimate the percentage of respondents or records that will result in usable, complete data records. If during the course of data collection supervisors note that the sample is not being obtained at the expected rate, decisions must be made quickly on how to change procedures or number of personnel to obtain the agreed-upon sample size. Failure to make such changes often extends data collection time, which leaves less time and money for data analysis and report writing.

During the *field edit* in our Whittier Narrows study, we discovered that our expectations about the number of subjects we needed were on the mark for most of Los Angeles County, but that we needed more telephone numbers to reach our goal of 200 interviews in the high-impact area. Consequently, an additional 274 telephone numbers were randomly generated. If we had not conducted the *field edit* we might not have known that our sample was seriously inadequate until we started analyzing our data.

QUALITY-CONTROL EDIT

The third edit is a *quality-control edit*. Here every item in the questionnaire or record abstraction form is checked for completeness, consistency, and clarity. When errors are found, the interview is referred back to the interviewer for clarification or reinterview. While the exact content of a quality-control edit varies for each research project, the following summarizes what should be included in a quality-control edit. Researchers must take each of the following steps:

1. Check household rosters to be sure they are correctly and fully filled out.
2. Check that data were collected from the correct record, respondent, household, or the like.
3. Evaluate all data submitted by data collectors to ensure their overall patterns of tallying responses and completion rates are in line with study expectations and respondent refusals are not significantly different from those of other data collectors.
4. Use call records to evaluate whether interviewers are varying their attempts to find respondents. Use similar methods to log and monitor data collection efforts of record abstractors and observers.
5. Resolve ambiguities in instrument use that can surface during data collection; for example, check that collectors explain disparities between the number of persons dependent on reported household income and the number of persons living in the household.
6. Check that missing data (e.g., don't know, inapplicable, refusal, missing) have been appropriately and consistently recorded.
7. Check whether precoded response categories for closed-ended questions are being used appropriately. If there are indications that problems exist,

42

this means that data collectors need further training or response categories need to be revised. Such revisions should be made quickly, even in the middle of a study.

8. Check that interviewers are following instructions and asking all specified probes for eliciting answers to open-ended questions. Similar procedures can be developed to monitor data gathering of observers and record abstractors.

9. Monitor mileage claims or telephone charges of data collectors. Such information can confirm or fail to support claims about work performed.

10. Record the time taken for data collection and evaluate significant deviations from it.

11. Be sensitive to data that are too perfect.

With the exceptions of items 10 and 11, all these points were discussed earlier in this chapter. Clearly, a data collector who consistently turns in questionnaires that are incomplete, inconsistent, and illegible, or who consistently obtains data from the wrong person or record, should be terminated. Similarly, interviewers who consistently obtain a high number of refusals should be terminated. Evidence that a data collector is much faster or slower than other data collectors also may be reason for evaluation and possible termination. Interviewers who complete interviews too quickly may not be giving respondents sufficient time to hear the questions or consider their answers.

The "perfect" data form also gives reason to pause. Human beings and the records they create are rarely completely consistent. When a data collector always turns in forms with no evidence of error on the part of the data collector or changes in responses by respondents, it is possible that the data collector "created" the data.

Similar kinds of problems may develop with self-administered questionnaires. Here the respondent, not the data collector, may be falsifying data. Respondents falsify data for many reasons; for instance, they may wish to present a more favorable image of themselves (e.g., by lowering age or raising income), they may not know or cannot accurately remember an item, or they may wish to please the interviewer or data collector. Whether the problem lies with the respondent or the data collector, the only way to determine whether such suspicions are valid is to ask a different data collector to reinterview the respondent or reabstract the record.

DATA ENTRY EDIT

The final manual edit is done as data are entered into the computer. This *data entry edit* serves as a check on the prior three edits, but some concerns are addressed here for the first time. For example, the respondents' descriptions of their jobs and workplaces are coded using the Census Bureau's *Alphabetical*

Index of Industries and Occupations. If these data need clarification, data collectors may be asked to recontact respondents; but obviously, as one gets further from the actual time of data collection, the ability to resolve problems declines and eventually data are lost.

Summary

While describing four stages of manual data editing, we have emphasized three points: Preliminary data editing should be done as close to the time of data collection as possible, to maximize the ability to make corrections while respondents and data sources are still available; data editing should include checks on the sample and its availability; and all data should be edited by more than one person. We suggest that, at minimum, the data collector, a supervisor, and a data entry worker should independently examine data for consistency, completeness, and clarity.

4. DATA ENTRY

Once data collection has been completed and checked, the process of data entry and cleaning starts. During data entry the verbal or numeric data collected using questionnaires, abstraction forms, or observations are entered into a computer, principally as numeric data "codes." These data codes (discussed in Chapter 2), together with labels and other attributes of the variables, constitute the data file. *Data entry* refers to the process of computerizing the data. Although other methods of data entry are briefly mentioned, only keyboard entry is considered in this chapter.

In the first section of this chapter we review how the evolution from punch cards to personal computers has changed the ways that computers are used in research studies. In the second section, we discuss the mechanics of computerizing the study data, beginning with definition of data file structure and variables, continuing with entry of the basic data values, and finishing with initial screening and cleanup necessary to ensure that the data are complete and correct. The last section discusses the training of data entry personnel.

Creating Computerized Data Files: Then and Now

One commonly thinks of statistical data analysis as the prime application for computers in research studies. Over the last two decades, however, changes in computers probably have had a greater effect on data entry than on statistical analysis. We will take a brief look at how such changes have created data processing advantages for the new computer-aided work patterns in contrast to the shortcomings of some old ways of thinking about data processing.

THE OLD WAY: BATCH PROCESSING

The Punch Card Legacy. Punch cards were developed for data processing long before electronic computers were invented. The key feature of punch cards was invariant positioning of data. Combinations of hole punches resulted in each card column representing a single alphanumeric character or digit. Thus one 80-column card could represent 80 consecutive characters or digits of data. Each variable was entered into a specific column or group of columns, creating what became known as *fixed-format* data. The early punch card systems placed a premium on simple, regular data formats and minimal input. Extra blanks, field-separator delimiters, and other syntactic aids to human readability frequently increased error problems with slow mechanical card readers.

The Early Computers. The early mainframe computers were big, finicky about operating environments, difficult to program, expensive to run, and difficult to maintain. A researcher took great care to prepare data and program instructions to minimize computer time, and jobs were fed to the computer as prepackaged "batches" by trained operators. In short, mainframe computer systems enforced an economy where computer resources were highly valued and rationed, and clerical resources for off-line data preparation were regarded as relatively cheap.

THE CONTEMPORARY WAY: COMPUTER-AIDED WORK

Beginning with the introduction of solid-state electronic components, the computer world changed radically. *Multiprocessing* and *time-sharing* capabilities allowed people to use the computers via *remote* keyboard terminals and display screens. Computers could now be used effectively to minimize overall production costs and to make things easier for workers who were not computer experts. Specifically, computers could be utilized to improve everyday error-prone human tasks such as data entry, as well as to perform difficult statistical computations.

The Desktop Personal Computer. The culmination (so far) of this revolution has come in the last decade. The desktop computer and the computer terminal connected to a midsize departmental computer are common office tools along with copiers, fax machines, and telephones. Workers routinely use spreadsheet, word-processing, and simple database programs for daily tasks. To take advantage of computer-aided work patterns, the developers of statistical analysis program packages have created data entry systems that use the PC in an interactive fashion, making data entry easier, quicker, and more accurate.

Expanding Horizons. Several advances suggest even easier times ahead for routine data entry operations. Computer-assisted interviewing techniques and scanners that read and enter documents directly into the computer will augment and, in some cases, replace keyboard entry of data. The increasing availability of mainframe-type relational database management systems on PCs will improve access to extensive bodies of data such as those needed by large, recurrent surveys. Perhaps most important for the PC user, the emergence of multitasking and windowing operating systems should speed up and ease the work of data entry, cleaning, and analysis.

We look next at the practical activities of defining data files, entering data, and cleaning out the errors.

Creating the Data File

Before data entry can begin (and ideally at the same time that data collection forms are designed), the researcher must decide how the data are to be organized. A data file can be simple—a few columns and rows of numbers—or an intricate collection of data values, definitions of variables, related data entry forms, and cleaning specifications. For a very small project, a researcher might opt to enter data into a table using a simple editing program. For a very large project or a continuing survey service, one may need an industrial-strength relational database management system augmented by custom editing features. We will cover the middle ground, concentrating on ways to create well-structured and documented data files of moderate size with standard data entry programs that are included in major statistical packages.

PACKAGE PROGRAMS FOR DATA ENTRY

One of the consequences of the broad acceptance of personal computers has been a proliferation of computer programs. We have chosen to illustrate our discussion with the data entry offerings from two major statistical program packages: SPSS Data Entry II (SPSS, 1987) and SAS FSP FSEDIT (SAS, 1987). In this chapter, we will refer to the data entry components simply as SPSS and SAS. BMDP, the third major statistical package we use in our data analysis illustrations, has a data entry product planned for release just prior to the appearance of this volume.

THE SHAPE OF THE FILE

Computerized data files can assume many forms; however, for most statistical analyses of study data, the appropriate form is a *rectangular* data file—essentially a table. Each horizontal line represents the data record for a specific case or subject, and each vertical field represents a particular variable for that case.

The variables are in the same order for each case. A rectangular data file is needed to run statistical packages such as SPSS, SAS, and BMDP, although the programs have some capability to change hierarchical files into rectangular ones.

Usually each *record* in a data file represents an individual case or person. The designation of what a record represents depends, however, on the *unit of analysis* for the study. If an individual person is the unit of analysis, then all the data for one person in the sample constitute one record in the data file. If the study is examining a sample of hospitals, school classrooms, or census tracts, then the unit of analysis is a hospital, a school classroom, or a census tract. (Sometimes a study has multiple units of analysis; for example, a household and each of the people in the household. In such studies, the researcher might set up multiple data sets or create hierarchical data sets. This book does not cover the alternative structures of complex files and problems associated with them.)

When we speak of a variable in rectangular data files or in tables, we are referring to a *field* of similar data items (age, for instance). A variable field may be as narrow as a single character, a group of digits, a dollar sign and decimal point for a money variable, or it may be an entire language phrase resulting from an open-ended question. Most numeric data items are converted to different forms in internal computer storage, not necessarily related to the printed width of the field. The implication, then, is that a rectangular file denotes a constant number of variable fields for successive cases or subjects (records) and not necessarily a constant number of punch card columns or bytes of computer memory space.

THE FORMAT AND CONTENTS OF THE DATA FILE

ASCII Files. The simplest type of data file has fields consisting of groups of digits or letters that are held in random-access memory (RAM) or stored on computer storage media (hard disks, floppy disks, tapes, and so on) in character image form as ASCII (American Standard Code for Information Interchange) character codes. (In mainframe computers another character coding, EBCDIC—for Extended Binary-Coded-Decimal Information Code—may be used.) The character image format does not have numeric digits converted into an internal binary form that is efficient for computation. Typically, file formats referred to as ASCII lack any data description information to define the types and names of variables, allowable value ranges, and so on. However, an ASCII file can be created and edited by any simple text editor program, is easily transportable from one program or computer to another, and is close to being a universal standard. Most of the common statistical packages, spreadsheet programs, word processors, and database managers can import and export ASCII file formats (often referred to as raw-data files). Sometimes ASCII files are referred to as DOS files on IBM-compatible PCs.

PC Spreadsheet and Database Files. Most research groups and PC users are familiar with spreadsheet programs such as Lotus 123 and database programs such as dBASE. These programs, therefore, are sometimes used for data entry, especially of small- to moderate-size study results. The data files created from these programs may include names for the fields (variables), format and field width information, and some coding of missing values. The regular file formats from these programs have in some cases become de facto standards for data interchange because of their widespread use, and the file formats of one program are often readable by the others.

The major statistical analysis programs make various provisions for input of data from these sources. For example, SPSS can read the regular files from several different spreadsheet and several database programs, taking in not only the raw data values for the variables but also variable names, data types, input field widths, and the like. SAS provides a means (DBF and DIF procedures) for converting back and forth between database and spreadsheet program formats and SAS data sets. BMDP does not accept input in the regular formats of spreadsheet, database, and word-processing programs, but suggests exporting ASCII (character image) output from those programs for input into BMDP. Variable names, types, and so on cannot be transferred directly.

Statistical Program System Files. The major statistical packages provide special versions of data files that encode additional information about the file along with the data values. In SPSS, for example, a *system file* contains the data items in internal binary format specific to the computer in use, a dictionary containing definitions of the variables, and even data entry forms, cleaning specifications, and skip values. In BMDP a somewhat comparable internal file format is known as a *BMDP file*, and in SAS as a *SAS data set*. These specialized files, the *SPSS system file*, for example, provide several advantages. They keep all of the related information, such as variable names, with the basic data so that it need not be entered again for successive statistical analyses. Such files provide the investigators with much of the information needed for a codebook of the data as described in Chapter 6. They also facilitate the use of the files by a number of investigators, since the documentation for the data is on-line. Furthermore, they keep the numeric data in an internal binary format for computational efficiency, whereby speed of computation is enhanced. Finally, they provide an easy way to enhance the data file with newly added derived variables, identification of missing values, transformations, and additional labels to be used in subsequent analyses.

Unfortunately, the formats and information included are unique to each of the proprietary statistical analysis program systems—that is, all of the information in an SPSS system file is not *directly* usable in BMDP or SAS programs, and so on. However, the major program systems provide some mechanisms for reading each other's files. For example, on mainframe computers, SAS release 6 can read SPSS and SPSS-X files, but, as of this writing, SPSS cannot read SAS release 6 files. SPSS can, however, read SAS release 5 files, which SAS release 6 has the capability of creating. DBMS/COPY provides for transfers on PCs. The ability to move from program to program may change in future versions; readers are advised to check with their local computer facilities.

Because the data are stored in a hardware-dependent binary format, it is not usually possible to use a system file from one type of computer in another. A BMDP file created on a PC will not be directly usable on a VAX or an IBM mainframe computer. The BMDP and SPSS statistical program systems provide for *portable* versions of their system files for export and import between different computer hardware systems, and for transfer between mainframes and PCs. SAS also has provisions for preparing programs and data files that can be used with SAS on different computers.

Major computer centers often have utilities that help in exchanging data between program system files. Software is available for PCs to accomplish many file transfers (for example, a commercially available program, DBMS/COPY, will transfer files among a wide selection of spreadsheets, database programs, and statistical packages), and books are available that discuss file formats and transfers (for example, see Poor, 1990). Nonetheless, the simplest procedure is to enter the data using a data entry package that is part of the statistical program system you intend to use.

DEFINING THE DATA FILE

In using the structured data entry programs (as provided in the major statistical packages), one begins by naming the file and then defining the variables. These defined variables are then used in the program to guide data entry operations. Using SPSS, for example, one starts with the *Files Branch* to name a data file, then uses the *Dictionary Branch* to define the variables to be included in the file. The definition of each variable is done in an entry window, as illustrated below, that prompts for the variable attributes. The attributes in the left column prompt the user by showing the kind of information that can be described during data entry. The middle column provides an example of information that a user might enter, while the right column in the illustration describes the options that are available for each attribute.

Attribute	*Example*	*Description*
Variable Name	**marital**	(up to eight characters)
Variable Label	**marital status**	(up to 60 characters)
Type of Variable	**numeric**	(**numeric** or **string**)
Variable Length	**1**	(max for input/display)
Decimal Places	**0**	(number, for display)
Display Mode	**edit**	(**edit**, **verify**, or **display**)
Missing	**9**	(up to three codes)

SPSS allows one to assign labels to specified values of a variable. For example, for the variable *marital*:

Value	Label
1	never married
2	married
3	formerly married
9	missing

When variables have been defined in this fashion, the data file is permanently documented in computer-readable form. These variable definitions are then available to guide data entry, to facilitate cleaning of the data file, to provide necessary information for statistical analysis, and to annotate displays and printouts of results. The various data entry programs handle null or missing values differently. Refer to the system manuals for detailed provisions for defaults and missing value codes.

Figure 4.1 shows a frequency distribution from the Whittier Narrows study computed using the SPSS statistical analysis programs, with and without variable and missing value labels. To understand and interpret the table in part A of this figure, the researcher would have to refer to a codebook or questionnaire. In contrast, the table in part B can be understood and interpreted directly. Here, the variable label indicates that this is the frequency distribution for Question 50, which asks about ethnicity. The value labels identify the various codes or categories of ethnicity. Although it is tedious to create variable and value labels, their existence saves a great deal of time during analysis. They also provide partial documentation for a data set. Thus we recommend that when such a capability exists, variable labels and value labels be created for *all* data.

The SAS data entry procedure uses operations generally comparable to those of SPSS for definition of data files and their variables, although the details and the particular variable attributes used differ. For instance, SAS allows specifying of maximum and minimum allowable values for a variable as part of the variable definition, while SPSS obtains this information as part of *cleaning specifications*.

ENTERING THE DATA

The contemporary concept of computer-aided work is evident in data entry operations. Using SPSS, for example (or SAS data entry equivalents), the user does not need to keep track constantly of the order of variables, the number of characters in a data field, or the number of decimal places to enter for a value. The next variable for which a value is to be entered is clearly highlighted on the display screen, and many common input errors will be detected and rejected by the computer program, which indicates that correction is needed. The major advance is that the user no longer needs to know, or care, about inconsequential detail in data entry. Whether

A. Variable Without Labels
V547

VALUE LABEL	VALUE	FREQUENCY	PERCENT	VALID PERCENT	CUM PERCENT
	1	563	81.6	81.6	81.6
	2	62	9.0	9.0	90.6
	3	46	6.7	6.7	97.2
	4	4	.6	.6	97.8
	5	13	1.9	1.9	99.7
	7	2	.3	.3	100.0
	TOTAL	690	100.0	100.0	

VALID CASES   690   MISSING CASES   0

B. Variable With Labels
V547   Q50-ETHNICITY

VALUE LABEL	VALUE	FREQUENCY	PERCENT	VALID PERCENT	CUM PERCENT
WHITE	1	563	81.6	83.4	
BLACK	2	62	9.0	9.2	92.6
ASIAN	3	46	6.7	6.8	99.4
NAT AMER	4	4	.6	.6	100.0
OTHER	5	13	1.9	MISSING	
REFUSED	7	2	.3	MISSING	
	TOTAL	690	100.0	100.0	

VALID CASES   675   MISSING CASES   15

Figure 4.1. Variable With and Without Variable Label and Value Labels

numeric values are right-justified, with leading zeros rather than blanks, is no longer a concern of the user; the program has accepted the significant value typed in, and properly incorporated it into the developing internal data file structure.

One example will help to illustrate this shift in functions between human operator and computer. In the past, when developing a coding frame (see Chapter 2), one might have agonized over whether to allow two digits or three for a variable code for a postcoded open-end response. If the computer is keeping track and incorporating the input data into one of the *system file* formats as entered, this concern is unnecessary. The internal binary format for the numeric value occupies the same amount of storage (typically 8 bytes) whether the code is 2, 3, or 15 digits.

Researchers have often avoided using shortcut techniques such as free-format input with field separators (comma or blank delimiters), elimination of nonsignificant leading zeros, and null entries for skipped variables. Their rationale has been that conversion of this abridged data entry information back into fully detailed fixed-format records would involve esoteric computer programming work or be fraught with error opportunities, and that visual proofing of the data as entered is error prone. The advantage of the contemporary data entry packages is that the data can be displayed or printed for user proofing at any stage in the operation—before and after cleaning, after range checking or transformations—in exactly the format used during input.

FORMS OR SPREADSHEETS?

The data entry programs discussed here allow alternative formats for data entry: a one-record-at-a-time mode generally known as a *form*, and a *spreadsheet* or *table* mode that directly represents the rectangular data file being created. SPSS allows instant switching back and forth between the modes. (With SAS the process of switching is somewhat less immediate, as the form and spreadsheet modes are implemented with different programs.)

The choice between these modes is in part a matter of personal preference, but the shape and size of the data file should be considered in the choice.

Spreadsheet. A tabular format for data entry where rows represent cases or records and columns represent variables is often called a spreadsheet. The spreadsheet entry mode requires no special setup and is efficient for small data files. The ability to see the input from previous records while entering new data can be helpful. If a data file has relatively few variables, scrolling left and right will not be required to view them all on the display screen in the spreadsheet mode.

Figure 4.2 presents an abbreviated example of spreadsheet data for three cases and seven variables using the questions given in Figure 2.2. Fields to the left of V92 or to the right of V97 are seen by scrolling the spreadsheet left or right on the computer display screen. Respondents with IDs 8002 and 2453 answered yes (coded 1) to V92 (Question 1), and the next four variables were skipped and coded 0 for "not applicable." ID 8910 answered no (coded 2) to V92 (Question 1) and, therefore, was asked Questions 1A-1C, which resulted in codes for V93-V96, and was then skipped past V97 (Question 2) to Question 8. V97 (Question 2) was coded 0 for "not applicable."

Form. The *form* mode uses the whole computer screen for the current case being entered. There are several arguments for using the *form* mode of input:

- An entry form can be structured to look like the original data collection instrument.

- Variables do not have to be entered in the order in which they were defined, if another entry order is useful.

- Large numbers of variables for each record can be accommodated easily with multiple-page forms. Flipping pages on the display typically is an easier and faster operation than scrolling a display left and right.

		Variable and Question No.					
ID	. . .	V92	V93	V94	(V95 | V96)	V97	. . .
		Q1	Q1A	Q1B	Q1C	Q1C	Q2
8002	. . .	1	0	0	0	0	1	. . .
.				→ skip			
.							
.							
2453	. . .	1	0	0	0	0	2	. . .
.				→ skip			
.							
.							
8910	. . .	2	5	19	1	0	0	. . .
.							→ skip to Q8
.							
.							

Figure 4.2. Example of Data Entry Spreadsheet Using Questions From Figure 2.2

- Long variables (such as from direct text entry of open-ended question responses) can be accommodated easily.
- Short coding comments and instructions can be included on the screen as prompts for the user.

Figure 4.3 presents an example of forms input using the first case from Figure 4.2. The information displayed on the screen corresponds to the data collection documents being read, with abbreviated text and code values, and explanatory notes or entry instructions added. The form may contain many pages (screens) to accommodate all of the variables for the data file, but the data entered on a set of pages represents a single case or respondent—equivalent to a single line on the spreadsheet in Figure 4.2. Here the data shown represent the respondent with ID 8002, also shown in Figure 4.2.

The two major statistical packages discussed in this chapter differ in how they implement *forms*. SPSS provides the features described here, tailored especially to the entry of survey and other research data. SAS provides similar features while allowing more options, but with more complexity.

SKIP-AND-FILL OPERATIONS IN DATA ENTRY

Particularly in survey studies, it is common to have branching sequences of variables in a data file (see Chapter 2). Given one response to a question, a more detailed sequence of follow-up questions is asked; otherwise, the detailed

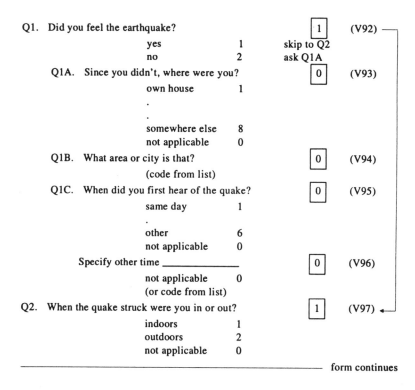

Figure 4.3. Example of a Data Entry Form Using Questions From Figure 2.2 With Data From Respondent 8002

sequence is skipped or an alternative sequence is pursued. At coding or data entry time the unasked questions need to be addressed, usually coded as "not applicable." The major statistical package data entry programs can be utilized in several ways to streamline handling of these skip-and-fill operations.

SPSS provides full support for skip-and-fill operations. For example, the entry of a particular predetermined code (e.g., 1 for yes) as the response to a variable causes the computer to move automatically to the first of a sequence of follow-up variables for entry. Entering a different response to the same question causes the program to skip over the follow-up variables and automatically enter predefined "not applicable" codes for them. SAS does not explicitly provide full support for skip-and-fill operations, but the user can approximate this capability through a series of programming operations.

CLEANING THE DATA FILE

Once the data set has been created, it must be cleaned. During cleaning, errors that occurred during data entry or that were not found prior to data entry are identified and corrected. The researcher checks the data for values that are out of range and for errors that show up as inconsistencies between variables.

Cleaning a data file involves a variety of checks. On small data files, many of these checks can be performed informally by a visual scan of a printout from the file, but for files with many records, many variables, skip-and-fill branching, or long string variables for open-ended text responses, a visual check is unproductive.

Range checking, checking variable values against predefined maximum and minimum bounds, is often done as a data screening or cleaning technique to catch spurious values or keyboard entry errors; for example, if 100 has been entered instead of 10.

SPSS provides for *cleaning specifications* that can be invoked *either* during data entry or, later, as a separate cleaning process for the data file. In addition to the range or bounds checking described above, cleaning rules can be formulated that are logical expressions making various assertions about the data (see Chapter 5). The cleaning process tests these assertions against each record in turn and produces a report that shows violations of the rules. SAS allows the definition of valid data ranges as part of the definition of variables, and provides an interactive error indication during keyboard input of data.

Comparable cleaning operations can be done after data entry with any statistical package program by running univariate statistical programs or procedures in which logical expressions (the cleaning rules) are applied to the data records as a *transformation* operation in which records with violations are thereby flagged for editing (see Chapter 5).

Consistency Checks Using Contingency Tables. Even when data appear clean following range checks, consistency checks may reveal errors. Part A of Figure 4.4 shows a cross-tabular table of two variables from Figure 2.2: V98 (Question 2A), "Where were you when the earthquake struck?" by V92 (Question 1), "Did you feel the earthquake?" (V92 and V98 are the variable names assigned when the data file was defined.)

Remember that this series of questions is in skip-and-fill format. A person who said yes to Question 1 (V92) *should* have been asked Question 2A (V98); a person who said no to Question 1 *should not* have been asked Question 2A. Thus there is something wrong with the data entered for the 5 respondents who are coded 1 on V92 and 0 on V98 and for the 7 respondents who are coded 2 on V92 and 1, 3, 4, or 7 on V98. We track down this problem by finding the identification numbers of these 12 cases, looking up their answers in the questionnaires, and correcting the computer file. Part B of Figure 4.4 shows the contingency table between the two variables after all the corrections were made.

A. Contingency Table Showing Inconsistencies

V92	COUNT	V98 NOT APP 0	OWN HOME 1	OTH HOME 2	WORK 3	SCHOOL 4	TRAV-ELING 5	PUB PLACE 6	OTHER 7	ROW TOTAL
YES	1	5	416	7	114	9	51	1	20	623 90.3
NO	2	60	3		2	1			1	67 9.7
	COLUMN TOTAL	65 9.4	419 60.7	7 1.0	116 16.8	10 1.4	51 7.4	1 .1	21 3.0	690 100.0

NUMBER OF MISSING OBSERVATIONS = 0

B. Contingency Table Showing Corrected Inconsistencies

V92	COUNT	V98 NOT APP 0	OWN HOME 1	OTH HOME 2	WORK 3	SCHOOL 4	TRAV-ELING 5	PUB PLACE 6	OTHER 7	ROW TOTAL
YES	1		420	7	114	9	52	1	20	623 90.3
NO	2	67								67 9.7
	COLUMN TOTAL	67 9.7	420 60.9	7 1.0	114 16.5	9 1.3	52 7.5	1 .1	20 2.9	690 100.0

NUMBER OF MISSING OBSERVATIONS = 0

Figure 4.4. Contingency Tables to Diagnose Inconsistencies Between Question 1 and Question 2A From Figure 2.2

Timing of Data Cleaning. The entire data set should be cleaned prior to analyzing any of the data. All too frequently, no effort is made to clean data, or data are cleaned in a piecemeal fashion as errors are discovered. Range checks can be done during data entry, or after data entry by running frequency distributions of all the variables in the data set. Errors usually can be spotted quite easily and, as we saw in part B of Figure 4.1, the addition of value labels for legitimate codes helps make illegal codes "pop out" in a frequency distribution. Consistency checks are more difficult to conduct, and it is more difficult to know exactly when to stop making them.

Cleaning of Longitudinal Data Sets. In some studies data collection occurs at multiple times over a period of months or years. Data cleaning in such studies is more complicated, and it is important to do it as soon as possible after each wave of data collection. It is particularly important to check demographic information or other information that should remain constant or change in predictable directions over time. For example, the respondent's gender, age, education, occupation, ethnicity, and number of children should either stay constant or change consistently over time.

There are, of course, situations in which legitimate changes do occur or reporting errors are made by the respondent. Respondents often forget about children who are away at college or in the military, sometimes falsify their own ages, and change their occupations or ethnic identities. Such cases are rare, however, and when these inconsistencies occur they must be checked and the discrepancy corrected, the data declared missing, the case dropped, or the reason for the discrepancy documented.

HOW CLEAN IS CLEAN?

Determining that the data file contains no out-of-range or inconsistent values does not mean that it contains no errors. An incorrect keystroke can result in a numeric value that is in the accepted range and for which no logical inconsistency exists. If a level of close-to-zero errors is desired, reentering the entire data file and comparing the results can be considered. The SPSS data entry program includes a "verify" mode in which the data being entered the second time are compared with those entered the first time. If the two values disagree, both values are displayed so that the data entry person can decide which to use. Alternatively, the data can be entered twice as if they were additional variables for each case. The order of entry of the cases should be identical. The resulting data set will have the same number of cases but twice the number of variables. Then, the first half of the variables are subtracted from the second half and any nonzero results are checked. Note that if the values entered the second time are identical to the first entry, all the differences should be zero. Obviously, the confidence in the data will be much greater if the data are verified, particularly for large data sets entered by unmotivated staff. It will double the cost of data entry, however, so careful assessment should be made of the extra cost versus the benefits of error-free data entry.

Training of Data Entry Personnel

Like data collectors, coders and data entry clerks must be trained and supervised. This is particularly important if coders and data entry clerks are hired only for those tasks. Such work tends to be repetitive and tedious, and it demands attention to detail. Persons who have no understanding of or interest in the outcome of the study frequently do not understand why accuracy and consistency are important in coding and data entry. We have found that full-time data entry personnel tend to make fewer entry errors than research assistants.

Many of the procedures used with data collectors can be modified for use in hiring, training, and supervising data processing personnel. Procedures to be used in coding and entering data should be reviewed in sequence and in detail. The researcher should have each person code and enter two or three "practice" forms. The practice forms should be selected or created to represent the kinds of problems expected during data entry.

Once actual coding and data entry begin, at least 10-25% of the work should be reviewed for accuracy. This can be done by use of available computer verification programs (e.g., SPSS and BMDP), by personal review of the work of individual data processors, or by having two data processors independently code or enter the same data and comparing their results. Any discrepancies must be examined and resolved. Data entry that involves a complex sequence of actions or that requires data processors to make judgment decisions should be monitored more frequently. In general, the coding and data entry associated with open-ended questions is more difficult than that associated with closed-ended questions. In large data sets with complex coding or data entry problems, it is sometimes advantageous to have a single person "specialize" in coding or entering certain kinds of data. Examples might include the use of the International Classification of Diseases to code information from hospital records or the use of the U.S. Census Bureau's (1992) *Alphabetical Index of Industries and Occupations* to code occupational status.

Even after careful instructions on the part of the researcher, problems surface during coding and data entry that are not anticipated. Coders and data entry clerks should be encouraged to watch for problems and to bring them to the attention of the researcher. If a problem is widespread or important, coding and data entry procedures should be modified and data already entered must be reviewed and, if necessary, corrected.

5. DATA PREPARATION FOR ANALYSIS

Once the data have been entered into the computer and a complete and documented data file is obtained, the data must be processed prior to analysis. For small data sets, data processing can be performed concurrently with statistical analysis, but for larger studies, it should be performed as a separate step. In the separate step, a data file of usable documented data is created that all the investigators on the project can analyze directly. This simplifies the entry of statistical instructions, because all the data processing steps are already completed.

One of the first steps in data processing (sometimes called data management) is to determine the *response* rate for the study and to decide if the sample obtained reflects the population from which it was taken. Subsequent steps include *data screening* for incomplete or missing data, possible *data imputation* for missing values, *outlier detection*, *transformations* to create more easily analyzed variables, *scale* evaluation, and *saving* the results in one or more working files and subfiles. The various computer program packages use similar data management methods, but the actual instructions vary. Here we discuss the methods, but do not give specific computer instructions; these can be obtained from the appropriate manuals. We assume that the reader has options equivalent to those found in SPSS, SAS, or BMDP program packages. To start the process, run a univariate statistical program such as EXAMINE or FREQUENCIES in SPSS, UNIVARIATE in SAS, or 2D in BMDP to obtain a simple data description on all the variables. This will list the number of missing values per variable, the maximum and minimum values for each variable, the number of responses in each category for nominal or ordinal variables, and summary statistics such as means, medians, and standard deviations.

Nonresponse

Data may be unavailable for two reasons (see Kalton & Kasprzyk, 1986). The first occurs when no information is available on a subject either because of refusal or because the subject (or the subject's record) cannot be found. We call this *nonresponse*. The second occurs when partial data are available from the subject but some items are missing. We call this *missing data.*

If there is appreciable nonresponse, investigators should attempt to evaluate how subjects with no data compare with subjects for whom data exist. One common check is to compare the demographic characteristics of the sample (age, gender, and so on) with those of the population from which it came. If the gender and age distribution of the population is known, the comparison is simple. If not, then census or other data thought to characterize the population are used. If it is determined that the sample obtained is not representative of the population, the magnitude of the difference should be assessed. For example, in survey samples women are often overrepresented. Typically, such discrepancies are simply reported, but the data from underrepresented groups (e.g., men) can also be weighted more in the analyses to approximate their representation in the population.

USE OF WEIGHTS

Weighting may be particularly important if results are to be used in projecting the need for services such as school or medical care. For example, if a community is considering building or relocating schools, projections as to the number, geographic location, and age distribution of children expected to attend school in the community must be as accurate as possible. In such cases, distributions on important variables in the sample should reflect the population, and the following formula for weighted sample means should be used (see Kalton & Kasprzyk, 1986, for an estimate of the bias of the unadjusted mean):

$$\bar{y}(w) = \sum W(j)\bar{y}(j)$$

where $W(j)$ denotes the proportion of the population in stratum j, $\bar{y}(j)$ denotes the mean of the subjects in stratum j in the sample, and $\bar{y}(w)$ denotes the overall weighted mean. This formula assumes that a simple random sample has been drawn. For further discussion, see Kish (1965) or Little and Rubin (1987). The major statistical packages allow for the use of weights.

Typically, the sample is divided into groups or strata using the variables (gender, age, and so on) on which response is anticipated to be dissimilar. The number of respondents and nonrespondents within each stratum is computed. Weights are computed proportional to the inverse of the response rate within each stratum (see Kalton & Kasprzyk, 1986). For example, suppose you obtained the following response by gender:

	Respondents	Nonrespondents	Sum
Male	100	60	160
Female	150	10	160
Sum	250	70	320

The response rate for males would be $100/160 = 0.6250$, and for females $150/160 = 0.9375$. The weights could be taken as $1/.625$ or 1.60 for males and 1.0667 for females, or could be adjusted further so that the sum of the weights equals the sample size. The adjusted weights are computed as

$$W(i) = w(i) \times N(r)/N(t)$$

where $w(i)$ is the original weight in the ith weighting stratum, $N(r)$ is the total sample size of responders, and $N(t)$ is the number of responders and non-responders. For males, we would have

$$1.60 \times 250/320 = 1.25$$

and for females 0.833. Since we have 100 males and 150 females in the sample, the sum of the weights is

$$100 \times 1.25 + 150 \times 0.833 = 250$$

(the sample size).

Logistic regression analysis provides another method of estimating weights. The existence or nonexistence of a response is treated as a dichotomous dependent variable and other variables are used to predict it (see Afifi & Clark, 1990; Hosmer & Lemeshow, 1989). If, for example, you have information on age, education, and gender *and* you can predict whether or not a person responded using these three variables, your respondents and nonrespondents differ on these characteristics. Logistic regression provides you with an estimate of the probability that a given subject's data will be missing. These probabilities can then be assigned as weights for all cases; cases that have missing data are given higher weights.

It has been our experience that the use of weights does not substantially change estimates of the sample mean unless nonrespondents are appreciably different from respondents and there is a substantial proportion of nonrespondents. Note that the use of significance tests with weighted data sets is not straightforward unless the weights are known to be without error.

Missing Data

For the second type of missing values, some data are available for all the subjects, but for certain subjects some data are missing. Such missing data will often be denoted in the computer files by a period or other symbol. Sometimes investigators distinguish among the different types of missing values, using responses such as "not applicable," "refused," "don't know," and "missing" (see Chapter 2).

All data sets should be examined for patterns of missing values. A small data set can be printed out and both *cases* and *variables* can be scanned for excessive missing values. If a subject has many missing values, the simplest procedure is to eliminate this case from the data set. The researcher may want to check the demographic characteristics of such subjects to see if there is something special about them. Variables (other than those legitimately skipped as "not applicable") that have many missing values probably should be eliminated. The objective is to reduce missing values to a minimum, scattered throughout rather than clustered in a few cases or variables.

When the data set is large, visual scanning is difficult and indirect methods of determining the patterns of missing values should be used. The major statistical packages can provide counts of the number of missing values by variable. SPSS and SAS allow you to rotate your data set so the variables become the cases and the cases the variables. You can then analyze the number of missing values per case. The BMDP AM program denotes missing values with an "M" and prints out the values that are either too small or too big; numerical values that are both present and within range are blank. This allows patterns of missing data to be discerned visually by scanning even quite large data sets. BMDP AM also provides the number of cases present by variable and by pairs of variables.

CASEWISE AND PAIRWISE DELETION OF CASES

Most statistical package programs allow multivariate analytical procedures to be done using either casewise or pairwise deletion of cases (see BMDP 8D or SPSS). Whenever possible, casewise (sometimes called listwise) deletion of cases is preferred. When casewise deletion of cases is used, only those cases that have data on *all* variables included in the analysis remain in the analysis. For example, if correlations were being computed between all pairs of five variables, only those cases with *no* missing data on *any* of the five variables would be included in the correlation matrix. This can result in an appreciable loss of cases if many variables are used. Suppose you wish to run a stepwise regression analysis that includes 25 variables. If 2% of the responses for each variable are missing completely at random, you will lose about 40% of your cases from the regression analysis.

When pairwise deletion of cases is used, the missing data for each pair of variables is examined. For example, if correlations were being computed between all pairs of five variables, the computer would be instructed to examine each unique pair. That is, if 100 cases in the study have no missing values on variables 1 and 2, those 100 cases are used to compute the correlation between variables 1 and 2. If, in contrast, 121 cases have no missing values on variables 1 and 3, those 121 cases are used in calculating the correlation between variables 1 and 3. As a result, each correlation coefficient conceivably could be calculated using a different sample size. With pairwise deletion, the typical correlation coefficient in a correlation matrix will be computed from a larger sample size than for casewise deletion. We recommend using this option *only if* the sample size is so small that it is critical to use all possible observations and the missing observations are missing at random, as discussed in the next section.

FILLING IN MISSING VALUES

In some instances you can go back to the individual subject or record and obtain information that fills in a missing value. This is recommended whenever feasible. Usually it is not possible, so you must either leave the value missing or fill it in using a procedure called *imputation*. Imputation procedures may be generally applicable to a variety of data or quite specific to a particular study. For example, in Chapter 2 we showed how an error in a "skip-and-fill" in the Whittier Narrows study resulted in some respondents not being asked for dollar estimates of the damage they experienced. These missing data were imputed by searching the data files for other subjects with similar types of damage, calculating the average amount of damage reported, and assigning the average to those for whom it was missing.

Before imputation is used, certain assumptions must be made about *how* the data are missing (Little & Rubin, 1987, 1990). Data can be missing completely at random (MCAR), missing at random (MAR), or nonrandomly missing. When

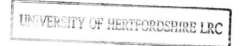

data are MCAR, the missing values are randomly distributed across all cases. For example, if one page of the data collection instrument was missing, answers for that page might not be obtained for one case. When data are MCAR, cases with missing values are assumed to be like cases with no missing values. This can be checked by dividing subjects into two groups according to whether or not they have missing data. Characteristics of the two groups can then be compared using procedures such as *t* tests that test for equal means across the two groups (see BMDP 8D). If data are MCAR, no appreciable differences should be found between the two groups on any of the characteristics tested.

More complex multivariate analyses can also be performed. For categorical data (nominal or ordinal), chi-square or log linear analysis can be used. If the sample size is small, these tests may have low power. Also, in performing such tests it is important to consider what variables are likely to be different between the two groups and not to perform tests on all possible variables or combinations of variables. For example, if a question was worded in a complicated manner or assumed sophisticated knowledge, nonresponse might be expected to vary inversely with subjects' education. In such a case the mean education of responders and nonresponders should be compared.

When data are MCAR, several imputation techniques can be used to replace the missing values. The simplest is to replace the missing value with the variable mean derived from all the cases that were not missing. This technique is used when no other variable is known to be highly correlated with the missing variable. For example, suppose your data included heights of children and some of the heights were missing. You could use the mean height of the other children (called mean substitution) as an estimate of the missing height, but your estimate would be improved by first fitting a regression equation where the dependent or outcome variable was height and the independent or predictor variables were age and gender. The data from the children with no missing values would be used to compute the coefficients for the equation. Once the equation was computed, it would be used to predict the heights of the children with missing values by combining their age and gender with the coefficients obtained from the equation. These predicted heights would then be entered into the data set. This would lead to less biased results than mean substitution. Using mean substitution or a regression equation to predict an imputed height is called a *deterministic* method.

One problem with the regression substitution technique described above is that everyone with the same age and gender who has missing data is assigned exactly the same height. In the above example, a height of 50 inches might be assigned to all 10-year-old girls whose height was missing in the data set when, in fact, the heights of 10-year-old girls with no missing data vary around 50 inches. This will also result in the variance of the dependent variable being underestimated. In recognition of this problem, some researchers add a residual value to the predicted value obtained from the regression equation. The added residual can be obtained by using a residual from a randomly selected complete case or by sampling from a theoretical distribution of residuals (see Kalton & Kasprzyk, 1986, for further information). When residuals are used, the method is called *stochastic substitution*. The objective is to obtain imputed values that are similar to those for children without missing data. This stochastic method can also be used with mean substitution. (For other methods of imputation, see Anderson, Basilevsky, & Hum, 1983; Little & Rubin, 1987.)

Generally, missing data are not randomly distributed across all respondents but may be missing at random within one or more subgroups. For example, male respondents may have more missing data, but within the group of male respondents, those with missing data do not differ from those who answered the question. Values can be imputed when the missing data are MAR, but the procedures used are more complicated. One such procedure is "hot deck" imputation, in which the answer given by an individual who did respond and who is similar to the respondent in other characteristics is substituted for the missing value (see David, Little, Samuhel, & Triest, 1986; Ford, 1983). Another method is maximum likelihood estimation (see Little & Rubin, 1990). The BMDP AM program can be used to obtain maximum likelihood estimates.

Finally, the missing values may not meet the assumptions of being missing at random. When data are missing because of refusals or don't knows, this rarely occurs randomly across the entire sample or within an identifiable subgroup. In such cases, it is difficult to make a theoretical case for imputation, though there are times when imputation is practical nevertheless. For example, when responses to only one or two items are missing in a scale that contains numerous items, we recommend imputing the values for these items. Techniques for imputation in scales will be discussed later in this chapter.

IMPLICATIONS FOR ANALYSIS

In general, most researchers do not perform imputation. It involves a considerable amount of time, and some journal reviewers distrust one or more of the procedures used. One reason for this distrust is that analyses of the combined imputed and actual data treat the imputed values as if they were actual data and tend to provide too optimistic estimates of the significance levels. If the true level is, say, 10%, the level including imputed values may come out to be 5%. Statistics are biased once missing values are replaced, although the extent of the bias may be minor if very little is replaced. For example, when mean substitution is used, the variance is underestimated unless a residual term is added. On the other hand, unless data are MCAR, serious biases can occur if data analyses are limited to only those cases with complete data, and large reductions in sample size may lead to serious reductions in the power of statistical tests.

The statistical packages offer options that make replacement of particular missing values with means or other values straightforward, as, for example, BMDP AM as noted above and SPSS for mean substitution.

In some studies it may be important to analyze data both with and without the missing values replaced, and then compare the results to make sure that the method of replacing missing values did not lead to appreciably different interpretations. Other analyses can be performed that highlight the effect of cases with missing values. For example, the researcher can create a 0,1 dummy variable that reflects whether each case does (1) or does not (0) have information on important predictor variables. This dummy variable can be considered a predictor variable. Other predictor variables for which complete data exist can also be chosen. Finally, new, interactive predictor variables can be created using statistical package programs. These interactive variables are obtained by multiplying the dummy variable by each of the predictor variables for which complete data exist. (For an example of creating an interaction variable, see Afifi & Clark, 1990, p. 232.) The resultant regression equation contains three kinds of predictor variables: the predictor variables for which complete data exist, the dummy variable denoting cases for which an important predictor variable is missing, and all interactions between the dummy variable and the predictor variables with complete data. The dependent variable used should be an important dependent variable for which no cases are missing. In essence, this amounts to testing whether there are significant interaction coefficients between group status (i.e., missing versus nonmissing) and the effects of the predictor variables on the dependent variable. If all the interaction coefficients are insignificant predictors of the dependent variable, it is argued that one can, with some confidence, generalize from the equation computed from the sample with the complete data to the population from which the sample was drawn. (We want to thank an anonymous reviewer for this suggestion.)

Outliers

Outliers are observations that appear inconsistent with the rest of the data set (see Barnett & Lewis, 1984). Outliers can be avoided to a large extent by using range checks in data entry programs (see Chapter 4) or can be identified by running a univariate statistical package program and checking results against acceptable values. If the values obtained appear unreasonable, the distribution of observations for the variable should be examined. When variables are nominal (categorical) or ordinal (ordered data), the process of checking univariate distributions against acceptable values is usually sufficient to identify outliers. The decision that an interval variable contains outliers is more complicated. In this section the detection of outliers for interval or ratio data is discussed.

Three methods are commonly used for identifying outliers. First, researchers rely on their knowledge of the variable under study and declare an observation an outlier if it is outside the range of common experience. For example, most physicians would question a systolic blood pressure of 400 or an age of 128. Second, many researchers declare an observation an outlier if it appears to them to be far removed from the rest of the data set. Suppose you had the following data set: 1, 2, 3, 4, 5, 7, 8, and 25. The 25 is "unlike" the other observations in order of magnitude. This kind of outlier often can be detected by examining the percentile distributions available from many univariate summary programs. Finally, there are formal statistical tests for outliers (see Barnett & Lewis, 1984; Dunn & Clark, 1987; Hoaglin, Mosteller, & Tukey, 1983). The formal tests generally assume that variables are normally distributed, and are quite sensitive to lack of normality.

Outlier detection has received a great deal of attention, particularly in the context of regression analysis. As a result, many statistical packages include almost too many statistics (see Afifi & Clark, 1990; Chatterjee & Hadi, 1988; Cook & Weisberg, 1982). Chatterjee and Hadi (1988) include a chapter on detection of multiple outliers, and Rousseeuw and van Zomeren (1990) discuss methods of detecting multiple outliers in multivariate point clouds.

When an observation is clearly an outlier and seems quite unreasonable, most researchers have little hesitation in deleting it. The ones that are difficult to decide on are those that appear to be unusual but are not impossible. For example, a woman can weigh 500 pounds. Should her weight be declared an outlier or not? One solution to this dilemma is to ask whether or not this person would be considered as part of the target population for which you wish to make inferences. If the answer is yes, her weight probably should be included. Another alternative is to do the analysis both with and without the questionable outlier.

Transformations of Data

Variable transformation is one of the major operations in data processing. Transformations are often used to collapse categories of nominal or ordinal data to obtain a smaller, more usable number of categories. If running a univariate statistical program shows that some of the categories have been chosen by very few respondents, it may be sensible to combine them with similar categories. For nominal data, any categories conceivably could be combined, but for ordinal data, only adjacent categories should be combined. The decision to collapse categories is a compromise between having too many categories with some chosen by very few respondents and collapsing so much that information is lost.

Some statistical procedures are more easily performed with dichotomous, two-category, or 0,1 data. Categorical data with three or more categories are often transformed to a series of dummy variables with only two outcomes (0 or 1) for use in multivariate analyses (see Afifi & Clark, 1990).

Transformations are also used to change the units of interval data, to sum or otherwise combine variables to create a scale or other summary score, and to summarize skip patterns. In longitudinal data, it is often necessary to make transformations on data that are collected at different times. For example, "change" scores such as weight loss are often computed by subtracting data collected at time 1 from data collected at time 2.

We will first discuss types of transformations and then how to use them to obtain new variables. Finally, we will discuss the use of transformations to normalize data.

ARITHMETIC TRANSFORMATIONS

One of the simplest operations is the arithmetic transformation. Suppose gender has been coded male = 1 and female = 2 and you desire to use it as a 0,1 variable so that odds ratios (see Reynolds, 1977) can be computed. Subtracting a 1 from the variable will make the desired transformation. Height might be measured in centimeters and you want to report it in inches, so you divide the measurement by 2.54. Interaction predictor variables are often created by multiplying two predictor variables together, as illustrated in the previous section. To avoid errors, all such arithmetic transformations of the data should be done in the computer rather than by hand calculator prior to data entry. SPSS, BMDP, and SAS manuals provide specific instructions on how to perform such arithmetic operations.

The arithmetic operations commonly available are addition (+), subtraction (−), multiplication (*), division (/), and exponentiation (**) (raising a variable to a power—for example, squaring it). The statistical packages perform arithmetic operations in the reverse order from that in which you learned them—exponentiation first, then division and multiplication, and finally subtraction and addition. Parentheses can be used to control the order of operations, since quantities inside parentheses are evaluated first. For example, in the combination "(y+6)**.5," the computer first sums y and 6 and then computes the square root of the sum. If the parentheses were missing, the computer would first take the square root of 6 and then add it to y. For "avercost=(costa+costb)/2," again the computer will combine the quantity in the parentheses first and then divide by 2. If the parentheses were missing, the computer would divide "costb" by 2 and then add it to "costa."

FUNCTIONS OF DATA

In addition to the arithmetic operators, SPSS, SAS, and BMDP have numerous *functions* that can be used in data screening, transformations, and statistical analyses. Commonly used functions include taking the log of a variable, computing the mean of a variable, determining the maximum and minimum of a variable, assigning random numbers, recoding dates, and generating cumulative distribution functions of common distributions such as the normal. These functions can be used in combination with the arithmetic operations. For example, "z=log(y+100)" would result in a new variable called z being computed from the log of the sum of variable y plus 100.

COMPARISON OPERATORS

The major packages have functions called *comparison operators* that can be used in transformations or for case selection. For example, categories can be collapsed using comparison or logical operators embedded in *if-then* statements. Commonly used comparison operators include the following:

Symbols	Statement	Examples
gt, >	greater than	age > 18
ge, ≥	greater than or equal to	age ≥ 19
lt, <	less than	age < 66
le, ≤	less than or equal to	age ≤ 65
eq, =	equal	age = 19
ne, ≠	not equal to	age ≠ 18
and, &	both or all true	age > 18 and age < 66
or, I	either true	age < 18 or age > 65

These operators compare two or more variables, constants, or functions. The computer checks the truth of the statement containing the operator for each subject. For example, if the statement was (age greater than 18), the programs will check each subject's age to see if a number greater than 18 is given. If the statement was (age greater than 18 *and* age less than 66), it would be true only for persons 19-65 years of age. If the statement was (age less than 18 *or* age greater than 65), it would be true if the subject was either younger than 18 or older than 65.

The comparison operators are used in what are called *if-then* or *if-then else* statements. The form of an if-then statement is as follows: If (this statement is true) then (take this action). For example, you could write:

if (age>18) then (use this subject)
if (educat=1 or educat=2) then (recode neweduc to 1)

The if-then statements are used to select subjects, to transform variables already in the data set (often for use in tables), to create new variables that are added to the end of the data set, to make dummy variables, to replace missing values with imputed values (see Afifi & Clark, 1990), and to perform consistency checks on the data.

The form of writing the if-then statements varies by statistical package, but the result is essentially the same. The else clause is added to simplify entry of actions that have numerous possible outcomes. For example,

if (educat=1 or educat=2) then (educat=1) else (educat=2)

transforms the variable *educat* to a 1 if it originally was a 1 or 2, and to a 2 if it was anything else.

Skip Variables. Transformations must be used to create variables that are suitable for analysis from skip-and-fill questions (see Chapter 4). Often a single variable is created from a series of questions. For example, alcohol usage is often determined by first asking respondents if they drink. If they answer no, they skip a series of questions on what they drink and how much, and are coded zero. For those answering yes, their intake of each type of drink is multiplied by the amount of alcohol contained in that drink, and then the amounts are summed over the types of drinks to provide a single variable giving daily alcohol intake.

After performing the transformations to change the scale of a variable, to collapse variables, or to adjust for skips, it is important to check the results to see that the transformations were done correctly. Checking is sometimes done by choosing a few examples from the data set and doing them by hand to see if the results are the same as those the computer produced. A more comprehensive method for nominal and ordinal data is to compute a two-way table of the original variable against the transformed variable. The results in the interior of the table will show how the original and transformed results compare for all the cases. This is particularly useful when complex comparative statements are used.

TRANSFORMATIONS TO ACHIEVE NORMALITY

Transformations are commonly used to achieve approximate univariate *normality* out of a skewed or nonnormal distribution. Many tests of hypotheses and confidence limits are based on the assumption of a normal or Gaussian distribution. If data are normally distributed, their histogram should be symmetric and bell shaped. Because the normal distribution can be written as a mathematical expression, it is possible to use formal statistical tests to decide if data follow a normal distribution. These formal tests are sensitive to outliers, so it is important to screen the data first and remove obvious outliers.

A normal distribution is symmetric about its mean and median. The sample median is the middle observation if the sample size is odd or the average of two middle observations if it is even. It is approximately equal to the 50th percentile. Symmetry implies that the difference between the median (50th percentile) and, for example, the 25th percentile (P25) should be approximately equal to the difference between the 75th percentile (P75) and the median. Percentiles divide a sample into 100 equal parts; they can be produced by the SPSS FREQUEN-CIES, SAS UNIVARIATE, or BMDP 2D program.

Two commonly used graphical methods for determining whether a distribution is approximately normal are to plot a histogram and check whether it is symmetric, or to obtain a normal probability plot and check whether it follows a straight line. Histograms and normal probability plots can be obtained from SPSS, SAS, and BMDP programs.

There are also several formal tests for normality. The commonly used Shapiro-Wilks's W test is available in SPSS EXAMINE, SAS UNIVARIATE, and BMDP 2D. While good for small samples, this test can also be used on larger samples. For very large samples, the Kolmogorov-Smirnov D is often used. This is available in SPSS EXAMINE and SAS UNIVARIATE.

The skewness statistic indicates how nonsymmetric a distribution is. Skewness will be close to zero if a distribution is normal. If a distribution has a longer tail to the right, the skewness will be positive. If a distribution has a longer tail to the left, the skewness statistic will be negative. When the data are skewed, it is usually to the right. It is important to screen the data first for unusually large or small values, since outliers can have a large effect on the skewness statistic. SPSS and BMDP provide information on the standard error of the skewness statistic so the user can test if it is zero. A distribution that has a skewness greater than 0.8 is noticeably skewed.

If the skewness is significantly different from zero, you might want to consider transforming the data to reduce the skewness and obtain a closer approximation to a normal distribution, as discussed next.

There are several strategies to determine the appropriate transformation. If the theoretical distribution of the data is known, there may be a transformation that is known to transform the raw data toward normality. For example, the square-root transformation is commonly used for data that follow a Poisson distribution. When the researcher does not know the theoretical distribution that the data follow, power transformations should be considered (Hoaglin et al., 1983; Tukey, 1977).

Power Transformations. Power transformations take the form

$$(X + A)^P$$

where X signifies the variable, A is a constant (often zero), and P is the power that is used. For example, if $A = 0$ and $P = \frac{1}{2}$, then the transformation computes the square root of the data. Raising X to a power less than 1 reduces large values of X more than small values of X. As a result, it "draws in" the long right tail. As a simple example, suppose we had six observations with observed values of 1, 4, 9, 9, 16, and 25. The median is 9 and the mean is 10.67. The difference between the smallest value and the median is 8, but the difference between the largest value and the median is 16, which indicates a possible skewness to the right. Similarly, for the mean we would have $10.67 - 1 = 9.67$ and $25 - 10.67 = 14.33$. If we take the square root of each observation we obtain 1, 2, 3, 3, 4, and 5, which are symmetric about the mean or median.

Values of P less than 1 are chosen if the data are skewed to the right; values of P greater than 1 are chosen if the data are skewed to the left. When data are skewed to the right, progressively decreasing the value of P progressively reduces the skew to the right. As you decrease P, the distribution becomes approximately symmetric and finally skewed to the left. Common values of P that are tried are $\frac{1}{2}$, 0, and -1. Since taking the logarithm of the data is conceptually equivalent to $P = 0$ (Tukey, 1977), taking the log of the data transforms the distribution more than taking the square root. Similarly, taking the inverse of the data ($P = -1$) transforms it more than the log. When the inverse is taken, usually a negative sign is put in front of the result so that the direction of the numbers stays the same. When data are skewed to the left, the data are most often squared ($P = 2$).

The constant A can be used to improve the results once P is chosen. For example, if the data are skewed to the right and a log transformation (either natural or base 10) improves the results, but not quite enough, and the inverse transformation is too great, subtracting a constant will have the effect of decreasing the skewness. If all positive numbers are to be maintained, the constant must be less than the smallest value of X. An alternative to subtracting a constant A would be to try values of P between 0 (the log transformation) and -1, say, $-\frac{1}{2}$. Often the constant is used to avoid in-between values of P that are difficult to explain. Use of a constant is also thought by some investigators to shift the data to values with a more natural zero point. To decrease the effect of the transformation, add a positive constant A. (See Afifi & Clark, 1990, for a graphical method of choosing P and A developed by Hines & Hines, 1987.)

It should be kept in mind that a transformation that works well on your sample may not necessarily be the best transformation for the entire population. This is particularly true for small samples. For this reason, many investigators choose common transformations that have been used by others such as the log or square root, if these work reasonably well on their sample. Any of the methods mentioned previously to determine if the data are normal can be used to evaluate the results.

Advisability of Transformation to Normality. The decision on whether to transform is dependent on what statistical analyses you expect to use, the degree of nonnormality, and the variability of the data. Some statistical procedures, such as logistic regression, do not assume normality. Some statistical tests are quite robust to (i.e., unaffected by) lack of normality.

If the coefficient of variation (standard deviation divided by the mean) is less than one-third (see Hald, 1952) or the largest observation divided by the smallest is less than two (see Hoaglin et al., 1983) the data frequently are not sufficiently variable to make it worthwhile to perform a transformation. In addition, some types of distributions can never be transformed to approximate normality, although they may be brought closer. For example, a distribution with positive numbers where the mode (most common value) is at zero cannot be transposed to yield a normal distribution.

Once data are transformed, all inferences and discussions of the transformed variable must be made in terms of the newly transformed values. In deciding whether to use transformations, the reader must remember that some persons have difficulty understanding how transformations affect data. As a result, they may not understand inferences or discussions that depend on the transformations you have performed.

Other Kinds of Transformations. Other transformations sometimes are performed after statistical analysis is started. For example, in regression analysis, data are often transformed to achieve a straight line or plane; in analysis of variance, transformations are frequently used to reduce the interaction mean square. The power transformations can be used in making these transformations (see Tukey, 1977). There are particular techniques that are useful with particular statistical analyses. Our advice is to consult a textbook that discusses tests of normality for the analysis you wish to use, and examine the output available in the various computer programs to help you decide what transformations to use.

Transformations often make it possible to use standard statistical tests and confidence intervals for regression analysis, discriminant function analysis, analysis of variance, and so on, so that nonparametric methods or robust statistical techniques are not necessary.

Scale Evaluation

Different authors use the term *scale* somewhat differently. Babbie (1973) defines a scale as the assignment of scores to response patterns among several items making up a scale. He defines an index to be the summation of scores assigned to specific items according to the responses of the subjects. Thus, by his definition, a Guttman scale would be a scale, but a Likert summation of scores would be an index. Most other authors would define scaling as the process of assigning numbers to the measurement of attitude. By attitude, we mean the degree of positive or negative affect associated with some object or stimulus. Here we will use the word *scale* to apply to either indexes or scales.

LIKERT SCALES

The most commonly used scale procedure is the Likert scale, and the evaluation of already constructed Likert scales will be treated here. The construction of Likert scales is discussed in McKennell (1977), and an introduction to the fundamentals of unidimensional scaling theory and construction is given in McIver and Carmines (1981; see also DeVellis, 1991). Other possible measures of attitude include the Guttman scale (see Torgerson, 1958), Thurstone (see Edwards, 1957), and the semantic differential (see Osgood, Suci, & Tannenbaum, 1957). In using a Likert scale, one is scaling the subjects, but in Guttman and Thurstone scales, the procedure includes scaling both the stimuli and the subjects, separately.

Typical Likert scales consist of from 4 to 40 items. For example, an item might state, "I have trouble concentrating on tasks." Respondents typically are asked to state the extent to which they agree with each statement using a 5-point scale. For example, "strongly disagree" = 1, "disagree" = 2, "undecided" = 3, "agree" = 4, "strongly agree" = 5. Items that are worded negatively must have their scores reversed. For a 5-point scale, this is achieved by subtracting the original value from 6. This is done so that 5 always signifies strong agreement or approval. The scale score is typically obtained by summing the scores (including the reversed ones) for each item.

The use of a Likert scale has many advantages over attempting to gauge opinion with a single question. The answers to a single item have been shown to vary with format or wording to such an extent that we recommend forming multiple items into scales if the attitude being measured is an important part of the study. Examples of Likert scales can be obtained from the literature (e.g., Chun et al., 1975; George & Bearon, 1980; Kane & Kane, 1981; McDowell & Newell, 1987; Reeder et al., 1976; Robinson et al., 1973, 1991; Robinson & Shaver, 1973; Shaw & Wright, 1967).

Characteristics of a Good Likert Scale. The characteristics that we want to find in existing scales include parsimony, minimal overlap with other constructs under study, high validity and reliability, unidimensionality or known dimensionality, and summated scores that can be assumed to be interval or ratio data. The interest in minimal overlap with other constructs is an important facet of parsimony. The inclusion of numerous long and similar scales has been shown to be dysfunctional (see Andrews, 1984).

It is essential to understand and define clearly the attitude to be measured. Bollen (1989) points out that most researchers assume that subjects' attitudes "cause" their responses to items (and not vice versa). He therefore calls the items "effect indicators," as they reflect the effect of an attitude. Therefore, there must be evidence or a clear rationale for the selection of items for a Likert scale.

High validity and reliability (see Bollen, 1989; Carmines & Zeller, 1979) are essentials of a good scale. In this section, we briefly define validity and then discuss methods for measuring reliability. It is often possible to find information in the literature on the reliability of an existing scale you wish to use. Even when information is available from past studies, you should check the scale yourself, especially if your respondents differ from those on whom the scale was developed. Generally, reliability is more easily assessed, is more frequently assessed, and is assessed prior to assessing validity. Demonstration that a measure is reliable does not ensure that it is valid.

Validity. A scale is valid if it measures what it is supposed to measure. Validity can be assessed in any or all of three main ways: (a) by seeing whether the summated scale score predicts behavior that is assessed separately from the scale (criterion-related validity); (b) by assessing whether the items included cover the universe of content thought to be important (comprehensiveness of item coverage, content validity)—here knowledge of the attitude being measured is crucial; and (c) by determining whether it is correlated with other measures as expected from theoretical considerations (construct validity). Assessing validity by simply computing the correlation between the scale score and another criterion requires that both be measured accurately; otherwise, the evaluation of validity becomes quite subjective. You will need to use a scale with items that have clear and consistent meanings that represent the attitude you wish to measure. Additional measures of validity are presented by Bollen (1989).

Reliability. In this context, reliability is the degree to which the results are consistent across time (test-retest reliability), data collectors (stability), and items of the scale (homogeneity or internal consistency). Reliability is defined as the ratio of the variance of the true score to the variance of the actual measured score. It lies between zero and one. Carmines and Zeller (1979) recommend that scales ideally should have a reliability of at least 0.80; however, many widely used scales have reliabilities in the 0.65 to 0.80 range. In regression analysis, if the dependent variable has low reliability, the estimates of the slope coefficients and the mean of the dependent variable are not biased but the variability of the estimates is increased. If the independent or predictor variables have low reliability, the estimates of the slope coefficients are biased in a downward direction. The estimate of the variability of the dependent variable is not changed, but the variability of the estimates of independent variables is increased.

The methods usually used to assess reliability relate to one of two purposes. The first is to make sure that the reliability of the scale is sufficiently high. The second purpose is to determine the effects of each item on reliability. These two purposes become intertwined in that the reliability can sometimes be increased by removing items.

If it is possible to administer the scale twice to the same subjects, reliability can be assessed by obtaining the simple correlation of the *test-retest* summated scores. This would seem the simplest method, but it is often not feasible. In a typical survey, retesting is not done. When it can be performed, questions remain concerning when to do it. If you wait too long, the subjects could change their attitudes, but if you do it too soon, the subjects may remember and try to repeat what they did before.

The most commonly used reliability measure is called *Cronbach's alpha.* After the researcher has reversed the coding of items where needed, Cronbach's alpha can be calculated either from the original item values or from standardized item values. The scores for standardized items have a mean of zero and a variance of one. We denote the first calculation as "raw-data alpha" and the second as "standardized alpha." Raw-data alpha is computed using the variance-covariance matrix computed from the item values, where the diagonal of the matrix contains the variance of each item and the rest of the matrix is composed of the covariances between all pairs of items. The variance-covariance matrix of the standardized scores is the correlation matrix. The process of calculating the correlations standardizes the original item values. In either case, using the variance-covariance matrix or the correlation matrix, the formula for alpha is as follows:

$$\alpha = \frac{P}{P-1}\left(1 - \frac{\sum \text{diag}}{\sum \text{all entries}}\right)$$

where P equals the number of items, *diag* denotes the diagonal elements of the matrix, and *all entries* denotes all the elements of the matrix including the diagonal. Alpha can vary from 0 to 1. Alpha increases as the size of the off-diagonal elements (covariances or correlations) increases relative to the size of the diagonal elements (variances). Since standardized alpha is calculated from the correlation matrix, the variances in the diagonal are always 1s, so their sum is simply P or the number of items. Increasing the number of items (P) also increases alpha if the average magnitude of the covariances or correlations stays the same. This happens because, as P increases, the number of off-diagonal elements increases faster than the number of diagonal elements.

The decision as to whether to use the raw-data alpha or the standardized alpha is complicated. Most researchers use summated scale scores computed from the raw data. As we mentioned in the section on transformations, when transformations are made on data inferences can be made only to the transformed data. In the case of Cronbach's alpha, when the standardized alpha is used inferences can be assumed to apply only to the standardized items; inferences cannot automatically be assumed to apply to the raw data for the population of persons from whom the sample of subjects was drawn. If it can be assumed that the population variances of the raw-data items are equal, then it can be assumed that standardizing the items makes no difference and that the results obtained with the standardized alpha also apply to the raw-data scale. If it *cannot* be assumed that the items have equal variances in the underlying population, then the raw data alpha should be used if raw-data scores are summed.

The researcher can use two procedures when attempting to test the validity of the above assumptions. First, he or she can examine the actual range and variances of the raw item scores in the sample. If it can be concluded that they are equivalent across items, it strengthens the researcher's confidence that the standardized alpha can be used. Second, the researcher can compare the standardized alpha to the raw-data alpha. The size of the two alphas will be similar if the sample variances are similar, but can be quite different if the sample variances are substantially unequal.

Alpha is equal to either reliability or a lower bound to reliability, depending upon the assumptions made. It provides a conservative measure of the true reliability. See Bollen (1989) for an informative summary of the assumptions made in the above measures of reliability.

Alpha can be computed from a covariance or correlation matrix output of a computer program, but the easiest way to obtain it is to use the RELIABILITY program in SPSS. This program will provide the overall standardized or raw-data alpha for your scale as well as numerous other useful statistics. It will also help you decide how to remove items from a scale if this is desired. Usually, well-known scales are used untouched, for comparability and other reasons. If, however, you desire to remove some items, one strategy for deciding which ones to remove is to examine the reliability of the scale with the candidate item removed. If the alpha goes up or stays the same, that item is a candidate for removal. The RELIABILITY program provides the value of alpha if each item and only that item is deleted from the scale. It also provides the correlation of each item with the corrected total score (that item removed) as well as other useful statistics. Each item should be positively and appreciably correlated with the corrected total score. If it is not, this may indicate that an item either does not improve reliability of the scale or measures something different from the majority of the items. An item that does not contribute to reliability or that pertains to a different attitude can be removed and the program rerun to search for additional candidate items.

Additional Evaluation Techniques. Another technique is to use the *conditional statements* to select subjects that score in the top 25% and bottom 25% on total score and to compute the average score for each item for both of these subgroups. An item that does not have a high average for the top 25% subjects or a low average for the bottom 25% of the subjects is not behaving consistently and could be considered a candidate for removal. Items can also be considered for removal if they have an appreciably smaller standard deviation than others in the scale, since this probably indicates that most respondents are heaping in only one or two categories.

It is also possible to divide the sample into subgroups based on gender or age. For research purposes, suppose that you would like the scale to be used in a similar fashion by males and females or young and old persons. It is not that you expect the same mean for males and females for each item, but that you prefer they use a similar frame of reference. The standard deviations and correlations of the items can be examined for each subgroup. You may be more interested in items that have a sizable standard deviation (not everyone answers the same) for each subgroup and similar simple correlations within each group. The RELI-ABILITY program can also be run on subgroups to gain further insight into the reliability of the scale.

Number of Dimensions. One concern that researchers have with Likert scales is uncertainty about their unidimensionality. Suppose half the items in a scale contribute to one dimension and the other half to another independent dimension. From the tests given previously, a researcher might miss the presence of the two dimensions, and certainly will not know what items belong to which dimension. Obviously, scales that measure along a single dimension are simpler to interpret. It may be, however, that overlapping dimensions are needed to measure the complexity of the attitude structure. See McKennell (1977) for further discussion of this and methods for deciphering the dimensions.

Several empirical methods are useful in deciding if several dimensions exist. One is simply to read the items and try to decide if they all fall along a single dimension. The second is to obtain the simple correlation matrix and examine it to see if two or more clusters of items exist that are highly intercorrelated within each cluster but uncorrelated or negatively correlated between clusters. The problem with the second approach is that while it is relatively simple to see the separate sets after the items have been ordered so that those within each cluster (or factor) are adjacent, it is very difficult to see when the items are all mixed up.

To deal with the problems described above, two statistical techniques, cluster analysis and factor analysis, have been recommended (see McKennell, 1977). These help to determine whether separate dimensions exist and what items belong to which dimension. If cluster analysis is used, you will want to run a program that clusters the *variables* and not the subjects, since it is the items that are being examined. The VARCLUS procedure in SAS and the 1M program in BMDP are suitable.

Factor analysis is more widely known and used (see Kim & Mueller, 1978, for an introduction to factor analysis). If the scale is strictly one-dimensional, you would expect to see a single principal component or factor explain a sizable proportion of the variance. If overlapping dimensions are present, several factors may emerge. We recommend the use of an oblique rotation, so that the separate factors are not forced to be uncorrelated, and factor scores be saved. The larger factor loadings will show which items contribute most to which factor. If the factors obtained (using an oblique rotation) are clearly uncorrelated and the items load on separate factors, the possibility of different dimensions should be explored. A scree plot can be used to decide upon the number of factors to consider. A second factor analysis of the factor scores can be performed to see if a single factor results (see Clark, Aneshensel, Frerichs, & Morgan, 1981, for an example of such an analysis). If a single factor is obtained, there is a basis to argue for an overall dimension composed of overlapping dimensions. SPSS, SAS, and BMDP will perform oblique rotations of the factors.

If one has an a priori hypothesis regarding the number of dimensions that underlie a scale, confirmatory factor analysis should be considered (see Long, 1983, for an explanation of the uses of confirmatory factor analysis).

Weighting Items. Another concern about using Likert scales is whether the items should be summed directly or differentially weighted prior to summing. Following Likert, most existing scales were developed and tested as undifferentiated sums of the items. It is simpler to make comparisons with past results if the items are treated the same way. Some researchers feel uneasy about this if a factor analysis of the items shows that the factor score coefficients (or factor loadings) are quite unequal; they may desire to use a differentially weighted sum or a factor score. If the factor analysis provides clear and understandable factors, use of the factor scores may be desirable. However, typically a high correlation will be obtained between summated and factor scores so that the simpler summated scores are preferred. One empirical approach is to do it both ways (summing the items and computing separate factor scores) and see which result is most useful in subsequent analyses.

Imputation of Missing Values in Likert Scales. It should be noted that methods of imputing missing values can also apply to Likert scales. Often a respondent will fail to answer only one or two items in a Likert scale with numerous items. There are several methods used to impute item scores. Some investigators will assign the average score for that item from those who did answer the item. Mean substitution is easily implemented in SPSS. Others treat it as an "undecided" and, for example, will assign a score of 3 on a 5-point scale. Some assign a score that reflects the subject's answers on other items. For example, suppose there were 6 items but a subject answered only 5, with a total score of 20. The subject's average score is 20/5 = 4; that average can be assigned to the missing item so the subject's summated score is 20 + 4 = 24. A more complex method is to perform a regression analysis predicting the missing item from other items, using values from subjects who answered all the items. Then, this regression equation is used to estimate the missing item using the method given in the section on missing values. If a respondent is missing most of the items, most investigators would declare the summated score to be missing. If one or more items have excessive missing values, the items should be examined for problems and possibly excluded.

Summary of Likert Scales. In checking Likert scales, usually a variety of methods are used until a consensus can be reached on how respondents are using the scale. The results from the cluster analysis should agree to a reasonable extent with the factor analysis. The items that cluster will likely load on the same factor. If time is limited and you are sure that the scale is unidimensional, use of the RELIABILITY program in SPSS may be all that is needed.

All scales are compromises. If your only concern is obtaining high reliability, this can be accomplished by making minor wording changes in the items during scale development until you obtain high between-item correlations. This, however, usually results in low validity. Conversely, developing a variety of items that covers the full range of content may lower the scale's reliability and result in multiple overlapping dimensions rather than a single dimension, though it may also lead to a scale with high validity.

In performing the previously mentioned checks on Likert scales, an interval scale is assumed both at the item level and in the summated scale that is created. Most of the statistics used (means, covariances, and correlations) require an interval scale. Although considerable discussion is given in Sonquist and Dunkelberg (1977) concerning the reasonableness of the summated score being an interval scale, at the item level, it is an assumption that is commonly made in order to use available statistics.

Creation of Subfiles for Analysis

When large data sets exist, subfiles often are created for particular analyses. For example, in surveys it is not unusual to end up with 600 to 1,000 variables. For a given research task, an investigator may wish to use only 15 variables. In order to save computer time it is useful to create a *subfile* with only the desired variables. Also, if numerous investigators are using the same data set and some are not closely connected with the project, it is often prudent to give each investigator an agreed-upon subset of the data rather than the entire data set. If errors are found in any of the subfiles, corrections must be made in the master file.

Investigators often create a *subfile of cases* when they have a very large sample size, and run though their proposed analyses on the smaller sample as a way of screening out obviously useless statistical analyses. The statements needed to run the statistical packages can also be edited and corrected using the smaller sample size. This saves computer time. For example, in a study of 45,000 birth certificates it makes sense to run preliminary analyses on a subsample. The three package programs have procedures for creating subfiles of variables or cases. In addition, the use of subfiles that are random samples of the total files can be useful for cross-validating results. SPSS, SAS, and BMDP provide options for taking random samples of the cases.

With cleaned, transformed, and documented working files, the investigators are finally ready to perform the needed statistical analyses and write their reports and articles.

6. A CHECKLIST FOR STUDY DOCUMENTATION

Documentation is a continuing process that starts at the conception of the study and provides an audit trail for all steps (and missteps) along the way. In earlier chapters we have stressed the crucial importance of good records and notes. Here we offer an annotated checklist of key points that should be documented. Data storage, disposal of collection forms, and placing the data in the public domain are briefly discussed.

Sample Design

Describe the population sampled, the method of sampling, sampling procedures and problems, and the final sample. If strata or clusters were taken, they also should be described. Record the names and characteristics of any sample-weighting variables used.

Data Collection Instrument

Keep copies of all data collection instruments that were used. Any nonobvious rationale for the inclusion of a variable should be noted. Document the origin and authorship of all materials adopted or adapted from the work of other researchers. Keep an annotated copy of the final instruments. Pretests and pilot tests should be described, together with summaries of the changes they inspired.

Data Collection Training and Procedures

Include instruction and training materials prepared for interviewers or data abstractors. Important topics include the objectives, funding, and sponsorship of the study, provisions for confidentiality, anticipated problems or questions the workers may face, and procedures for quality control.

Coding of Data

Document carefully and explicitly all codes assigned to data gathered from interviews, records, observations, and so on. For precoded data collection instruments an annotated copy of the instrument is valuable, but may lack some needed information. Before the use of the newer data entry systems, codebooks were written that included each variable's number, name, location, format (written in fixed-format notation, such as F3.1), and information about how data were coded. Now, the needed portion of codebooks comes from the data entry program as described below. In addition, either references or reasons for coding decisions may need to be kept. Special problems should be noted.

Data Entry for Computerized Files

At minimum, the documentation must describe fully the variables that are included in the data set. The description might include names, the correspondence between the computerized data codes and the original data items, and the formats and statistical program linkages of the computer-stored data files. Without this documentation, a raw-data file is useless because there is no "key" to explain the location of data or the meaning of the data included in the file. Information should be kept about both the cleaning status of the data and the process by which data were cleaned. Include information about the range of acceptable values for each variable and the kinds of consistency checks that have been made between variables.

Data entry programs developed for the major statistical analysis packages now provide much of this information in computer-readable form as a by-product of the data file definition and data entry actions. Printouts of this information, suitably annotated by hand or with a word-processing program, can serve as excellent documentation.

Data Processing That Precedes Analysis

Document how missing values and outliers are handled, and keep a record of what transformations are used and how scales are checked. These actions modify the field-collected data in ways that facilitate statistical analysis and influence research conclusions. The actions taken, the problems they serve to correct, and any underlying assumptions must be documented in detail, and the order of execution noted. Annotated statistical program instructions provide an efficient way to do this.

Frequency Distributions for All Study Variables

These are sometimes referred to as "master frequencies." A copy should be available to all users of the data set.

Archives of Data Files

Archive copies of the data should be transferred to removable media (magnetic tape, floppy diskettes, removable hard-disk cartridges, or the like) for safekeeping away from the computer system. Multiple backups are recommended, since tapes and disks can either be defective or become defective over time. It is prudent, also, to create a more general form of the file for safekeeping. This maximizes one's ability to transfer the data and subsequent analyses to other computer hardware systems or to another statistical package. If the original data entry produces a raw-data file to which variable labels, definitions, and so on subsequently are added using one of the statistical packages, both the raw data and the additional information should be stored in computer-readable form.

Researchers often keep hard copies of raw-data files (if the data set is not too large), with verbatim answers to any uncoded, open-ended questions, keyed to the respondents' identification numbers.

After Data Processing and Analysis Are Finished

DISPOSAL OF DATA COLLECTION FORMS

A policy should be established and executed for disposal of original field data. The creation of full and timely documentation allows data collection forms to be destroyed. We prefer shredding of data collection forms rather than storing them for three reasons: (a) Storage can require large amounts of space, (b) preserving the confidentiality of stored documents is difficult, and (c) the certainty that the original documents will be destroyed creates an incentive for timely and complete data entry and cleaning.

Proper and timely destruction of data collection forms is particularly important when data are collected that reveal either illegal or potentially embarrassing behavior on the part of respondents. In even the most secure locations and even when researchers think all possible identifying information has been stripped from the data set, confidentiality protection for study data is not absolute, since access often can be obtained through subpoena. Proper and timely destruction of data forms reduces this risk.

MOVING DATA INTO PUBLIC DOMAIN

As Sieber (1991) notes, while "openness is a familiar idea in scientific research, . . . until recently, openness in science has meant publishing one's methods and results" (p. 1). The norms are beginning to change in this regard. Issues such as the high cost of original data collection, widely publicized incidents of research fraud, improved technology for storing and inexpensively distributing large data sets, and increased recognition that it is important to replicate analyses, particularly when findings are new or controversial, are contributing to increased data sharing.

The National Academy of Sciences, many professional associations, major funding agencies, journals, and universities are now encouraging, recommending, or requiring that researchers make raw data available to others. No single policy has been established, so groups differ in the specifics of their recommendations, but all provide exceptions or mandate protection for data sets in which individuals can be identified. When data are collected under federal contract, "the Contractor grants to the Government . . . a paid-up, non-exclusive, irrevocable worldwide license in such copyrighted data to reproduce, prepare derivative works, distribute copies to the public, and perform publicly and display publicly by or on behalf of the Government" (Commerce Clearing House, 1991). The National Science Foundation (1989) explicitly requires that data collected under grants be made available to other researchers "at no more than incremental cost and within a reasonable time," while the Public Health Service requires that data be made available to the federal government (U.S. Department of Health and Human Services, 1990). The *American Journal of Public Health* (1991) requires that authors retain data for at least three years and make it available to the editor on request. Many professional associations have developed policies regarding the form and timely dissemination of research findings and data sets and the protection of human subjects within research settings. Often these have been incorporated in formal codes of ethics (e.g., American Sociological Association, 1988) or supervised by standing committees of the professional association such as the American Psychological Association's Committee on Standards in Research (e.g., Grisso et al., 1991).

While some data sets are shared through informal networks, data increasingly are being placed in archives such as those run by the Institute for Social Science Research at UCLA and the Interuniversity Consortium for Political and Social Research (ICPSR). The process of placing data in a publicly accessible archive raises "increasingly complex questions concerning . . . data ownership, authorship, the responsibility for sharing data, balancing the rights of academic freedom versus the need for informed supervision, and determining the timing and method for releasing 'sensitive' results to the public" (Grisso et al., 1991). Nonetheless, we recommend that data sets be moved into archives as soon as they have been cleaned and documented, and preliminary analyses have been completed. Sometimes it is appropriate to ask that data sets be archived with restricted access for some period of time following the completion of data collection, but we feel that such restricted access should not exceed five years. When a data set is moved to archives, the researcher must be sure that full documentation accompanies the data set and that all identifying information is stripped from it. Groups such as ICPSR have protocols to assist the researcher in ensuring that data are archived appropriately (see Geda, 1991; Stephenson, n.d.). For more information on the history and current status of data sharing in the social sciences, we recommend Sieber (1991).

REFERENCES

ADAMS, R. N., and PREISS, J. J. (1960) Human Organization Research: Field Relations and Techniques. Homewood, IL: Dorsey.

ADAY, L. A. (1989) Designing and Conducting Health Surveys: A Comprehensive Guide. San Francisco: Jossey-Bass.

AFIFI, A. A., and CLARK, V. (1990) Computer-Aided Multivariate Analysis (2nd ed.). New York: Van Nostrand Reinhold.

ALWIN, D. F. (ed.) (1991, August) Research on Survey Quality. Special issue of Sociological Methods and Research, Volume 20.

American Journal of Public Health (1991) "Information for authors." Vol. 81: 134-138.

American Sociological Association (1988) "Code of ethics." December 2.

ANDERSON, A. B., BASILEVSKY, A., and HUM, D. P. J. (1983) "Missing data: A review of the literature," pp. 415-494 in P. H. Rossi, J. D. Wright, and A. B. Anderson (eds.) Handbook of Survey Research. New York: Academic Press.

ANDERSON, B. A., SILVER, B. D., and ABRAMSON, P. R. (1988a) "The effects of race of the interviewer on measures of electoral participation by blacks in SRC national election studies." Public Opinion Quarterly 52: 53-83.

ANDERSON, B. A., SILVER, B. D., and ABRAMSON, P. R. (1988b) "The effects of the race of the interviewer on race-related attitudes of black respondents in SRC/CPS national election studies." Public Opinion Quarterly 52: 289-324.

ANDREWS, F. (1984) "Construct validity and error components of survey measures: A structural modeling approach." Public Opinion Quarterly 48(2): 409-442.

BABBIE, E. R. (1973) Survey Research Methods. Belmont, CA: Wadsworth.

BAILEY, K. D. (1987) Methods of Social Research (3rd ed.). New York: Free Press.

BARNETT, V., and LEWIS, T. (1984) Outliers in Statistical Data (2nd ed.). New York: John Wiley.

BOLLEN, K. A. (1989) Structural Equations With Latent Variables. New York: John Wiley.

BOONE, M. S., and WOOD, J. T. (1992) Computer Applications for Anthropologists. Belmont, CA: Wadsworth.

BRADBURN, N. M. (1983) "Response effects," pp. 289-328 in P. H. Rossi, J. D. Wright, and A. B. Anderson (eds.) Handbook of Survey Research. New York: Academic Press.

BRADBURN, N. M., SUDMAN, S., and Associates (1979) Improving Interview Method and Questionnaire Design. San Francisco: Jossey-Bass.

BREWER, J., and HUNTER, A. (1989) Multimethod Research: A Synthesis of Styles. Newbury Park, CA: Sage.

CAMPBELL, B. (1981) "Race of interviewer effects among southern adolescents." Public Opinion Quarterly 45: 231-244.

CARMINES, E. G., and ZELLER, R. A. (1979) Reliability and Validity Assessment. Beverly Hills, CA: Sage.

CHATTERJEE, S., and HADI, A. S. (1988) Sensitivity Analysis in Linear Regression. New York: John Wiley.

CHUN, K. T., COBB, S., and FRENCH, J. R. P., Jr. (1975) Measures for Psychological Assessment: A Guide to 3,000 Original Sources and Their Applications. Ann Arbor: University of Michigan, Institute for Social Research, Survey Research Center.

CLARK, V. A., ANESHENSEL, C., FRERICHS, R., and MORGAN, T. (1981) "Analysis of effects of sex and age in response to items on the CES-D Scale." Psychiatry Research 5: 171-181.

Commerce Clearing House, Inc. (1991) Federal Acquisition Regulation (FAR), Subchapter A—General, Part 1, Federal Acquisition Regulations System. Chicago, IL: Commerce Clearing House.

CONVERSE, J. M., and PRESSER, S. (1986) Survey Questions: Handcrafting the Standardized Questionnaire. Sage University Paper series on Quantitative Applications in the Social Sciences, 07-063. Beverly Hills, CA: Sage.

CONVERSE, P. E. (1970). "Attitudes and non-attitudes: Continuation of a dialogue," pp. 168-189 in E. R. Tulte (ed.) The Quantitative Analysis of Social Problems. Menlo Park, CA: Addison-Wesley.

COOK, R. D., and WEISBERG, S. (1982) Residuals and Influence in Regression. New York: Chapman & Hall.

COTTER, P. R., COHEN, J., and COULTER, P. B. (1982) "Race-of-interviewer effects in telephone interviews." Public Opinion Quarterly 46: 278-284.

DAVID, M., LITTLE, R. J. A., SAMUHEL, M. E., and TRIEST, R. K. (1986) "Alternative methods for CPS income imputation." Journal of the American Statistical Association 81(393): 29-41.

DEROGATIS, L. R., and SPENCER, P. M. (1982) The Brief Symptom Inventory (BSI). Riderwood, MD: Clinical Psychometric Research.

DEVELLIS, R. F. (1991) Scale Development: Theory and Application. Applied Social Research Methods, Volume 26. Newbury Park, CA: Sage.

DILLMAN, D. A. (1978) Mail and Telephone Surveys: The Total Design Method. New York: John Wiley.

DUNCAN, O. D., and STENBECK, M. (1988) "No opinion or not sure?" Public Opinion Quarterly 52: 513-525.

DUNN, O. J., and CLARK, V. A. (1987) Applied Statistics: Analysis of Variance and Regression (2nd ed.). New York: John Wiley.

EDWARDS, A. L. (1957) Techniques of Attitude Scale Construction. New York: Appleton-Century-Crofts.

FAULKENBERRY, G. D., and MASON, R. (1978) "Characteristics of nonopinion and no opinion response groups." Public Opinion Quarterly 42: 533-543.

FIECK, L. F. (1989) "Latent class analysis of survey questions that include 'Don't Know' responses." Public Opinion Quarterly 53: 525-547.

FINK, A., and KOSECOFF, J. (1985) How to Conduct Surveys: A Step-by-Step Guide. Beverly Hills, CA: Sage.

FLEISS, J. L. (1981) Statistical Methods for Rates and Proportions (2nd ed.). New York: John Wiley.

FLEISS, J. L. (1986) The Design and Analysis of Clinical Experiments. New York: John Wiley.

FORD, B. L. (1983) "An overview of hot-deck procedures in incomplete data," pp. 185-207 in W. G. Madow, I. Olken, and D. B. Rubin (eds.) Sample Surveys, Vol. 2: Theory and Bibliographies. New York: Academic Press.

FREY, J. H. (1989) Survey Research by Telephone (2nd ed.). Newbury Park, CA: Sage.

GEDA, C. L. (1991) "The Inter-University Consortium for Political and Social Research." American Economic Association Newsletter (March): 16-18.

GEORGE, L. K., and BEARON, L. B. (1980) Quality of Life in Older Persons. New York: Human Sciences Press.

GRISSO, T., BALDWIN, E., BLANCK, P. D., ROTHERAM-BORUS, M. J., SCHOOLER, N. R., and THOMPSON, T. (1991) "Standards in research: APA's mechanism for monitoring the challenges." American Psychologist 46: 758-766.

HALD, A. (1952) Statistical Theory With Engineering Applications. New York: John Wiley.

HALL, E. T. (1966) The Hidden Dimension. Garden City, NY: Doubleday.

HINES, W. G., and HINES, R. J. O. (1987) "Quick graphical power: Hyphen transformation selection." American Statistician 41: 21-24.

HOAGLIN, D. C., MOSTELLER, F., and TUKEY, J. W. (eds.) (1983) Understanding Robust and Exploratory Data Analysis. New York: John Wiley.

HOSMER, D. W., and LEMESHOW, S. (1989) Applied Logistic Regression. New York: John Wiley.

HYMAN, H. H. (1972) Secondary Analysis of Sample Surveys: Principles, Procedures, and Potentialities. New York: John Wiley.

JOBE, J. B., and LOFTUS, E. F. (eds.) (1991) Cognition and Survey Measurement. Special issue of Applied Cognitive Psychology, Volume 5.

KALTON, G., and KASPRZYK, D. (1986) "The treatment of missing survey data." Survey Methodology 12(1): 1-16.

KANE, R. A., and KANE, R. L. (1981) Assessing the Elderly: A Practical Guide to Measurement. Lexington, MA: Lexington.

KEANE, T. M., CADDELL, J. M., and TAYLOR, K. L. (1988) "Mississippi Scale for combat-related posttraumatic stress disorder: Three studies in reliability and validity." Journal of Consulting and Clinical Psychology 56(1): 85-90.

KIECOLT, K. J., and NATHAN, L. E. (1985) Secondary Analysis of Survey Data. Sage University Paper series on Quantitative Applications in the Social Sciences, 07-053. Beverly Hills, CA: Sage.

KIM, J. O., and MUELLER, C. W. (1978) Introduction to Factor Analysis. Sage University Paper series on Quantitative Applications in the Social Sciences, 07-013. Beverly Hills, CA: Sage.

KISH, L. (1965) Survey Sampling. New York: John Wiley.

LITTLE, R. J. A., and RUBIN, D. B. (1987) Statistical Analysis With Missing Data. New York: John Wiley.

LITTLE, R. J. A., and RUBIN, D. B. (1990) "The analysis of social science data with missing values," pp. 374-409 in J. Fox and J. S. Long (eds.) Modern Methods of Data Analysis. Newbury Park, CA: Sage.

LONG, J. S. (1983) Confirmatory Factor Analysis. Sage University Paper series on Quantitative Applications in the Social Sciences, 07-033. Beverly Hills, CA: Sage.

McDOWELL, I., and NEWELL, C. (1987) Measuring Health: A Guide to Rating Scales and Questionnaires. New York: Oxford University Press.

McIVER, J. P., and CARMINES, E. G. (1981) Unidimensional Scaling. Sage University Paper series on Quantitative Applications in the Social Sciences, 07-024. Beverly Hills, CA: Sage.

86

McKENNELL, A. C. (1977) "Attitude scale construction," pp. 183-220 in C. A. O'Muircheataugh and C. Payne (eds.) Exploring Data Structures, Vol. 1: The Analysis of Survey Data. New York: John Wiley.

MILES, M. B., and HUBERMAN, A. M. (1984) Qualitative Data Analysis: A Sourcebook of New Methods. Beverly Hills, CA: Sage.

National Science Foundation (1989) Notice 106 (April 17). Washington, DC: Government Printing Office.

OSGOOD, C. E., SUCI, G. J., and TANNENBAUM, P. H. (1957) The Measurement of Meaning. Urbana: University of Illinois Press.

PATTON, M. Q. (1990) Qualitative Evaluation and Research Methods. London: Sage.

POE, G. S., SEEMAN, I., McLAUGHLIN, J., MEHL, E., and DIETZ, M. (1988) "'Don't Know' boxes in factual questions in a mail questionnaire: Effects on level and quality of response." Public Opinion Quarterly 52: 212-222.

POOR, A. (1990) The Data Exchange. Homewood, IL: Dow Jones-Irwin.

PRESSER, H., and SCHUMAN, H. (1989) "The measurement of the middle position in attitude surveys," pp. 108-123 in E. Singer and S. Presser (eds.) Survey Research Methods: A Reader. Chicago: University of Chicago Press.

REEDER, L. G., RAMACHER, L., and GORELNIK, S. (1976) Handbook of Scales and Indices of Health Behavior. Pacific Palisades, CA: Goodyear.

REESE, S. D., DANIELSON, W. A., SHOEMAKER, P. J., CHANG, T. K., and HSU, H. L. (1986) "Ethnicity-of-interviewer effects among Mexican-Americans and Anglos." Public Opinion Quarterly 50: 563-572.

REYNOLDS, H. T. (1977) Analysis of Nominal Data. Sage University Paper series on Quantitative Applications in the Social Sciences, 07-007. Beverly Hills, CA: Sage.

ROBINSON, J. P., RUSK, J. G., and HEAD, K. B. (1973) Measures of Political Attitudes. Ann Arbor: University of Michigan, Institute for Social Research.

ROBINSON, J. P., and SHAVER, P. R. (1973) Measures of Social Psychological Attitudes. Ann Arbor: University of Michigan, Institute for Social Research, Survey Research Center.

ROBINSON, J. P., SHAVER, P. R., and WRIGHTSMAN, L. S. (1991) Measures of Personality and Social Psychological Attitudes. New York: Academic Press.

ROUSSEEUW, P. J., and VAN ZOMEREN, B. C. (1990) "Unmasking multivariate outliers and leverage points." Journal of the American Statistical Association 85: 633-639.

SCHUMAN, H., and CONVERSE, J. M. (1989) "The effects of black and white interviewers on black responses," pp. 247-271 in E. Singer and S. Presser (eds.) Survey Research Methods: A Reader. Chicago: University of Chicago Press.

SCRIMSHAW, S. C. M., and HURTADO, E. (1987) Rapid Assessment Procedures for Nutrition and Primary Health Care. Los Angeles: University of California, Latin American Center Publications.

SHAW, M. E., and WRIGHT, J. M. (1967) Scales for the Measurement of Attitudes. New York: McGraw-Hill.

SHEATSLEY, P. B. (1983) "Questionnaire construction and item writing," pp. 195-230 in P. H. Rossi, J. D. Wright, and A. B. Anderson (eds.) Handbook of Survey Research. New York: Academic Press.

SIEBER, J. E. (ed.) (1991) Sharing Social Science Data. Newbury Park, CA: Sage.

SINGER, E., FRANKEL, M. R., and GLASSMAN, M. B. (1989) "The effect of interviewer characteristics and expectations on response," pp. 272-287 in E. Singer and S.

Presser (eds.) Survey Research Methods: A Reader. Chicago: University of Chicago Press.

SONQUIST, J. A., and DUNKELBERG, W. C. (1977) Survey and Opinion Research: Procedures for Processing and Analysis. Englewood Cliffs, NJ: Prentice-Hall.

SPRADLEY, J. P. (1980) Participant Observation. New York: Holt, Rinehart & Winston.

STEPHENSON, E. (n.d.) Retention and Archiving of Survey Material. Los Angeles: University of California, Institute for Social Science Research.

STEWART, D. W., and KAMINS, M. A. (1993) Secondary Research: Information Sources and Methods. Applied Social Research Methods, Volume 4. Thousand Oaks, CA: Sage.

SUDMAN, S., and BRADBURN, N. M. (1982) Asking Questions. San Francisco: Jossey-Bass.

Survey Research Center (1976) Interviewer's Manual (rev. ed.). Ann Arbor: University of Michigan, Institute for Social Research, Survey Research Center.

TORGERSON, W. S. (1958) Theory and Methods of Scaling. New York: John Wiley.

TUKEY, J. W. (1977) Exploratory Data Analysis. Reading, MA: Addison-Wesley.

TURNER, R., NIGG, J. M., and HELLER PAZ, D. (1986) Waiting for Disaster: Earthquake Watch in Southern California. Berkeley: University of California Press.

U.S. Bureau of the Census (1970) 1970 Census, Industry and Occupation Coding Training Manual. Washington, DC: Government Printing Office.

U.S. Bureau of the Census (1992) 1990 Census of Population: Alphabetical Index of Industries and Occupations. Washington, DC: Government Printing Office.

U.S. Department of Health and Human Services. (1990) Public Health Service, PHS Grants Policy Statement. DHHS Publication (OASH) 90-50,000 (rev.). October 1. Washington, DC: Government Printing Office.

U.S. Office of Management and Budget (1990) Data Editing in Federal Statistical Agencies. Prepared by Subcommittee on Data Editing in Federal Statistical Agencies, Federal Committee on Statistical Methodology, Statistical Policy Office, Office of Information and Regulatory Affairs, Office of Management and Budget. Washington, DC: Government Printing Office.

VAN DUSEN, R. A., and ZILL, N. (eds.) (1975) Basic Background Items for U.S. Household Surveys. Washington, DC: Social Science Research Council, Center for Coordination of Research on Social Indicators.

WEBB, E. J., CAMPBELL, D. T., SCHWARTZ, R. D., and SUCHREST, L. (1966) Unobtrusive Measures: Nonreactive Research in the Social Sciences. Chicago: Rand McNally.

WEBER, R. P. (1985) Basic Content Analysis. Sage University Paper series on Quantitative Applications in the Social Sciences, 07-049. Beverly Hills, CA: Sage.

WEEKS, M. F., and MOORE, R. P. (1981) "Ethnicity-of-interviewer effects on ethnic respondents." Public Opinion Quarterly 45: 245-249.

WEINBERG, E. (1983) "Data collection: Planning and management," pp. 329-358 in P. H. Rossi, J. D. Wright, and A. B. Anderson (eds.) Handbook of Survey Research. New York: Academic Press.

RELEVANT SOFTWARE MANUALS

BMDP Data Entry (1991).

BMDP Statistical Software Manual, Vol. 1, for 1990 Software Release (see Chapter 2, "Data").

88

DBMS/COPY.
SAS IBM 370 Formats and Informats.
SAS/FSP Guide, Version 6 (1987) (data entry).
SAS Procedures Guide, Release 6.03 (1988).
SAS Language Guide for Personal Computers, Version 6 (1987).
SPSS Data Entry II for the IBM PC/XT/AT and PS/2 (1987).
SPSS/PC+ V2.0 Base Manual (1988), by Marija J. Norusis. Chicago: SPSS Inc.
SPSS/PC+ Update for V3.0 and V3.1 (1989).

ACKNOWLEDGMENTS

We would like to thank A. A. Afifi, Beverly Cosand, Philip Costic, Ralph Dunlap, Eve Fielder, Virginia Flack, Carolyn Geda, Linda Lange, Corrie Peek, Susan Sorenson, Elizabeth Stephenson, Terri Walsh, Mel Widawski, and two readers from Sage Publications for their helpful comments and assistance on earlier drafts; Welden Clark for invaluable assistance with Chapter 4; Gloria Krauss for clerical assistance; and Margie Norman, Gloria Krauss, and Ralph Dunlap for editing assistance. Data used in examples were collected and processed with funds from the National Science Foundation (No. 62617 and BCS-9002754), the Natural Hazards Research and Application Center (Purchase Order 494933C1), the Earthquake Engineering Research Institute (EERI M880411), the National Center for Earthquake Engineering Research (Purchase Order R34779), and the Southern California Injury Prevention Research Center under funds from the Centers for Disease Control (No. R49/CCR903622).

SURVEY QUESTIONS   PART II
Handcrafting the
Standardized Questionnaire

JEAN M. CONVERSE

STANLEY PRESSER

PREFACE

This book is based on the premise that surveys must be custom-built to the specification of given research purposes. Yet it is unrewarding to be told, always, that writing questions is simply an art. It is surely that, but there are also some guidelines that have emerged from the collective artistic experience and the collective research tradition. We have arranged these ideas in three classes, or concentric circles, which progressively narrow to the specific design task, and we have written this book in three chapters to match.

Chapter 1 bears on general strategies culled from examples or experience of question-crafters and the findings of empirical researchers. In one sense, this material is a litany of cautions, offering more general perspectives than specific procedures. We hope that Chapter 1 presents something of the judicial or "research temper" as applied to survey questions.

Chapter 2 focuses on specific empirical findings. In recent years, there has been renewed research into question design and question effects, and much has been learned about how some questions tend to "behave." But the implications of this research for actual practice are not always clear. In this chapter we have selected those research findings that seem to us to have fairly direct applicability.

Chapter 3 tries to zero in on the actual task at hand. It is about pilot work and pretesting and making use of the advice of experts—critics, colleagues, and especially interviewers. It is commonplace that all survey questions must be pretested, but there is no commonly shared "tradition" about how to go about it. We have found only a very few references bearing on the subject. In this chapter we hope to contribute to the building of such a tradition.

Throughout this book we draw upon our own research experience as well as upon the published literature and the experience relayed by colleagues. Because we have had more personal experience with face-to-face and telephone interviewing than with written questionnaires, we make few extensions to that third mode of administration. Our experience is focused in still another way. We are most familiar with questionnaires designed for use with the broad American public—national cross-section samples drawn by the Institute for Social Research, or samples of the greater Detroit metropolitan area by the Detroit Area Study (both of the University of Michigan). We have had only a very little experience with surveying the well educated or intensely motivated such as college students, legislators, social scientists, political activists, and medical patients; some of the cautions that we urge in Chapter 1, especially, may well not apply to questionnaire design for these special groups.

Who will find this book of value? We hope that it will be useful to practitioners trying to handcraft their own questionnaires, and to students, and instructors in graduate and undergraduate teaching of survey research and social science methods. For professional survey researchers with years of practical experience and a rich knowledge of the research literature, this book can only remind rather than instruct.

We are grateful for the interest and editorial criticism of Howard Schuman, the original prime mover of this project. We also thank Tracy R. Berckmans, Robert M. Groves, Lee Sigelman, Charles F. Turner, Sage Publications editors John L. Sullivan and Richard G. Niemi, and two anonymous reviewers for their many good suggestions. These counselors are of course innocent of all failings that remain in the book.

1. STRATEGIES OF EXPERIENCE AND RESEARCH

The Enduring Counsel for Simplicity

Surveys and polls have become a staple of American cultural life in the course of the past 40-50 years. There are now burgeoning archives of survey data—banks of questions, whole studies to be replicated, imitated, or adapted to new purposes—but models of ideal question practice are nevertheless still hard to come by. Replication itself may be a weak reed. Even if we carefully select questions that have been used before, we cannot be sure that the original questions were good ones in the first place; and even if they were, new bugs may have gotten into old questions, as language and the world moved on.

We are better advised to start with two more general perspectives: the experience of master question-writers and the general strategies distilled by empirical researchers (these people are sometimes one and the same). Just as these social scientists cannot anticipate all the varied *functions* of the research that we plan, so they cannot instruct us unerringly in our question *forms*. Their insights will often be rather general and we will have to make such applications as we can to the research at hand.

We find convergence in their counsel, nonetheless. Question-crafters tend to speak of the need for simplicity, intelligibility, clarity. The experimental researchers, striving for more abstraction, tend to refer to "task difficulty" and the properties of questions that are likely to add to "respondent burden" (Babbie, 1973; Bradburn, 1983; Bradburn and Sudman, 1979; Hoinville and Jowell, 1978; Kahn and Cannell, 1957; Kornhauser and Sheatsley, 1976; Maccoby and Maccoby, 1954; Payne, 1951; Sheatsley, 1983; Sudman and Bradburn, 1982). But these two sets of preoccupations are highly overlapping with similar implications for the handcrafting of survey questions. They both point to the fact that questionnaires are often difficult to understand and to answer. As Sheatsley (1983: 200) observes,

> Because questionnaires are usually written by educated persons who have a special interest in and understanding of the topic of their inquiry, and because these people usually consult with other educated and concerned persons, it is much more common for questionnaires to be overwritten, overcomplicated, and too demanding of the respondent than they are to be simpleminded, superficial, and not demanding enough.

This means, in turn, that writing sufficiently clear and "simple" questions is hard-won, heavy-duty work for survey researchers. It requires special measures to cast questions that are clear and straightforward in four important respects: simple language, common concepts, manageable tasks, and widespread information.

SIMPLE LANGUAGE

Speaking in common tongues

Speaking the common language means finding synonyms for the polysyllabic and Latinate constructions that come easily to the tongue of the college educated. One need not, usually, say "principal" because "main" will do as well. "Intelligible" is rarely as good as "clear" or "understandable." "Intuitive" (or "counterintuitive") has taken a leading place in the special vocabulary of social scientists, but it is a pretentious choice if "feeling" carries essentially the same meaning.

Although the number of syllables in a question is not a perfect indicator of the complexity or the difficulty of words, it is a good place to start being wary. One may want to check suspicious words against published frequency counts of American vocabulary, to try to cut "elevated" language down to the size of the plainer-spoken alternative (Carroll et al., 1973; Dahl, 1979; Kučera and Francis, 1967). These volumes have stringent limitations, however, for they tally the literal appearance of a word, not the frequency of its use in all its special meanings. We have learned more from talking, listening, and pretesting than from reference books of this kind.

Must questions be written in standard English? Yes, almost always, but not necessarily standard *written* English or a grammar teacher's special tongue. The standard may be *spoken* English, for indeed in the face-to-face and telephone interview, these questions will be spoken by an interviewer. We feel that it is legitimate to violate certain conventions of written English if the pure construction sounds stilted or pretentious. For example, other writers on question design have recently made use of this item: "Physical fitness is an idea the time of which has come" (Fink and Kosecoff, 1985: 38). For our part, we would either use the unadulterated cliché, "an idea whose time has come," or abandon the item. But these details are finally matters of taste. There is consensus on the broader view that questions should be in straightforward language—not chatty, overfamiliar, or cast in some subculture's slang.

Must questions be short?

The counsel to keep questions short has been qualified by research and experience of recent years. In 1951, Payne was convinced that one should aspire to asking questions that numbered no more than around twenty words (Payne, 1951: 136). Under some conditions, however, length appears to be a virtue. In an experimental study of health measures, for example, more symptoms were reported by respondents when longer questions were asked. In the standard version, respondents were asked such questions as, "What medicines, if any, did you take or use during the past 4 weeks?" In a redundant version, questions were lengthened with "filler" words designed to add no new information as in this example: "The next question is about medicines during the past 4 weeks. We want to ask you about this. What medicines, if any, did you take or use during the past 4 weeks?" (Henson et al., 1979; Laurent, 1972).

It is not yet entirely clear what is going on in these experiments. The additional material spoken by the interviewer may stimulate the respondent to talk more, and this additional talk may aid the respondent's recall too (Sudman and Bradburn, 1982: 50-51). On the other hand, the extra material may simply give the respondent more time to think; and there is indeed ample evidence that interviewers tend to go too fast (Cannell et al., 1979).

These results about longer questions are evocative but still somewhat ambiguous. One should consider the use of redundancy now and then to introduce new topics and also to flesh out single questions, but if one larded all questions with "filler" phrases, a questionnaire would soon be bloated with too few, too fat questions. In any case, the more important strategy may be attacking the issue of interviewer pace directly and instituting special training to slow interviewers down.

In other cases, long questions or introductions may be necessary to communicate the nature of the task. In the so-called feeling thermometer used by the National Election Study (NES), each specific question is brief:

Our first person is Jimmy Carter.
How would you rate him using the thermometer?

But the introduction is a massive 140 words:

I'd like to get your feelings toward some of our political leaders and other people who are in the news these days. I'll read the name of a person and I'd like you to rate that person using this feeling thermometer. You may use any number from 0 to 100 for a rating. Ratings between 50 and 100 degrees mean that you feel favorable and warm toward the person. Ratings between 0 and 50 degrees mean that you don't feel too favorable toward the person. If we come to a person whose name you don't recognize, you don't need to rate that person. Just tell me and we'll move on to the next one. If you do recognize the name, but don't feel particularly warm or cold toward the person, you would rate that person at the 50 degree mark [Miller et al., 1982: 86].

Despite its length, the thermometer question seems to be clear to respondents because of the familiar image of this measuring device.

These long questions cannot be faulted as generically "bad examples," for they have been put into useful service. Beginners writing their own, original questions are probably well-advised nonetheless to heed Payne's counsel for brevity. The best strategy is doubtless to use short questions when possible and slow interviewer delivery—always—so that respondents have time to think.

Some avoidable confusions

Double vision. Counsel against using the "double-barreled" question is ubiquitous. One form of the offender is usually pretty easy to spot ("Do you think women and children should be given the first available flu shots?"), and we need not discuss it further. Another form has often been identified with the problem of "prestige," when a policy issue is identified with a public figure, for example, President Reagan's policy on Nicaragua. Such a question has two attitudinal objects—the president and the policy—so it too can be considered a less obvious form of the double-barreled question. It may be treated as two separate questions, in a split sample comparison, or it may be considered an indissoluble double stimulus, in which the policy is not fully identifiable without the association of the president.

Double *negatives*, however, are much to be avoided; they can introduce a needless confusion and they can creep in unobserved. Consider this Agree/Disagree item:

Please tell me whether you agree or disagree with the following statement about teachers in the public schools:

Teachers should not be required to supervise students in the halls, the lunchroom, and school parking lots.

Agree   Disagree

One may Agree that teachers should not be required to do this kind of duty outside of the classroom. But the Disagree side gets tangled, for it means "I do not think that teachers should not be required to supervise students outside of their classrooms"—that is, teachers should be required. Such a question can slip into a list when investigators have not read aloud and *listened* carefully to all the questions in the series. Such difficulties raise the issue, which we discuss in Chapter 2, of whether or not Agree/Disagree items should be used at all. But if they are considered essential, one should try to cast them as positive statements.

Implicit negatives—mispronounced. It is also possible that the negative meaning conveyed by words such as *control, restrict, forbid, ban, outlaw, restrain, oppose,* lends itself to confusion. If these "restrictive" words get attached to questions involving positive notions about freedom and liberty, it may not be clear whether respondents are for restricting *free* trade or restricting *trade.* One should be on the lookout for this kind of problem, even though little research bears directly on the point and written illustrations of it may not be compelling. It may seem far-fetched, for example, that words so opposite in meaning as these two might be confused:

- Do you favor or oppose a law *outlawing* guns in the state of Maryland?
- Do you favor or oppose a law *allowing* guns in the state of Maryland?

Still, it is important to remember that when respondents are listening to questions, not reading them, they are entirely reliant on what interviewers say, and if a key word *is* mispronounced or mumbled by an interviewer, it will probably be misheard or misinterpreted by the respondent. The experience of monitoring telephone interviews can—and should—make investigators vigilant to anticipate the likelier distortions and avoid them, if possible, by choosing words that are more difficult to confuse.

Overlong lists. The use of printed aids in the personal interview is probably a good deal more common than it was in early days of survey research. Respondents now are often given a "show card" to read that spells out the alternatives to a question. Certainly anything as complex as Kohn's (1969) list of thirteen qualities that might be considered desirable in a child—such as:

- that a child has good manners
- that a child has good sense and sound judgment
- that a child is responsible

—would typically be designed for simultaneous presentation in two forms: oral presentation by the interviewer and silent reading by the respondent. It is often the case that even simpler sets of four or five alternatives such as Very Often, Frequently, Seldom, and Hardly Ever will be read aloud by the interviewer and also made available in written form on a card or a small booklet for the respondent's reference. This is highly desirable practice. It is not helpful for illiterates, to be sure—and interviewers should be trained to be sensitive to that situation—but it seems to represent a convenient review for everyone else. We know of no research on the point but common sense appears to have made "show cards" a common technique.

Dangling alternatives. Asking response alternatives before introducing the topic itself, such as "Would you say that it is very often, frequently, seldom, or hardly ever that. . . ." is a difficult construction; it demands that the respondent keep these unattached alternatives in mind before knowing what topic to fix them to. The subject matter must come first; then the respondent can consider matters of degree or frequency: "How often do you and your husband disagree about spending money: very often, frequently, seldom, or hardly ever?" is the preferred order.

COMMON CONCEPTS

Making questions conceptually clear may be the most difficult assignment for social scientists, for they are usually rather charmed by abstract thinking in the first place, and then are trained in its pleasures. They lose touch with how difficult abstractions can be if one is not accustomed to moving them around in the mind. Mathematical abstractions tend to be difficult for the general public—and even for some people who are highly educated by not in mathematics or statistics.

"Variance" for instance—survey researchers would not think of asking the general public questions about variances or standard deviations. They know perfectly well that the concept of an average, or a mean, is much more widely understood than the concept of variability about that mean, or measures of dispersion. (Even statistically inclined baseball fans, avid about batting averages, are less likely to understand short-term variability in batting performances, and will cheer the streaks and boo the slumps.) Although survey researchers wisely avoid variance, they occasionally use concepts that are no less difficult.

Rates of change, for instance, bear on concepts that are formalized in calculus—not the stuff of everyday culture. This question was asked of a national sample in recent years:

Compared to a year ago, do you feel the prices of most things you buy are going up faster than they did then, going up as fast, going up slower, or not going up at all [Harris and Associates, 1970: 157]?

Mark that this is not simply asking whether or not prices are going up. It asks the respondent to compare the rate at which prices are going up this year with the rate they went up last year. Note too that although the question is full of short words—there is not a real polysyllable in it—it is still a very difficult question. It was duly answered by almost everyone in the national sample—only 2% said that they were Not Sure; 72% said that prices this year were going up faster than last year—and probably because respondents simplified it to comment not on comparative rates but simply current rise of prices.

There is a little evidence that even concepts that seem a good deal easier, such as percentages and proportions, are not handled well by much of the general public. In a study by Belson (1981: 244-245), respondents were asked what meaning they had given to various questions, such as "What proportion of your evening viewing time do you spend watching news programmes?" Only 14 of 53 respondents understood proportion as "part," "fraction," or "percentage." About one third of the others interpreted the term in a broadly quantitative sense (such as how long, how many hours, how often). A larger group interpreted the question to tap other dimensions entirely—*when* they watched, *which* programs, even which channel. Belson suspects that a substantial proportion of people do not understand the meaning of the word itself, and that another set, who probably do understand it, tend to avoid the difficulty of working it out.

That sounds like a splendid reason for not asking such a question. There is enough work for respondents to do in totting up their own total listening behavior (assuming that it is quite regular) and then adding up the news programs—without asking for a proportion, too. Far better to ask the respondent two or three simpler questions, on total listening time and on news-listening, on this order:

- In the past week, (SINCE DATE OR DAY) how many hours did you watch television in the evening?
- Did you spend any of that time watching any news programs? (IF YES) How many hours did you watch news programs?

And let investigators calculate the proportion themselves!

MANAGEABLE TASKS

Meaning: the fact/attitude divide

Is it easier for respondents to answer questions of personal fact—questions bearing on their own experience and behavior—than to respond to questions about opinions and attitudes? From a common-sense standpoint, it might seem so. Questions of personal fact, after all, refer to a physical or social reality: whether one is married or not married; whether one went to work yesterday or stayed home in bed with the flu; what one's job is and what paycheck it yields; and so on.

In recent years, survey questions of "fact" have come under new scrutiny, as the boundary between facts and attitudes has been shown to be sometimes a vague and permeable one. For example, as Smith (1984b) has pointed out, ethnicity is often left to the respondent's own subjective definition ("What do you consider your main ethnic or nationality group?") because respondents may have a large collection of birthplaces in their genealogy or lack the relevant information. Being unemployed is another example of a subjectively defined fact, for it incorporates the notion of "looking for work," a phrase that might mean anything from pounding the pavement to looking out the window. The measure of unemployment used by the federal government's Current Population Survey includes any of these activities—anything, in fact, except "nothing"—so it is the respondent who defines what "looking for work" means.

"Facts" of this sort can hardly be distinguished from attitudes, and may be prey to the kinds of ambiguities of meaning and frame of reference that attitude questions are. Recent work for the National Crime Survey shows ambiguities in the definitions of crime, for example. In an experimental study designed to broaden respondents' frame of reference for criminal victimization, a debriefing was held with respondents. They were presented with six different vignettes and asked whether or not each one was "the type of crime we are interested in, in this survey." Results showed that the experimental questionnaire had been effective in certain respects but was not wholly successful in matching respondents' and investigators' definitions of reportable crime. For example, the theft of an office typewriter from "Mary's" desk at work was included by about 90% of respondents, although this was not considered in scope by the investigators because the survey was to cover only personal and household belongings. On the other hand, assault by

"Jean's" husband—he slapped her hard across the face and chipped her tooth—was not deemed a crime by about 25% of the respondents (Martin 1986: 32-33). The current attention to spouse and child abuse turns on the last point especially: The effort to give criminal status to behaviors that have been excluded from that definition when the victims were family members (Cowan et al., 1978; Skogan, 1981).

As Martin (1986: 4) points out, however, ambiguity and subjectivity cannot be eliminated entirely from crime reporting:

> For all classes of [National Crime Survey] crimes, there is a gray area of ambiguous events for which "victims" may be uncertain about what happened (e.g., whether an article was lost or stolen) or what was intended (e.g., whether a broken window was the result of vandalism or attempted burglary). . . . Especially as measured in a victimization survey, the presence of threat rests on victim interpretation of offender intent.

Meaning: the inherent difficulty of shared definitions

Providing a common frame of reference is not an easy task, and ensuring that respondents use it is tougher still. What the researcher offers the respondent as a frame of reference may not be one that the respondent commonly uses, and it may be difficult for the respondent to put on the researcher's angle of vision, like a pair of glasses with the wrong prescription. What "family" is to mean, for instance, may have to be specified lest respondents vary in their frame of reference from their immediate family to their far-flung extended family. (For that very reason, a researcher may abandon "family" entirely in favor of "people living in the household.") "The neighborhood" may also have just such an elastic character. Even if a researcher labors to define it ("we mean the houses in this block" or "the people living three blocks in every direction") the respondent may persist in thinking about the "neighborhood" however he or she always does. Whether these floating definitions really matter or not will depend on a lot of things—the construct, the research purposes, the population being sampled, the range of effective ambiguity—but one is not comfortable simply assuming across the board that these ambiguities *never* matter.

It is our impression that it used to be more common than it is now to arm interviewers with highly detailed definitions, such as "By 'family' we mean . . . " or "If the respondent asks how far the 'neighborhood' extends, say . . . . " It has been repeatedly pointed out by field supervisors that it is not interviewers who need to know the full definition of the question—it is respondents. Anything that an investigator wants respondents to hear or assume should be included in the question itself, so that *all* respondents will be exposed to it. We think this has been good counsel. We suspect, in any case, that these detailed instructions tucked into interviewer manuals are likely to be lost in the shuffle and the more of them there are, the worse it probably is. (We know of absolutely no research on this point.)

How one establishes clear definitions for shared meaning is not at all obvious in any general sense, nor is any general prescription likely. One simply has to keep on the lookout for any data or experience that may help, and one must keep trying to *gather* such data. For large-scale surveys, it seems inevitable that one will always be approximating, chipping away at ambiguity. If we are commonly reminded that our definitions are usually too vague or sloppy, it is also appropriate to remember that we can also err in expecting an unrealistic degree of exactness.

In a recent symposium on question wording, for example, the pursuit of the too-narrow was apparent. An experienced investigator reminded his peers that they must continue to get out into the field, themselves, lest they lose very valuable firsthand information; and he told of his own experience of ringing a doorbell at a home where the family watching television happened to be in full view. The person who proved to be his respondent was not in the livingroom when he rang the bell. She had gotten up and gone into the kitchen for a moment during the commercial, and came back into the livingroom just as he was ushered into the house. In the course of the interview, he asked her what she had been doing when the doorbell rang, and she said, "Watching television."

The point of the vignette was that for this particular study, which had to do with the watching of the *commercials*, when the woman went into the kitchen, she was no longer "watching television" from the investigator's standpoint (Webb, 1982: 63). From the woman's point of view, she was indeed watching—not every second, not without momentary deviations or interruptions, but watching nevertheless. The researchers wanted a more literal-minded account, but would they have been pleased to hear an account of this sort?

When the doorbell first rang, I was lifting my left foot and putting it ahead of my right foot. Or no, perhaps not. I rather think that I was lifting my right foot. . . . But when the doorbell *finished* ringing. . . . But I'm not really sure now. I may be mixing things up.

They probably wanted an account of mindful attention, not just eyes only, in any case. The respondent's very sensible "approximation" may well be the most precise estimate we can expect to get in the naturalistic setting of the household survey.

Recall of the past

If survey researchers were guided entirely by a concern for valid descriptive data, they would focus on *the current, the specific, the real* (Turner and Martin 1984, I: 299); it is increasingly apparent that memory questions in general tend to be difficult. Recalling an event or behavior can be especially difficult in any of several circumstances: if the decision was made almost mindlessly in the first place, if the event was so trivial that people have hardly given it a second thought since, if questions refer to events that happened long ago, or if they require the recall of many separate events. This is obvious enough, but some consumer surveys, for example, still ask a profusion of extremely detailed questions about the properties of a motor oil or a hair dye, and ask respondents to introspect intensively about why they bought one brand or another.

One is on safer ground asking about major life events that are likely to have been important or *salient* to the individual, but there is evidence that recall of even "important" events either fades with time, or requires specific cues to bring them into focus at the time of an interview. Hospitalizations, for instance, are presumably nontrivial events for most people, but recall of hospitalizations has been shown to erode with time (Cannell et al., 1979: 8). To enhance validity of the reporting of the past, five techniques have been recommended: (a) bounded recall, (b) narrowing of the reference period, (c) averaging, (d) landmarks, and (e) cueing. The first four address more directly the problem of dating events than the problem of remembering events at all. Only the fifth, cueing, tackles more directly the problem of forgetting the event itself. We shall consider each one briefly in turn.

Bounded recall addresses overreport due to "forward telescoping." There is quite good evidence that if one asks respondents about events in the last six months, they may actually see "beyond" that and include events that happened earlier (Neter and Waksberg, 1965), which of course creates overreporting. Bounded recall establishes a baseline measure in an initial survey. Then in a subsequent panel reinterview, one inquires about events that have happened since that first interview. This thoroughgoing strategy is of course available only to those with the resources to mount a panel study.

Sudman and his associates (1984), however, have recently used specific bounded recall periods in a single interview. For example, respondents were asked about health behavior in the previous calendar month and then were asked about the same events in the current calendar month. In an experimental design using this type of bounded recall, reports of illness were reduced by 7%-20%. The results were not compared to validation data, but they suggest a reduction in telescoping.

The effort in recent years to *narrow the reference period* for survey reporting is a welcome corrective, in general. Researchers probably used to require far too much, asking questions with an unexamined assumption that most people kept marvelously minute mental records of what and how much they ate, drank, walked, drove, bought, coughed, worried, or thought. As Turner and Martin (1984, I: 297) point out, long reference periods for measuring victimization are virtually "worthless if the answers are to be treated as factual." It is common now to reduce the reference period to six months or less. For certain events, at least, one can narrow the time period of interest to the very immediate past, such as last week, or yesterday. Rather than asking, "Do you get regular physical exercise? (IF YES), How many hours of physical exercise do you usually get in a week?" one can zero in on a narrow time period and ask, "Did you get any physical exercise yesterday?" And if yes, "How much?" By the time the study has been completed, that "yesterday" will sweep across several weeks, perhaps even months, and estimates will have to be analyzed with that range in mind, especially if the activity is one that varies seasonally. One may also want to determine whether or not this refers to "typical" or habitual experience.

One can correct for such variability by asking respondents to "*average*." In research into college students, Schuman and his associates (1985: 958, 965) asked students about their time-use in a single day and a "typical" day in this sequence:

> The next few questions are about studying. First, apart from time spent in class, how much time, if any, did you study *yesterday*? By studying, we mean reading or any other assignment, writing, or review done outside of class.

Was that amount of time typical of the time you spent studying on *weekdays* during the past week or so?

(If No) What *was* the typical amount of time you spent studying on *weekdays* over the past week or so?

A similar sequence was then asked about week*ends*, because students' activities differ in the two periods. The investigators found that the "typical" or "averaging" question was more useful than the "single day" question because it took account of fluctuations in study time over the academic term.

The use of *landmarks* to aid dating is an experimental strategy that looks promising. Loftus and Marburger (1983) report positive results in experimental use of "landmark" events ("Since the eruption of Mt. St. Helens, has anyone beaten you up?") and major holidays such as New Year's Day to anchor the timing of other events. A similar technique using a calendar showing all major holidays of the year has been used as an aid in dating personal life events (DAS, 1985).

Providing *cues* to memory is still another strategy that is largely experimental. The purpose of cues is to stimulate recall by presenting a variety of associations. It recognizes the fact that because human memory uses a great variety of coding schemes to store information, what appears to be a "forgotten" event may be perfectly accessible if the correct storage file is tapped.

The victimization research that we have discussed set out specifically to stimulate recall of "crime" by describing concrete events. Instead of asking respondents if they had experienced "assaults," for instance, one item asked if anyone had used force against them "by grabbing, punching, choking, scratching, or biting." One purpose of this concreteness was to circumvent the premature aborting of memory search that is likely when a respondent has a (false) feeling of having nothing to report (Martin, 1986: 3-4). The cueing approach resulted in a 65% increase in victimization report, but the increase had to be discounted for events that were out of scope, events that happened before the six-month reference period, and other errors. The net increase, ranging from 19% to 39% (Martin, 1986: 64) is still impressive, but the results suggest that we cannot be entirely confident that more reporting is necessarily better reporting, as we often assume in assessing surveys of health, crime, and other kinds of behavioral data.

Results for both landmarks and cueing are not yet entirely clear or replicated extensively enough to suggest exactly how to activate memory most effectively, but the data on telescoping and forgetting continue to argue the need for new techniques.

Hypothetical questions

If we ask a hypothetical question, will we get a hypothetical answer—as some lighthearted critics have warned? Perhaps not, but the counsel of experience and research suggests that asking most people to imagine what if—what might have happened in their lives if things had been otherwise, or what they might do if—confronts them with a special task that is likely to be difficult. If the respondent is to take the mission seriously, it takes a good bit of imaginative projection as well as some time to mull over the possibilities. Certain survey objectives may cry for the use of hypothetical questions but it is well to be sure that it is a real necessity. When we ask hypothetical questions hoping to tap some underlying attitude, we know very little about what respondents actually have in mind when they answer. There appears to be only a little research on the point (Smith, 1981). It seems likely that respondents repair to their own personal experience when they have any, and yet if most people are trying to use their own experience, perhaps one can ask them about it directly.

There are instances in which hypothetical questions can nevertheless be valuable for certain research objectives. They usually represent an effort to *standardize* a stimulus because actual experiences range so widely, and the investigator does not know what set of experiences the respondent is bringing to the question. They can also be used in an effort to tie attitudes to some realistic contingencies. For example, people can be asked to imagine cost/benefit trade-offs. Would they favor such and such governmental program if it meant that their income tax would go up? Would they favor a tax cut if it meant that such and such service would go down? Would they favor X foreign policy if it meant that young men would be drafted in Y large numbers? And so on. Hypothetical questions provide no guarantee that respondents will feel the full force of political or economic realities, but they can try to add some realism to political rhetoric.

Hypothetical questions, nevertheless, are not easy and they deserve hard scrutiny before use. If one thinks that hypothetical questions are essential, ask them, but consider two other strategies as well: (1) Append to the battery on hypotheticals at least one question on actual experience, if possible; (2) more important, probe at least one of the hypotheticals for the respondent's frame of reference in answering the question. We are all in need of these kinds of data.

WIDESPREAD INFORMATION

Gallup's (1947: 687) early work on public information occasionally dramatized the widespread distribution of ignorance on certain topics. In the late 1940s, for example, Gallup Poll respondents were shown a map outlining the United States and asked to point to 10 of the best-known states (New York, California, Texas, and so on). That only 4% of Americans with a grade school education could locate all 10 states may not be surprising but those with at least some college education did not fare much better: only 8% could do so.

The finding that political information and interest are thinly distributed in some national groups has become a commonplace in research circles, but it was actually a discovery of survey research. Journalists and other educated observers who gathered their impressions from highly involved elites regularly exaggerated the knowledge and involvement of the broad public—and probably still do. Newcomers to survey research are also likely to assume that their own interests are mirrored in the general public. It can be very instructive to consult current poll and survey data on the broad public's level of information and interest.

When respondents know little about a subject, can one fill in some of the gaps on the spot? Investigators sometimes try, as in questions of this sort: "As you probably know, Honduras is right next to Nicaragua . . . " What the investigator presumably means is something like this:

> You probably don't really know this fact, or at least some people don't, or you may need reminding, so let me tell you that Honduras is right next to Nicaragua so that I can ask you the next question about military operations on the border between the two countries.

Most people probably cannot seize upon and use complex new information that quickly. The people who need instructions about where Honduras is are probably not entirely clear about where Nicaragua is, so the new information that these countries are neighbors may not be very illuminating, nor instant opinions on military implications very useful. As Nisbett et al. (1982) observe of experimental work with college students, "information is not necessarily informative."

Try it yourself. How ready are you with an opinion on this question, asked in a Harris survey in 1973:

I'd like to describe to you a new kind of insurance plan that would minimize the risk involved in investing in the stock market. You might want to read along with me on this card. (HAND RESPONDENT CARD "N.") According to this plan, you would be free to choose any stocks that you want to buy from an approved list of Blue Chip stocks like U.S. Steel, AT&T, or General Motors. An absolutely reliable company would guarantee to buy back the stock from you after ten years, but not earlier, for what you paid plus any gains in the value of the stock since you bought it. If the value of the stock decreased during the ten years you would still get back your original investment and the company, not you, would bear the loss. The price you would pay for this insurance against loss would be the dividends on the stock. This means that you would give up any dividends the stock would pay during the ten year period in exchange for this guarantee against loss.

If you wished to leave this insurance plan before the ten years were up, you would be free to do so and could sell the stock for the current market price. If the stock had increased in value, you would profit. If it declined, you would bear the loss, if you left the plan before the ten years were up. For leaving the plan, however, you would have to pay some charge like one or two years of dividends, which would vary according to how long you'd been in the plan. Remember, the firm offering this plan is absolutely reliable and the plan would be guaranteed by a major reputable insurance company. If such a plan were available, under which you would give up dividends on your stock in exchange for insurance against any loss on the money you put in, how interested would you be in participating in it—would you be definitely interested, do you think you might be interested but would like more information, do you think you would probably not be interested but would still like more information, or would you definitely not be interested at all [Harris, 1974]?

This question was asked not of stockbrokers or insurance agents but a national cross section. If respondents cannot be expected to learn complex new material in the course of a survey question, the example should suggest that some survey questions are—impossible.

Some Interesting Complexities

The counsel to simplicity neglects three interesting, more complex approaches to question design. We will discuss them here briefly not because either experience or general research strategy gives us much guidance into their application but because their use raises important questions. We will consider, in turn, factorial design (using vignettes), ranking scales, and magnitude estimation scales.

Factorial surveys use vignettes or "stories" in the study of judgment, decision-making, or attribution processes. The vignette itself is not new to survey research, but its design and randomization by computer program is. The following example is adapted from Alexander and Becker (1978: 94):

> Mr. Miller is a salesman who works for you. He comes into your office one morning to tell you that he has been drinking on the job. Miller is white, about 22, has been working for you for three months, and shows an average performance record.

The vignette factors are then varied—Mr. Miller becomes a Ms., age 56, black, an employee of 20 years, with an outstanding work record, and her drinking on the job has been observed by a trusted coworker. Respondents are asked to explain how they feel about each concrete instance.

When we vary dichotomies on even six variables, as in this example (sex, age, race, length of employment, work performance record, and source of information), 64 (2 to the 6th power) possible vignette combinations result—and many more factors would be of interest as well. The question-writing chores for such factorial designs begin to look rather daunting. Computer programs are designed not only to reduce these mechanical labors but also to randomize the combinations of factors and reduce these combinations to those of greatest analytic interest (Alexander and Becker, 1978: 96).

Factorial surveys have some very attractive features. To respondents, vignettes offer concrete, detailed situations on which to make judgments rather than the demand for abstract generalizations. Even though the questions are hypothetical, vignettes reduce the need for respondents to be insightful and conscious of their own thought processes. And one can construct vignettes to disentangle multicollinearity of the real world, where, for example, more expensive houses will also tend to be the larger houses, in better repair, located on more attractive lots, and so forth (Rossi and Anderson, 1982: 22).

Much of the early work in factorial surveys has been conducted with special samples, such as specific occupational groups and college students, but two 1986 surveys will be of special interest because they use factorial survey design with samples of the general public: the metropolitan cross-section of the Detroit Area Study, and the national cross-section of the General Social Survey of the National Opinion Research Center. Two features are common to both surveys. The number of vignettes is limited (to 15 in one case; to two groups of 10 in the other) on the basis of pretest evidence that beyond this number respondents tended to become fatigued or bored. These vignettes are also presented as self-administered sections in a survey that is otherwise face-to-face. This has the advantage of being less monotonous in delivery than oral pretest presentation seemed to be, but it has the counterpart disadvantage that interviewers cannot assess the degree of respondents' comprehension, or probe for ambiguity, or offer clarification. (Mellinger et al., 1982, used oral presentation in their vignette study of risk-benefit dilemmas in biomedical research and concluded that respondents' comprehension was adequate to the complex task.)

Methodological work is not yet widely available on various important issues. How does the task difficulty of vignettes compare with that of other survey questions? How do respondents view the task? How much of the information, which is rather densely packed into these vignettes, is actually absorbed by the respondent? (How much of the information is indeed "informative"?) What is the practical limit on the number of factors that can be varied? Are there context effects of the kind that we sometimes observe in traditional survey questions? Or effects from the order of presentation of the story elements? (See Chapter 2.) This is a tall order for research findings, which we cannot fill even for many, more conventional approaches to survey measurement, so it is hardly surprising that newer techniques such as factorial surveys have not yet inspired much of this kind of investigation. But the lack should make for caution, for we do not know much yet about how factorial surveys behave.

Ranking scales have a longer history in survey research. In the early 1920s, as distinguished an experimental psychologist / market researcher as Daniel Starch (1923: 197) presented respondents with ranking scales that now look towering. For example:

What do you consider the most important in buying boys' and children's clothing:

Material	Comfort
Durability	"Wear like iron"
Union made	Price

Style	Reputation of the firm
Tailoring	Fit
"Satisfaction or money	Maker's guarantee
back" guarantee	Merchant's guarantee

And Starch asked respondents to rank all 13 items in the order of importance.

Tasks of this scope were soon seen to be much too difficult (Franzen, 1936: 6) and in our own time, rank orders of this size are all but invisible in the literature. Shorter rankings are not uncommon—lists of four or five, for example—as well as partial rank orders such as Kohn's list of qualities desirable in children. Kohn (1969) also presents respondents with thirteen items, as it happens, in the question we have already noted:

- that a child have good manners
- tries hard to succeed
- is interested in how and why things happen, etc.

But respondents are given the simpler task of choosing, first, the three most desirable qualities and then one of that set that is most desirable of all. (They are also asked the same selection sequence for the least desirable qualities.) Kohn has used the ranked measures in an influential study of parental values, in which bipolar values of self-direction and conformity are found to be associated with higher and lower occupational status, respectively. It is widely agreed that rankings, even of this modified form, are more difficult than rating scales. The latter do not require choices among items; they take less time; and they can also be administered readily over the telephone in a way that long rank orders cannot, for they usually require "show cards." Ranking, nevertheless, is not without advantages. Among other things, the very fact that ranks are more difficult may help elicit the appropriate effort from respondents. It is worth asking, nevertheless, whether or not ranking is easy *enough* to be used in cross-section samples and whether or not results from it are comparable to those from rating scales.

Alwin and Krosnick's (1985) split sample experiments deal with these issues. First, they find that the relative importance given the qualities is very similar with rankings and ratings. Both measures also show the same "latent" dimensions, self-direction, and conformity. But they do *not* show the same relationships to predictor variables. Self-direction is positively correlated with education and income when rankings are used but not when ratings are used. As Alwin and Krosnick observe, the ranking technique may force a contrast between self-direction and conformity by asking respondents to make choices that they may not otherwise make. Ranks may measure not only the latent dimension of contrast between self-direction and conformity but also the very "ability to see logical contrast in the list of ranked qualities" (Alwin and Krosnick, 1985: 549).

This finding raises a very basic issue. When we ask questions that are widely acknowledged to be difficult ones, such as rank ordering, how are we to interpret observed relationships to education? Is this a "real-world" finding, or one that is compromised by artifactual properties because the highly educated bring something special to the task itself? Or should an artifact of this sort be considered a social fact? *Ratings* are not without their problems too, and indeed Krosnick and Alwin (forthcoming), in further work, conclude that, on balance, rankings still have more to recommend them for the study of values than ratings do. But these findings and their recent evidence of primacy and recency effects in the administrations of the Kohn lists suggest that we need much more guidance from research to understand question effects from the use of ranking scales.

Magnitude estimation scales are a third, more complex, technique of interest. They represent contemporary efforts to adapt to the measurement of social opinion the kinds of ratio scales developed in psychophysical measurement. Some social scientists have been drawn to this kind of scaling in frustration at the limits posed by the ordinal measurement of so much survey work: the loss of information when categories arbitrarily constrain the range of opinion; and the loss of precision in applying to ordinal measurement statistics appropriate to interval levels of measurement. Magnitude scaling of attitudes has been "calibrated" through numeric estimation and physical line-length estimation of physical stimuli such as light and sound.

The application of numeric estimation to social opinions is shown in this example (Lodge, 1981: 19):

I would like to ask your opinion about how serious YOU think certain crimes are. The first situation is, "A person steals a bicycle parked on the street." This has been given a score of 10 to show its seriousness. Use this situation to judge all others. For example, if you think a situation is 20 TIMES MORE serious than the bicycle

theft, the number you tell me should be around 200, or if you think it is HALF AS SERIOUS, the number you tell me should be around 5, and so on. . . .
COMPARED TO THE BICYCLE THEFT AT SCORE 10, HOW SERIOUS IS:
A parent beats his young child with his fists. The child requires hospitalization.
A person plants a bomb in a public building. The bomb explodes and 20 people are killed . . .

And so on.

In "line production," respondents are asked to draw lines that correspond to ratio judgments of the same kind, as in this example:

Some people believe that we should spend much less money for defense. Others feel that defense should be increased. And, of course, some other people have opinions in between.

Compared to the government's present level of defense spending, do you think we should increase defense spending, keep it about the same as now, or decrease defense spending [Lodge, 1981: 63]?

Then respondents are asked to draw a reference line to show what the government is currently spending on defense, and then to draw a response line to indicate how much the respondent favors an increase or decrease in defense spending. (In this use, the line is intended to represent a measure of intensity with which respondents hold their opinions, not the amount of increase or decrease in spending that they want.)

Magnitude scaling has shown some interesting results. Lodge (1981: 77) reports work showing an increase of 12%-15% in variance explained from the use of magnitude over ordinal scaling. In more recent work, Norpoth and Lodge (1985) report the successful use of magnitude scaling in a study of sophistication and intellectual structure of political attitudes. But the technique also poses some special problems. For instance, respondents must be given instruction and practice in making proportional judgment so that investigators can be sure that respondents have the competence to do so and are not reverting in their social opinion scales to the ordinal judgments so commonly used in surveys. Can people handle the tasks of numeric estimation—if, as we have been warned in other studies, many people shy away from such numeric tasks as calculating proportions? Are there any special precautions that we might take to make use of the interesting properties of these measures without incurring unduly heavy tasks for the respondent or unacceptable losses of information? We have little information about such questions. There has been little methodological work into magnitude scaling, perhaps because there are some special costs and burdens in undertaking the design at all.

Although these more complex techniques have considerable interest and potential usefulness in survey research, there is much about them that we do not yet understand. We are better guided, for now, by the counsel of experience or general research strategy that we have reviewed in this chapter, and by the findings of experiment, to which we now turn in Chapter 2.

2. THE EXPERIMENTAL EVIDENCE

Informal knowledge and personal experience have played a larger role in the design of survey questions than formal results from split sample experiments, probably because the implications for practice from such experiments are not always clear. Yet, important practical guidance can be drawn from experimental findings, especially those of the last decade or so. In this chapter we begin with some specific implications from the research literature and then turn to a number of general lessons.

Specific Questions
Are Better Than General Ones

The goal of standardized measurement is central to survey research. For the reasons we have noted, it has been considered essential to keep the wording of questions constant across respondents. But, of course, even the same question sometimes means different things to different people. Recent research indicates that this is particularly likely with general questions. The more general the question, the wider the range of interpretations it may be given. By contrast, wording that is specific and concrete is more apt to communicate uniform meaning.

The advantages of specificity can be seen in an experiment carried out by Belson and Duncan (1962) on British newspaper and magazine readership. A question that presented respondents with a list of periodicals and asked them to check those they had looked at the previous day was compared with one that asked respondents simply to list the newspapers and magazines they had looked at the previous day.

The most striking difference between forms was in the proportion mentioning *Radio Times*, a publication similar to the American *TV Guide*. More than five times as many people mentioned it on the checklist as on the other form (38% versus 7%). Apparently, some people thought of *Radio Times* as a magazine, but others did not. On the version where periodical titles were not mentioned, these different understandings affected people's answers. On the checklist, this extraneous source of variation was avoided, and a more consistent measurement across respondents was obtained.

The Belson and Duncan study also points to a second advantage of specificity. In addition to more precise communication of question intent, specificity aids respondent recall. Although the *Radio Times* difference was far and away the largest, the checklist produced higher readership estimates for every publication. Unaided, respondents had difficulty recalling all the magazines and newspapers they looked at yesterday. Seeing a list of possibilities helped them remember. (The lack of validation data means we cannot definitively rule out the possibility that people exaggerated their reading on the checklist, yet the pattern of results makes this unlikely. For example, the form differences were much smaller for newspapers than for magazines, as one would expect given that newspaper reading is a daily activity and thus easier to recall than less regular magazine reading.)

The virtues of specificity are by no means limited to items about behavior. A series of experiments on the measurement of happiness demonstrates the same point for attitude questions (Turner, 1984). The experiments varied the order in which these two questions were asked:

- Taken altogether, how would you say things are these days: would you say that you are very happy, pretty happy or not too happy?
- Taking all things together, how would you describe your marriage: would you say that your marriage is very happy, pretty happy or not too happy?

The first question is very general. It asks about unspecified "things." People may answer in terms of different combinations of their health, job, marriage, and so on. This probably explains why answers to the general question are affected by whether it is asked before or after the marital happiness question. Either of two processes may occur: When the marriage question is asked first, respondents' feelings about their marriage may suffuse their judgment about life in general; alternatively, answering the marriage question first may lead respondents to subtract that topic from the second question bearing on things in general.

The specific question on marital happiness, on the other hand, is not vulnerable to this order effect. Respondents answer the marital happiness question the same way, regardless of whether it comes before or after the general happiness question (Turner, 1984). Its greater specificity apparently makes its interpretation less subject to influence from factors like question placement. It is the meaning of more abstract, less definite items that are particularly prone to such problems (Kalton et al., 1978; Smith, 1981).

One further disadvantage of general items is worth mentioning. Responses to general attitude items are poorer predictors of behavior than responses to specific attitude questions. Indeed, the more specific an attitude item, the stronger the connection between attitudes and behavior. Thus, for example, an attitude question about open housing laws was a better predictor of willingness to sign petitions about the issue than a series of questions measuring general racial prejudice (Brannon et al., 1973).

Despite this catalogue of weaknesses, general questions cannot be ruled out entirely. They have their uses when a "global" measure is of analytic interest; when there is not the time or space to ask about *everything* in specific detail; and when the comparison of general and specific views is itself of interest.

When to Leave It Open and When to Close It

A widespread criticism of closed questions is that they force people to choose among offered alternatives instead of answering in their own words. Yet precisely because closed questions spell out the response options, they are more specific than open questions, and therefore more apt to communicate the same frame of reference to all respondents.

This advantage of the closed form is demonstrated in the results of an experiment on work values that compared the following two questions (Schuman and Presser, 1981):

People look for different things in a job. What would you most prefer in a job?

People look for different things in a job. Which one of the following five things would you most prefer in a job—work that pays well; work that gives a feeling of accomplishment; work where there is not too much supervision and you make most decisions yourself; work that is pleasant and where the other people are nice to work with; or work that is steady with little chance of being laid off?

On the open form, many respondents said "the pay" was the most important aspect of a job. There was evidence that some of these individuals meant "high pay" whereas others meant "steady pay." But both kinds of answers were expressed in the same words, making it impossible to separate the two. The closed form solved this problem. Individuals of the first sort chose "work that pays well," whereas those of the second type chose "work that is steady." Thus building distinctions into the answer categories can more accurately tap differences among respondents than letting people answer in their own words.

Of course, this will only be true if the response categories have been appropriately designed. In another open-closed experiment, people were asked what they thought was the most important problem facing the nation (Schuman and Presser, 1981: 86). As the survey began, the U.S. was hit with an unexpected natural-gas shortage. This was reflected on the open version, where 22% said the "energy shortage" was the most important problem. On the closed version, designed without knowledge of the energy problem, there was hardly a trace of concern about the shortage, over 99% choosing one of the five offered alternatives (unemployment, crime, inflation, leadership quality, and breakdown of morals and religion). Thus when not enough is known to write appropriate response categories, open questions are to be preferred.

A second area in which open questions have been shown to be better than closed ones is the measurement of sensitive or disapproved behavior. Bradburn and Sudman (1979) compared open and closed estimates of drinking and sexual activity, both of which are known to be underreported in surveys. The closed questions had the response categories, "never, once a year or less, every few months, once a month, every few weeks, once a week, several times a week, and daily," The open questions, of course, had no response categories. In every case (beer, wine, liquor, petting, intercourse, and masturbation), reported frequencies were significantly higher on the open form. Apparently, the presence of the low-frequency categories on the closed form makes people less willing to admit to higher frequencies.

There are other special purposes for which open questions are better suited than closed items (to measure salience, for example, or to capture modes of expression). But in most instances, a carefully pretested closed form is to be preferred for its greater specificity.

Offer a No Opinion Option

The typical survey question incorporates assumptions not only about the nature of what is to be measured, but also about its very existence. "The trouble is," as Katz (1940: 282) perceived early in the development of public opinion measurement, "that the polls have often assumed that because a problem is of practical importance or of political interest, therefore there is a public opinion on the problem which can be measured."

This problem is intensified by the standard survey practice of not including "don't know" or "no opinion" as a response option mentioned in the question. Experimental research shows that many more people will say "don't know" when that alternative is explicitly offered than when it is not. Such filtering for no opinion generally affects from about an eighth to a third of those interviewed (Bishop et al., 1980a; Schuman and Presser, 1981).

The size of the effect is partly a function of the way in which the don't know option is offered. Making the filter a separate question (example A) has a larger effect than simply including "no opinion" as one of the response options (example B).

(A) Here is a statement about another country. Not everyone has an opinion on this. If you do not have an opinion just say so. Here's the statement: The Russian leaders are basically trying to get along with America. Do you have an opinion on that? (IF YES:) Do you agree or disagree?

(B) Here is a statement about another country. The Russian leaders are basically trying to get along with America. Do you agree, disagree, or do you not have an opinion on that?

Likewise, "Have you thought much about this issue?" is a stronger filter than "Do you have an opinion on this?" (Schuman and Presser, 1981).

Even when asked *un*filtered questions, however, most survey respondents do not mindlessly give opinions when they do not have them. About 70% of American adults volunteer "don't know" to unfiltered items about plausible sounding but obscure or fictitious issues (Bishop et al., 1980b; Schuman and Presser, 1981). On the other hand, some respondents apparently do manufacture opinions on the spot, and thus filtering for "don't know" is a good practice.

Filtering is especially important toward the beginning of an interview to make clear to respondents that no opinion is a legitimate answer. Doing so at the outset, as well as training interviewers to accept "don't knows," should also reduce the need—and monotony—of filtering routinely throughout an interview.

Omit the Middle Alternative and Measure Intensity

Survey researchers disagree about whether or not middle alternatives should be included in the wording of questions. Moser and Kalton (1972: 344) argue that "there is clearly a risk in suggesting a noncommittal answer to the respondent." Yet as early as 1944, Rugg and Cantril (1944: 33) argued for offering the middle alternative "in that it provides for an additional graduation of opinion."

Split sample experiments indicate that the resolution of the issue is important, as results depend on whether or not the middle ground is provided. It is not unusual for 20% of those interviewed to *choose* a middle alternative when it is offered although they would not *volunteer* it if it were not mentioned. Strikingly, however, this tends to have a limited impact on the distribution of responses in other categories. This is illustrated in various experiments carried out by Schuman and Presser (1981). For example:

Should divorce in this country be easier or more difficult to obtain than it is now?		Should divorce in this country be easier to obtain, more difficult to obtain, or stay as it is now?	
Easier	28.9	Easier	22.7
More difficult	44.5	More difficult	32.7
Stay as is (volunteered)	21.7	Stay as is	40.2
Don't know	4.9	Don't know	4.3
Total	100.0%	Total	100.0%

Although the size of the middle category is very different on the two forms, the ratio of "easier" to "more difficult" is essentially unaffected by form. Holding aside the middle answers and the don't knows, about 40% say "easier" and 60% "more difficult" on both forms.

Who, then, are the respondents affected by the presence of a middle category? Intensity is the major characteristic that distinguishes them from those who give the same answer regardless of question wording. Offering a middle position makes less difference to individuals who feel strongly about an issue than it does to those who do not feel strongly.

These results suggest a solution to the middle alternative wording problem. Do not explicitly provide the middle category, and thereby avoid losing information about the direction in which some people lean, but follow the question with an intensity item, thus separating those who definitely occupy a position from those who only lean toward it.

How to Measure Intensity

The measurement of intensity is useful not only as a follow-up for items with logical middle positions, but for attitude questions generally. Strength of feeling has been shown to predict both attitude stability and attitude constraint. Thus strength measures can identify respondents who will be more consistent over time as well as more consistent between topics (Schuman and Presser, 1981; Smith, 1983).

Asking questions about intensity or centrality may also enhance our understanding of the nature of public opinion on an issue. In the late 1970s, for example, Americans were fairly evenly split in response to a question about whether or not a married woman should have access to a legal abortion, but this distribution concealed very different strengths of feeling on the two sides. Opponents of abortion were six times more likely than "pro-choice" advocates to say that they felt extremely strongly about the issue (Schuman and Presser, 1981: 246). Without the strength of feeling data, an analyst would have been more apt to misinterpret the even split between abortion proponents and opponents. (The so-called "mushiness index" is another way of getting at this dimension of public opinion; see *Public Opinion*, 1981.)

Two of the most commonly used intensity indicators are "strongly agree, agree, disagree, or strongly disagree" items (example A) and seven-point scales labeled at either end by opposing positions (example B).

(A) Now I'm going to read several statements. Please tell me whether you strongly agree, agree, disagree, or strongly disagree with each. "It is much better for everyone involved if the man is the achiever outside the home and the woman takes care of the home and the family." Do you strongly agree, agree, disagree, or strongly disagree?

(B) Some people feel the federal government should take action to reduce the inflation rate even if it means that unemployment would go up a lot. Others feel the government should take action to reduce the rate of unemployment even if it means that inflation would go up a lot. Where would you place yourself on this scale?
    Reduce Inflation   1 2 3 4 5 6 7   Reduce Unemployment

These approaches confound extremity, a dimension of attitudinal position, with intensity, how strongly a position is felt. Although intensity and extremity may frequently covary, individuals may hold an extreme position with little feeling, or invest a middle of the road position with considerable passion. Without separate questions for position and intensity (e.g., following a question about direction of opinion with an item like "How strongly do you feel about that—extremely strongly, very strongly, somewhat strongly, or not at all strongly?"), it is not possible to disentangle these dimensions.

Use Forced-Choice Questions, Not Agree-Disagree Statements

One of the most popular forms of attitude measurement is the agree-disagree statement. It is also the form that has come under most attack by methodologists. The approach suffers from "acquiescence response set"—the tendency of respondents to agree irrespective of item content. Consider this pair of items:

It is hardly fair to bring children into the world, the way things look for the future.

Children born today have a wonderful future to look forward to.

Although these items seem completely contradictory, Lenski and Leggett (1960) report that about a tenth of their sample agreed to both, a finding echoed in the results of split sample experiments.

Moreover, acquiescing is related to education. Its incidence is greatest among individuals who have had little schooling. Consequently, the use of agree-disagree items may distort conclusions about the relationship between education and opinion, as in the following example (Schuman and Presser, 1981: 223):

	Years of Schooling		
	0-11	12	13+
Would you say that most men are better suited emotionally for politics than are most women, that men and women are equally suited, or that women are better suited than men in this area?			
Percent "men better suited"	33	38	28
Do you agree or disagree with this statement: Most men are better suited emotionally for politics than are most women.			
Percent "agree"	57	44	39

The forced-choice form of this item shows that there is essentially no relationship between education and opinion about women in politics. (The difference between groups does not exceed sampling error.) On the agree-disagree version, by contrast, there is a clear relationship, less-educated respondents being more likely to give the traditional answer. But this is due to the greater tendency of the less educated to acquiesce, not to a real difference in attitudes toward women.

More generally, forced-choice items are more apt to encourage a considered response than are agree-disagree statements. Taken by itself, "The government should see to it that everyone receives adequate medical care," may have a plausible ring to it. Asked alone, "Everyone should be responsible for their own medical care," also may seem sensible. Thus for most purposes, the better survey item is, "Should the government see to it that everyone receives adequate medical care, or should everyone be responsible for their own medical care?"

The Problem of Question Order

Survey respondents are sensitive to the context in which a question is asked, as well as to the particular words used to ask it. As a result, the meaning of almost any question can be altered by a preceding question. Consider the item, "In general, do you think the courts in this area deal too harshly or not harshly enough with criminals?" In most contexts, respondents will interpret "this area" to mean a geographical location. Yet a very different meaning can be conveyed by asking the question in this context:

- Do you think the United States should forbid public speeches in favor of Communism?
- In general, do you think the courts in this area deal too harshly or not harshly enough with criminals?

In a pretest using this sequence, some respondents thought that the courts item referred to judicial treatment of public speeches advocating communism.

As a general rule, however, items affect one another mainly when their content is clearly related, as in the marriage and general happiness example discussed earlier (where one object subsumes the other), or when the answer to one question has an obvious implication for the answer to another. Thus fewer people say their taxes are too high after being asked a series of items about whether government spending should be increased in various areas (Turner and Krauss, 1978). Similarly, more people say America should let Soviet journalists into the U.S. if they have just been asked if the Soviet Union should admit American journalists (Hyman and Sheatsley, 1950).

In each of these examples, some respondents bring their answers to an item into line with what they have said to another item. One way to think about this is in terms of consistency. Another way of looking at it is in terms of salience. Earlier questions may make some experiences or judgments more salient or available to the respondent than they otherwise would be. This appears to have happened in an experiment on measuring crime (Cowan et al., 1978). A questionnaire that asked only factual items about whether the respondent had been criminally victimized in the last twelve months was compared with one that was prefaced by a series of attitude items about crime. People reported significantly more crime on the version preceded by the attitude questions. Answering the attitude items apparently stimulated memories of actual criminal events, although it is of interest to note that the differences occurred mainly for the more frequent, less serious kinds of crime.

Notwithstanding these examples, it should be emphasized that numerous experiments with related questions show no context effect. Thus, to take one instance, evaluations of President Nixon's job performance were unaffected by whether they followed a question about his possible impeachment (Hitlin, 1976). Many similar instances of order having no effect may be found in Schuman and Presser (1981).

Unlike the wording decisions we have reviewed, however, there are almost no experimentally based general rules to order questions. Before there was systematic study of the matter, experienced researchers recommended that general questions be asked *before* specific ones, in a "funnel" sequence (Kahn and Cannell, 1957). The research we reviewed earlier on general and specific items supports this intuition. Otherwise, in the case of attitudes, even where context is shown to have an effect, it is frequently unclear that one order is better than another. Instead, each order may reveal a different facet of the issue being studied.

Wording Effects: Potentially Important But Unpredictable

The most basic finding from research on question wording is a double edged one: Even small changes in wording can shift the answers of many respondents, but it is frequently difficult to predict in advance whether or not a wording change will have such an effect. "Forbid" and "allow," for example, are logical opposites, and thus substituting one for the other in the question "Do you think the United States should [allow/forbid] public speeches against democracy?" might easily be assumed to have no effect. Yet it turns out that many more people are willing to "not allow" such speeches than are willing to "forbid" them. On the other hand, referring to something as "bad and dangerous" would seem to load a question and thus have a noticeable impact on respondents. In fact, the following two items yielded identical results:

- There are some people who are against all churches and religion. If such a person wanted to make a speech in your (city/town/community) against churches and religion, should he be allowed to speak, or not?

- There are always some people whose ideas are considered bad or dangerous by other people. For instance, somebody who is against all churches and religion. If such a person wanted to make a speech in your (city/town/community) against churches and religion, should he be allowed to speak, or not?

About two-thirds of American adults were in favor of free speech on both forms (Schuman and Presser, 1981: 289-290).

Similar results are not uncommon. Consider this pair of examples from experiments conducted at the outset of the Second World War (Rugg and Cantril, 1944: 44):

(A) Do you think the United States will go into the war before it is over?

Yes 41%   No 33%   Don't Know 26%

(B) Do you think the United States will succeed in staying out of the war?

Yes 44%   No 30%   Don't Know 26%

Despite the apparently trivial change in wording, respondents were clearly affected. In the following pair of questions, however, there is a substantial change in wording without any effect at all.

(A) Some people say that since Germany is now fighting Russia, as well as Britain, it is not as necessary for this country to help Britain. Do you agree or disagree with this?

Agree 20%   Disagree 72%   No Opinion 8%

(B) Some people say that since Germany will probably defeat Russia within a few weeks and then turn her full strength against Britain, it is more important than ever that we help Britain. Do you agree or disagree with this?

Agree 71%   Disagree 19%   No Opinion 10%

Results like these demonstrate the subtleties and complexities inherent in language. They show that respondents tend to be constrained by the exact words of a question—as well they should be. (If we got the same answers no matter what wording we used, survey research would have no scientific basis at all.) Such results also indicate the importance of not basing conclusions on results from a single question. In this regard, four approaches deserve wider use.

CREATE SPLIT SAMPLE COMPARISONS

Wording experiments need not be confined to methodological research, but can be built into all surveys, at least for some items. Experiments of modest scope can be purchased at a minor increase in clerical costs. Multiple questionnaires are not needed, as one can simply construct a set of skip patterns for the different question wordings, and establish a random procedure by which the interviewer is directed to one or the other. This is a very easy matter with Computer Assisted Telephone Interviewing but even without the computer it may be straightforwardly accomplished by a procedure in which every other listing, after a random start, is designated A or B, leaving nothing to interviewer choice.

The risk accompanying wording experiments is learning that two forms of the "same" question are not equivalent. This reduces the sample size, as one would no longer be justified in combining these experimental apples and oranges in the analysis. If the experiment turned on a central question, this could be a sore loss. From a scientific perspective, of course, it might be a sorer loss if one *failed* to uncover these qualifications, ambiguities, or differences.

USE OPEN FOLLOW-UPS TO CLOSED QUESTIONS

Probes of closed questions provide another window on the meaning of items and an efficient way of combining some advantages of both open and closed questions. In the 1983 Detroit Area Study of attitudes and experiences regarding welfare, for example, a substantial majority endorsed the proposition that "Government is trying to do too many things that should be left to individuals and private businesses." Of the sample, 72% agreed that the government had taken on too many functions—at least this is what the investigators had meant by the question. When agreeing respondents were asked the follow-up question, "What things do you feel should be left to individuals or private businesses?" over a quarter could not answer at all. They could not think of anything "offhand" or "didn't know." Others said "Taxes are too high" or inveighed vaguely against government ("Government shouldn't be messing into things all the time—I'm for freedom"). Probing for the respondent's meaning revealed the flaws of what may have been an overly intellectual question. Thus the answers to open follow-ups can provide valuable guidance in the analysis of closed questions.

USE RANDOM PROBES

One can invest the time available for probing a few key questions and ask them of everyone. Or one can ask probes contingently of a subset of people who respond in certain ways, as in the case of those who agreed to the antigovernment item. Another approach is to spread a net of follow-up questions more thinly and widely, asking each respondent a small number of probes distributed randomly over the entire questionnaire.

In Schuman's design (1966) the interviewer probes nondirectively after the respondent has selected an alternative to a closed question, in wording of this sort:

• Could you tell me a little more about what you mean?
• Could you say more about what you have in mind?
• I see—could you give me an example?

The interviewer does not select the questions to be probed; rather, the questions are selected in advance of the interview by a random procedure, and marked on the questionnaire.

The random probe can be used extensively to provide a sample of follow-up answers for an entire questionnaire or more selectively for a subset of questions. Either way, it is valuable for three purposes: First, to pinpoint items that were particularly troublesome for respondents; second, to identify respondents whose understanding of the questionnaire was imperfect enough that they probably contributed mainly error to the study; and third, as a qualitative aid to interpretation.

This last use is illustrated in a study of black attitudes conducted by Schuman and Hatchett (1974). In analyzing the item "Generally speaking, do you feel (blacks/Negroes) have more, less, or the same duty as whites to obey the law?" it was expected that those who answered "less" would show higher than average scores on alienation. They did, but curiously, so did those who said blacks had "more" duty to be law-abiding.

Responses from the random probe indicated that this latter group interpreted the question in terms of blacks' greater need (rather than "duty") to be law-abiding because of racial discrimination:

• Whites can get away with things Negroes can't.
• Negroes have to be more careful.

In this context, the higher alienation scores for respondents who believed blacks had more duty to be law-abiding were not surprising.

ASK MULTIPLE QUESTIONS ON A TOPIC

The knowledge that any one survey item may be beset by a host of extraneous influences unique to it has led survey researchers to scale or index construction. It is probably fair to say, however, that the faith that scales can overcome the defects of single questions is not as strong as it once was. For one reason, scales can actually compound wording or form effects. If agree-disagree items, for instance, are prey to acquiescence, a battery of such items will amplify the distortion.

For another reason, scales may be bent out of shape by change over time. Items that correlate highly with each other at one point may move in different directions over time, as in this example from the National Election Study. As the graph shows (see next page), 3 of the 4 measures moved together quite nicely, rising in the 1950s and declining in the 1960s, suggesting that they each tapped some general facet of political efficacy. The fourth item, however, went its own way, rising consistently across the tide. Philip Converse (1972) interprets this as a response to the political activity of the 1960s, which featured not only voting but demonstrations, marches, and so on. More to our purposes here, he draws a methodological moral (p. 329):

> This is an interesting case . . . of a scale deemed unidimensional by Guttman criteria in 1952, one component of which has pulled out of line rather markedly in response to phenotypic events in a subsequent period. Our analysis of these trends would have been greatly muddied if we had proceeded with the composite scale taken as a whole.

So there is no real reprieve. Investigators wisely seek multiple and scaled measures but there is no guarantee they will remain scales. They may be scattered by the winds of change into component or single items that require individual interpretation. Yet single questions survive, too, for the simple reason that one can never, in a single survey, incorporate multiple measures of *everything*.

Multiple measures are nevertheless the strategy of choice. Relying on single questions makes it difficult to uncover complexity. Using multiple indicators makes it easier to discover where or how our understanding of the world is inadequate. The study of political party identification is an instructive case in point. For decades, party identification was seen by political scientists as simply the sense of attachment felt toward one of the parties, and was measured as follows:

- Generally speaking, do you usually think of yourself as a Republican, a Democrat, an Independent, or what?

128

- IF REPUBLICAN OR DEMOCRAT: Would you call yourself a strong (Republican/Democrat) or a not very strong (Republican/Democrat)?
- IF INDEPENDENT: Do you think of yourself as closer to the Republican or Democratic Party?

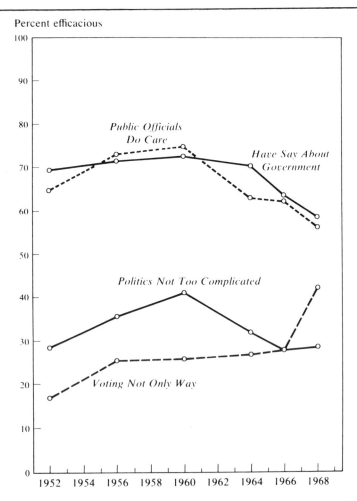

Percent efficacious

NOTE: From "Human Meaning of Social Change," edited by Angus Campbell and Philip Converse. Copyright © 1972 by the Russell Sage Foundation. Reprinted by permission of Basic Books, Inc., Publisher.

Figure 1: Trends in Responses to Political Efficacy Items, 1952-1968

This measurement approach assumes that people can identify with only one party and that political independence is nothing more than the absence of identification with a party. Recent research suggests that these assumptions are unjustified. In an analysis of 1980 national data, for example, Weisberg (1980) reports that a fifth of those classified as strong partisans by the traditional measure thought of themselves as Independents *as well as* party supporters. Results like these are leading to a reconceptualization of party identification as involving separate attitudes toward at least four objects: political parties in general, the Republican party, the Democratic party, and political independence. Thus to quote Weisberg (1980):

> Some people might be Independents because they dislike both parties, while others might be Independents because they like both parties equally, and still others might be Independents because they positively value political independence. Indeed, some people might consider themselves both Republicans (or Democrats) and Independents, particularly if they generally support Republican issue stands but feel that one should vote on the basis of issues rather than party labels.

Many if not most of the issues asked about in surveys are as complex as party identification. Consider, for instance, the debate about gun control. When Americans are asked if they favor banning private ownership of guns, a large majority expresses opposition. By contrast, when they are asked if they favor a law requiring a police permit before purchasing a gun, an equally large majority expresses support (Wright, 1981). These results reveal some of the complexity of attitudes toward this issue. Americans favor certain forms of gun control and oppose others. Asking multiple items not only facilitates the discovery of these contingencies and qualifications but makes the analyst less likely to fall into the trap of reporting a single number as representing public opinion on an issue.

As a general strategy, therefore, one should look for questions that cast light at different angles. In using multiple measures of this sort, we are not aspiring to experiment. Rather, we are trying to escape the confines of any single question to a richer context of inquiry—the prime objective of the two kinds of counsel we have so far considered, the lore of experience and the evidence of systematic experiment, as well as that of the one to which we turn in the next chapter, the continuous exploration of pretesting.

3. THE TOOLS AT HAND

Every questionnaire must, finally, be handcrafted. It is not only that questionnaire writing must be "artful"; each questionnaire is also unique, an original. A designer must cut and try, see how it looks and sounds, see how people react to it, and then cut again, and try again. Handcrafting a questionnaire involves successive trials, which we shall consider here in two stages: exploration and pretesting.

Exploration

The crafting of a questionnaire involves intellectual preparation of all sorts, well prior to the exploration we consider here. One must have a clear set of research purposes, knowledge of work on the problem that has already been conducted ("the literature" bearing on concepts and data), and some lively notions of how a survey could shed some new light. How should one start on the preliminary work of actual questionnaire design? We recommend starting out by consulting two kinds of people with special expertise.

EXPERTS AND INSIDERS

Professional experts

An exploratory study should take investigators out beyond their own academic or industrial subculture, to new "experts"—ones with differing counsel if at all possible. If investigators consult only the like-minded, they are likely to constrict the intellectual range of their inquiry and to give the *appearance* of bias. Academic researchers do not often have to contend with the kind of publicity that election pollsters face routinely, but when they do, they are much better prepared if they have already absorbed criticism from cultural strangers or even political "enemies." The recent attack on the Ladd-Lipset surveys of American academics by Serge Lang, a mathematician, is a complicated matter and doubtless a rare event, but Lang's charges of bias should serve as a cautionary tale to make survey researchers of all kinds more sensitive to varying interpretations of their questionnaire (Ladd and Lipset, 1976; Schuman, 1983). Survey questions, finally, must *seem fair* to people of widely different viewpoints—people one will meet, at the last, in a cross-section sample of the general population.

More important still, differing perspectives and experiences can turn up new information. Consider the finding that on three issues concerning federal government action on social policies, *conservatives* endorsed federal intervention almost as often as the sample as a whole did. The questions were of this form:

- Do you agree or disagree that the *federal government* ought to help people get medical care at low cost? [Turner and Martin, 1984, I: 82-83.]

The poll directors concluded that conservatives seemed to be moving to the left. The North American Newspaper Alliance was skeptical, however, and commissioned a split-ballot experiment that asked the "federal government" wording to half the sample, and to the other half substituted "private enterprise." The results showed that most people also favored intervention by private enterprise, and a comparable majority of *liberals* favored it, too.

Were conservatives moving to the left and liberals moving to the right? The split-ballot experiment suggested another hypothesis entirely: The public might be more concerned with getting action on these problems than with the issue of who took responsibility. This may be another illustration of agree/disagree problems that we noted in Chapter 2, but the important point for our present purposes is that the results were generated by the suspicion of bias. It is useful to be faced with these suspicions while one's questionnaire is still under construction, by intensive interviewing of professional experts on the other side of some intellectual or political fence.

Cultural insiders

Exploratory inquiry can involve "in depth" interviews with members of the target population, and it is the conviction of McKennell (1974), among others, that it should. He is skeptical of the practice of taking attitude items from "the literature," because they often represent other professionals' impression of what people in general think about things, with almost no validation by work with people in general themselves. At this exploratory stage, there is little prospect of formally *sampling* the target population, but interviewing even a few individuals can enrich the researcher's perspective. Another useful procedure is to assemble somewhat more formally the insiders of a given subculture in a "focused discussion group." This can be of special value when a target population is likely to have special perceptions, problems, and idioms that may be relatively foreign to the investigator—youth culture, gambling, drugs, prisons, and so on.

Because survey questions are now so abundant, it is the more difficult to proceed in the spirit of McKennell's (1974: 33) advice and undertake one's work "like an anthropologist approaching an alien culture, and regard one's own background and established frames of reference as a positive hindrance." Unfortunately, most of us are probably all too likely to neglect this preliminary phase of exploration and move quite directly to writing new questions and borrowing others from the survey literature.

BORROWING QUESTIONS FROM OTHERS

Large-scale surveys are now so common in American cultural and scientific life that survey questions have accumulated in a truly mountainous supply. Easy access to many survey questions is possible through various published compilations of survey questions. Early in the process of designing a questionnaire, one should consult these data, for they are very likely to save time and effort. Here we list nine that we have found most useful:

- Converse, Philip E., Jean D. Dotson, Wendy J. Hoag, and William H. McGee III (eds.), *American Social Attitudes Data Sourcebook 1947-1978* (Cambridge, MA: Harvard University Press, 1980).

- Gallup, George, *The Gallup Poll: 1935-1971* 9 vols. (New York: Random House, vols. 1-3, 1935-1971; Wilmington, DE: Scholarly Resources, Inc., vols. 4-9, 1972-1981).

- Hastings, Philip K. and Jessie C. Southwick (eds.), *Survey Data for Trend Analysis: An Index to Repeated Questions in U. S. National Surveys Held by the Roper Public Opinion Research Center* (Roper Public Opinion Research Center, 1974).

- Martin, Elizabeth, Diana McDuffee, and Stanley Presser, *Sourcebook of Harris National Surveys: Repeated Questions 1963-1976* (Chapel Hill: Institute for Research in Social Science, University of North Carolina Press, 1981).

- Miller, Warren E., Arthur H. Miller, and Edward J. Schneider, *American National Election Studies Data Sourcebook 1951-1978* (Cambridge, MA: Harvard University Press, 1980).

- National Opinion Research Center, *General Social Surveys 1972-1985: Cumulative Code Book* (Chicago: NORC, 1985).

- Robinson, John P., Robert Athanasiou, and Kendra B. Head, *Measures of Occupational Attitudes and Occupational Characteristics* (Ann Arbor, MI: Institute for Social Research, 1969).

- Robinson, John P., Jerrold G. Rusk, and Kendra B. Head, *Measures of Political Attitudes* (Ann Arbor, MI: Institute for Social Research, 1968).

- Robinson, John P., and Phillip R. Shaver, *Measures of Social-Psychological Attitudes* (Ann Arbor, MI: Institute for Social Research, 1973, rev. ed.).

Need we pretest these tried and true questions? It's a good idea, for two reasons. First, because language constantly changes, and we may catch some of these changes only if interviewers listen carefully and relay respondent comments. For example, interviewers for the National Election Study reported new meanings given this question:

- Do you think the people in Washington are smart people who know what they are doing?

This item had been used in the 1960s as one of several indicators of confidence in government. At the time of the Watergate scandals in the 1970s, however, new meaning was given to the question, as certain respondents volunteered wryly, "Oh yeah, those guys know what they're doing, all right—they're plenty smart."

Were *many* people supplying a cynical new context for "smart people"? There is rarely a means of knowing from pretests. These vignettes from the field nevertheless serve as a reminder that survey questions can weather and age with time, and some should be retired from replication. Pretesting of borrowed items is important, for a second reason, because the meaning of questions can be affected by the context of neighboring questions in the interview, as we have noted in Chapter 2.

Pretesting: Strategies, Purposes, and Phases

Pretesting a survey questionnaire is always recommended—no text in survey methods would speak against such hallowed scientific advice—

but in practice it is probably often honored in the breach or the hurry. There is never the money nor, as deadlines loom, the time, to do enough of it. There is a corollary weakness that the practice is intuitive and informal. There are no general principles of good pretesting, no systematization of practice, no consensus about expectations, and we rarely leave records for each other. How a pretest was conducted, what investigators learned from it, how they redesigned their questionnaire on the basis of it—these matters are reported only sketchily in research reports, if at all. Not surprisingly, the power of pretests is sometimes exaggerated and their potential often unrealized.

STRATEGIES OF DESIGN

A given pretest scheme projects a set of expectations for respondents, and variations in these change the character of the pretest. The design can change by whether or not respondents know that it is a pretest and by the role that interviewers play.

Respondents' awareness: participating and undeclared pretests

We term it a "participating" pretest when respondents are *told* that this is a practice run, and are asked to explain their reactions and answers. This design opens some doors of information and closes others. It opens the possibility, for example, of asking very detailed probes about each question, phrase by phrase, even key word by word.

- "What did the whole question mean to you? How would you say it?"
- "What did ＿＿ make you think of?"
- "What was it you had in mind when you said ＿＿＿?"

Because there is no need to simulate an actual interview, one can also ask respondents to react to different wordings of the same basic question.

- "Consider the same question this way: ＿＿＿."
- "How would you answer that question now?"
- "You said ＿＿＿. Would you feel differently if I said ＿＿＿?"

With this "intensive" design, one can examine a few questions in great detail. Not a large number, or the questionnaire as a whole. The participating strategy may limit the range of possible respondents as well, because it is probably of greatest interest to people who are accustomed to surveys, reflective and confident about their own opinions and mental processes, sensitive to nuances of language, as well as willing to give up time and thought to help social scientists. Narrowed down to this subset, investigators may find themselves relying on that familiar source of forced labor—colleagues, friends, and family.

One interesting study of pretesting used respondents from the broader public (convenience samples of store customers and a random sample of households) in a variant on the participating pretest (Hunt et al., 1982). The findings raise important doubts about whether or not the general public should be asked to serve as actual judges of survey questions. In a short written questionnaire, ten questions were designed to represent five well-known faults, such as questions with incomplete alternatives, as in "Do you vote Republican or Democrat?"; and questions with inappropriate vocabulary, such as "Do you think that the current inflation is demand based or cost based?"

The researchers felt that they built in "blatant" errors and asked their subjects "to be critical," but most of their respondents found nothing much to complain about. The missing alternative error was by far the most visible: a third of the 146 respondents commented on the problem, which is probably about the proportion who needed the main missing alternative, "Independent." Inappropriate vocabulary was noticeable to a somewhat smaller group, but "loaded words," "double-barreled" questions, and ambiguous questions were virtually unnoticed by almost everyone. This rare and welcome research on the pretest suggests that respondents are not very critical or sophisticated about survey questions, even when invited to be, and their counsel may not be a very good guide to practice. (Many respondents probably answer survey questions out of basic civility and politeness). Their actual *answers*, nevertheless—their interpretations and misinterpretations of investigators' intent—are likely to be illuminating.

In what we call the "undeclared" pretest the respondent is not told that this is a questionnaire under construction, and the interviewer plays it straight. Here one can indeed probe *some* of the questions for respondents' frame of reference and meaning, but not with the intensity or exhaustiveness permitted in the participating strategy. In this more "extensive" design one can test more questions and do so in a mode closer to the final questionnaire. The best strategy is probably to begin with a participating pretest, then move to an undeclared one.

The interviewers' responsibilities

The role of interviewers in the pretest can also vary, especially in the degree to which the role is structured. Some investigators who do pretesting themselves prefer the freedom of improvising questions on the spot during a first pretest. Very skilled interviewers can be instructed to do the same thing, keeping a close record of the exact questions they asked, or tape-recording the whole encounter. The degree of structure can also vary within the same pretest, with a few key staff researchers free to depart from a structured schedule to explore leads on the spot, and most interviewers constrained to test the questionnaire as written. In another variant, all interviewers can ask some unstructured questions at the end of a standardized interview (Belson, 1981).

THE PURPOSES OF PRETESTS

The confident comment that a certain question "has been pretested" implies, first, that pretesting is a permanent state of grace—once pretested, always pretested. This in turn implies that a pretested question can be pulled out of one questionnaire and simply patched into another without losing its pretesting credentials. Neither assumption is safe. "Pretested for what?" is the appropriate query, for there are some very specific purposes. Consider these ten, the first four of which are tests for specific questions:

- variation
- meaning
- task difficulty
- respondent interest and attention

The last six bear more on the questionnaire as a whole:

- "flow" and naturalness of the sections
- the order of questions
- skip patterns

- timing
- respondent interest and attention, overall
- respondent well-being

We shall consider the two groups in turn.

Testing questions

Variation. Testing items for an acceptable level of variation in the target population is one of the most common goals of pretesting, and it is probably this purpose that people usually have in mind when they say that a question "has been pretested." Questions that show a 95/5 or 99/1 distribution of Yes/No may represent descriptive findings of capital importance if, for example, they mean that 95% of a population has learned to read and write, that 1% is at risk for a certain disease, or the like. Often, however, one is on the lookout for items showing greater variability that will be useful in detecting subgroups of people or clusters of attitudes of analytic interest. One rarely has enough pretest cases to be at all confident, but very skewed distributions from a pretest can at least serve as warning signals.

Meaning. For this purpose, the fact that an item has been used in a published study may not tell whether it was ever fully pretested for meaning; or whether the meaning intended by the investigator was shared by most respondents at the time; or if so, whether it *still* is. If the original source was a written questionnaire administered to college students, it should be considered with special suspicion, and duly pretested for its applicability to a general population. The literature offers some colorful examples of confusion—"profits" taken for "prophets" is a classic—and other pretest vignettes provide other merry examples: "heavy traffic in the neighborhood" meaning trucks to investigators and drugs to respondents; "family planning" meaning birth control to investigators and saving money for vacations to other people (Berckmans, 1985). One woman of whom we recently asked family social-class level—"poor, working class, middle class, etc."—told us that her family wasn't really very sociable. How many people brought quite a different meaning to "social class" than the one we intended? Very few, as we happily learned from pretest results, but it was worth checking.

Testing the meaning of questions is probably the most important pretesting purpose. It may nevertheless be the most neglected because it can require such extensive probing, as in Belson's ambitious tests of questions. He administered, first, a short questionnaire to four small quota samples of approximately 50 each on the subject of television, using questions of a sort that he found in frequent use by a set of market researchers. The day after the interview, a specially trained interviewer returned to conduct a second intensive interview on the meaning of the questions.

On the face of it, the results are appalling. In no case did all respondents bring to every part of the question the approximate meaning intended by the investigator. For the highest scoring question, 50% of the sample interpreted all parts of the question within acceptable meanings. In the lowest-scoring question, *nobody* did. The average, overall, was an unimpressive 29%. The fact that Belson selected problem questions, however—types that he expected to confuse respondents— makes his findings a little less grim.

Belson's findings, nonetheless, carry two very important messages. First, the meaning that investigators intend for many questions actually used in surveys is often not the meaning that respondents apprehend. Respondents do not necessarily even *hear* every word of the question, much less assume the definitions that the investigator has in mind, or fully understand the concepts. Although a question presents the word "impartial," for example, perhaps the "im" gets lost and the respondent hears a synonym for biased, or perhaps the word "impartial" itself is an unfamiliar one (Belson, 1981: 76-86).

Second, respondents nevertheless answer most questions because, as Belson (1981: 371) writes,

> When a respondent finds it difficult to answer a question, he is likely to modify it in such a way as to be able to answer it more easily.

This is the first of 15 hypotheses that Belson distills from his results. For our reading, it is the most important and the most general of them all, and in fact many of the others could be subsumed under it. Respondents probably modify questions, for the most part, not because they are lazy or want to hide their ignorance, or even because surveys project a demand to be opinionated, as Riesman and Glazer (1948) cogently observed over 35 years ago. People seem to answer questions, most importantly, because they expect survey questions—or at least survey interviewers—to be sensible; people *think* they heard the question properly; or the part of the question that is meaningful takes on more salience or vividness and they answer that part; or they take the parts that are meaningful and reassemble a different question from them and answer that. In sum, respondents probably *transform* obscure questions into ones that seem sensible from their standpoint as they strain for meaning.

Task difficulty. A question can be hard to answer even though the meaning is entirely clear if the respondent has not previously packaged the information in the way the question demands. "How many pounds of coffee have you consumed this past year?" may be an answerable question for some very methodical shoppers, but most of us do not total up our consumption of coffee by the year, or even by the pound, and our estimate in these terms would probably be quite unreliable. The literature about "non-attitudes" should help us avoid asking respondents things they know little about (Converse, 1970; Smith, 1984a)—but it continues to be easy, nevertheless, to ask people questions we want to know rather than ones they are able to answer.

Take a recent DAS question:

- How important has it been to you to have more money than your parents had—very important, somewhat important, or not very important?

From a few follow-up probes, we learned that the question triggered people's ruminations about the importance of money itself ("money doesn't buy happiness," and so on) often without reference to their parents' fortunes, as if the question had read:

- How important has it been to you to have more money? . . . Very important, somewhat important, or not very important?

It seems to have been an evocative question for people who had been very poor as children; for others who had no such vivid memories, however, the whole idea may have been quite new. A few of our respondents volunteered just that. "Why I never thought of it before—I guess I'd have to say Not Very Important."

There are two morals to the money story. One turns on retrospective measurement itself, which is rarely recommended, because it is known that recall even of dramatic events can be fragile: People may forget the event itself or they may misremember the time at which the event occurred. And yet retrospective measures are sometimes essential. We asked a number of retrospective questions in this particular study, without illusion that we were getting exact measures of the past; for reasons connected to the analysis we were willing to take the risk of rough approximations.

There are, indeed, such times when any "rules" of question writing will be bent, because at the time it seems rather a matter of Hobson's choice. In this case, however—and this is the second moral—we did not pretest this question well enough. It was only on the final questionnaire that we picked up a smattering of evidence that many people had not organized the past or compared it with the present in quite the way we were assuming. Had we gotten the cues earlier, we might well have added an open-ended probe to the question on the final questionnaire to distinguish systematically the people for whom the question was a meaningful one. Or dropped the question.

Respondent interest and attention. This is an aspect of pretesting that ordinarily seems to get rather short shrift. Investigators are rather prone to forgetting that not everyone brings the same fervent interest to their topic that they do. Interviewers usually know whether respondents seem interested or stimulated by the questionnaire, and should be asked to report systematically on this dimension, at least to note questions that respondents found especially interesting and especially dull.

There is little research to support such caution. In fact, the proposition that survey data deteriorate when respondents' attention and interest flag markedly is one we take largely on faith and the evidence of fatigue effects in learning experiments. There is some recent suggestive evidence that such things hold in surveys, too. In a self-administered questionnaire, Herzog and Bachman (1981) asked some fairly large sets of questions in the same format; as many as 23 items were grouped together with a four-point choice ranging from Strongly Agree to Strongly Disagree. This format would probably have been more monotonous and deadly in a personal interview than in this paper-and-pencil questionnaire, but there was evidence of a "fatigue" effect toward the end of the question sets, as respondents tended to check the same alternative, no matter what the question.

Still, research into fatigue or boredom effects in surveys is rare—and it is a more complicated matter than the sheer length of time required by the questionnaire. Sharp and Frankel's (1983) recent study shows that length of the interview is experienced by respondents as a negative factor but is not in fact predictive of their willingness to participate in subsequent interviews. In the design of questions, investigators usually try to avoid the wearing repetition. They make of their surveys something of a pastiche, one kind of questioning and then another; a bit of so-and-so's format, and something in another style. This is an aspect of survey design that is guided by mysterious matters: the "art" of writing and especially arranging survey questions to keep respondents' attention and interest. Varying the format is important. In personal interviews, one can do this not only by using different kinds of oral questions but also by using some "show cards" or a small booklet that lists answer alternatives and some self-administered questions, but on the telephone one's choices are more restricted. Here, especially, one must pretest carefully for a desirable balance between the benefits of question variety and the "start-up" costs of explaining a new question format.

The first four objectives that we have discussed bear especially on the testing of *questions*. Another set of purposes that we turn to now bears more on the *questionnaire as a whole*. We should not put too fine a point on this distinction, for in every phase of pretesting, one is tinkering with the wording and form of specific questions and also trying to cast the overall shape of the questionnaire. Still, there is a difference in emphasis. One cannot really test the questionnaire as a whole until the basic sections are chosen and arranged in a given order, with the wording of many questions cast in more or less final form. So the pretesting objectives for the questionnaire tend to come second.

Pretesting the questionnaire

"Flow" and naturalness. Testing the "flow" of the questionnaire is such a matter of intuitive judgment that it is hard to describe or codify. One can at least be guided by one crucial caveat: Reading is not enough. One must listen to the questionnaire, over and over, hearing it as interviewers actually deliver it, trying to hear it as respondents do, always mindful that they will *not* have the print in front of them to review and clarify the meaning. What respondents hear is what they get, and every question probably comes anew to respondents, with a certain "surprise" quality.

The interest and clarity of the questions and a "sensible" arrangement probably contribute more to a coherent flow than any very elaborate transitions from section to section. Transitions can be simple and brief, such as "Now I am going to ask you some questions about your job . . . " or even the vague preparation, "Now I have some questions on a different topic . . . " These are not very elegant transitions, but in our experience they do not have to have nor should there be many of them. One wants a few (redundant) words that slow things down enough for the interviewer and the respondent to turn a corner to another subject— now and then, when without a transitional phrase changes seem too sharp.

The order of questions. The positive guides to the order of questions are few, and bear only the credentials of common sense. The proposition that one should open the questionnaire with "interesting" questions, for instance, seems like a good idea—assuming of course that one has tested questions for their interestingness.

Frey (1983: 103-105) offers more specific counsel that in telephone interviewing, especially, the initial questions should be items directly related to the topic of the interview expressed in the introductory statement, as in this example:

> Hello. This is _____ calling from the Telephone Survey Center of the University of Nevada, Las Vegas. We are conducting a survey of Nevada residents on their opinions and perceptions of the quality of life in the state. . . .
>
> First, I would like to ask how you feel about Nevada as a place to live. Do you consider it Very Desirable, Somewhat Desirable, Somewhat Undesirable, or Very Undesirable?

Frey suggests following this with an open-ended "Why" question of this sort: "What specifically do you find (desirable/undesirable) about living in Nevada?" to allow the respondent "to find his or her 'telephone voice.'" His basic point about the opening question is that if the introduction has successfully aroused the respondent's interest, it can be just as quickly deflated by a question unrelated to the announced topic, such as "Did you vote in the last national election?" or "What is your race?" Because we know that respondents' answers to open-ended questions tend to be more terse on the telephone than they are face-to-face (Groves and Kahn, 1979), finding a "telephone voice" may be of some special value. We would nevertheless urge caution in using open-ended questions with any frequency at the beginning *if* the questionnaire is basically closed, for one is "training" the respondent in the questionnaire from the very outset. In addition, open questions can sometimes be quite demanding, and tasks at the beginning of the interview should be easy ones that do not tax or discourage the respondent.

It is common practice to put "background" questions at the end of the interview. This ritual reflects, most of all, the sensitivity of income questions, which are the most vulnerable to refusal. If respondents are offended by being asked their income, at least their negative reaction appears late in the questionnaire. Most background questions are not really sensitive, however, and they are usually fairly easy for the respondent to answer and can be something of a welcome set of questions if earlier questions have been fairly demanding.

It may not be necessary, however, to move all background questions to the end of the questionnaire just because the income questions may belong there. Putting some background questions up front can be of use if the survey topic bears closely on the individual's own life history and experience, and the approach of the questionnaire is largely chronological. Moreover, if the interview is broken off before completion, some basic background information has been obtained. NORC's General Social Survey divides background questions between the beginning and the end of the interview for these reasons.

Skip patterns. Questionnaires must be pretested not only for the usual typographical errors, but for the logic and format of skip patterns, which can be very complex. If the skip patterns are incorrect or ambiguous, interviewers may vault over various questions or even whole sections and leave unanticipated holes in the data. Defective skip patterns should be caught before pretesting so that pretest interviewers can concentrate on the questions and the respondents' reactions rather than having to struggle against bad skips to get the questionnaire read at all.

The best way of proofreading the skip patterns is to turn the task over to several individuals, each of whom follows the route for a certain "scenario," such as these:

(A) The respondent was born in Mexico in 1947 and came to the U.S. in 1966. This is her first marriage; her husband had two children by a previous marriage, who are now living with R and her husband. She first voted in the 1976 national election . . .

(B) The respondent, age 56, has worked at an automobile assembly plant for 11 years as manager of the shipping department. He is married, without children. He and his wife have recently bought into an investment partnership that is buying real estate in Florida, and they hope to retire there when he is 62 . . .

Dividing up the labor in this way is useful for finding logical errors in the skip patterns. People who are sophisticated about surveys in general but uninformed about this one are especially valuable for this assignment, for they will duly follow the road signs of the questionnaire. Staff members who have been involved in designing the study may tend to go where they are "supposed" to go whether the skip directs them there or not.

It is important to think of the questionnaire as a road map, and consider its graphics accordingly. If the skip pattern is at all ambiguous visually, an interviewer may take the wrong route; and then confident that this is the correct way, never carefully read that instruction again. The clearest instructions are strong arrows, lines, outlines, very boxy boxes, with no fine print and no extraneous instructions at all.

Timing. It is ordinarily useful to ask interviewers to time each part of the questionnaire, section by section. That face-to-face survey interviews should average no more than a scant hour is a norm of practice with little grounding in experiment, though it has a long tradition in the 50-minute hour of clinical therapy and college classroom instruction. Beyond that time, one begins to worry about respondent fatigue, interview break-off, and initial refusal if respondents know the expected length. For telephone interviewing, the norms are for shorter times.

Respondent interest and attention, overall. Interviewers should be encouraged to notice and report on respondents' interest in the study. The problem may indeed be that the whole questionnaire is simply too long, and, if so, there is probably no better remedy than going back to the cutting board. Two other prescriptions should be considered, as well: new content and task variety.

Investigators will be loath to give any room to "throwaway" questions (without prospective analytic value) just because respondents might like to talk about them. With field costs so high, this is luxury beyond the typical research purse. Yet it is also foolish to expect respondents to have high motivation and sustained attention for a questionnaire that does not take much account of their interests. We do well to consider the questionnaire now and then from the respondents' perspective: Where is it lively and responsive? Where is it slow going? Can we go a little further to meet them halfway? Can we add anything that serves our own analytic direction and also brightens the way for respondents? At the least, we may have to place some questions strategically to perk up lagging interest.

The liveliest questionnaires in our ken move respondents from one activity to another, as they proceed through the questionnaire. Respondents are asked a set of Yes/No questions, perhaps; then a group of questions involving one choice from a list of, say, five options; then they are asked several questions in which they rate their own feelings on a scale; then they choose between one idea or the other. And so on. The variety of the answering task has been designed to engage the respondent's active attention. This characteristic can be pretested, by asking interviewers to make systematic observations of respondents' interest, and by asking respondents to report their reactions for themselves. Task variety cannot captivate respondents if the subject matter itself is irretrievably difficult or dull, for content itself appears to be far more telling. Questionnaires bearing on people's own experiences, life histories, and health are predictably more interesting to most people than an exclusive focus on attitudes or information. But when investigators want to explore topics that are not likely to be of widespread appeal, task variety may well be of special importance.

Respondent well-being. In our time surveys have burgeoned far beyond the original realms of political polling. Survey interviewers are now admitted into realms of privacy and sensitivity, to ask questions about alcoholism, drugs, crime, heterosexual and homosexual experience, marital satisfaction, divorce, abuse, the death of children, loneliness, mental illness, depression, suicide, physical handicaps, widowhood, terminal illness, religious experience, anxiety, and faith. The litany is long. Survey researchers have proved a voracious lot, with a huge appetite for information about people's lives and experiences.

Are people sufficiently protected from possible injury in this research process? Requirements that surveys offer "informed consent" to their respondents and undergo "human subjects review" by their institution represent an effort to protect respondents from any untoward effects. There are real problems and dilemmas in these efforts, however. In surveys contracted by and for the federal government, for example, questionnaires themselves are reviewed, and this means that they must be put in final form months before the field work is started, which is a major block to the research process. In the university, on the other hand, a "human subjects review" of the overall research proposal is usually undertaken months before a questionnaire is even designed; it is our impression that there is unlikely to be any review of the final questionnaire at all.

In the academic setting, who can say that a questionnaire is distressing respondents, leaving them feeling worse about themselves or their lives than the interviewer found them? If that happened, would the investigators know? Who would tell them? Is it anyone's responsibility to find out?

In our own experience, interviewers have sometimes taken that role. In a recent project, long-term and very skilled professional interviewers insisted that the questionnaire needed major redesigning. The topic was psychological depression, and interviewers reported that the pretest was *depressing* people with its exclusive focus on life's bad news and symptoms of mental illness. The design had included only those life events hypothesized to predict depression—the tragic and troubled and stressor events. The interviewers' intelligent reports and impressive experience finally prevailed: The questionnaire was duly redesigned to allow some upbeat features, such as the inclusion of some good life events and questions about how respondents had coped with their problems. The happy ending is that after the document went through *five* pretests, both respondents and interviewers registered great satisfaction with the study: a real favorite.

We have no hard data to support these moves. We were personally convinced that the problem was a real one by the particular interviewers' experience, arguments, concern—and talent. The experience pointed up the fact that some professional interviewers bring a personal involvement and a professional commitment to the well-being of respondents. When this is combined with personal self-confidence, broad professional experience, and good judgment, their advocacy on behalf of the respondent can be of enormous value to the quality of a survey. Some student interviewers, even though less experienced, bring equivalent talents and sensitivities. But temporary interviewers, who are on deck for a single study, even if they have advanced training in other fields, will usually lack that special advocacy of the respondent.

PHASES OF PRETESTING

Pretests represent a "qualitative" stage in the quantitative survey enterprise, with N's nothing like what they should be for quantitative evidence. For small pretests, numbering 25-75 cases, is it really worth coding the data and hand-tallying or grinding out marginal distributions? Yes—at the upper ranges, anyway. On rare occasions, marginal distributions can provide a measure of support for certain "hunches," and diminish one's confidence in others. And they can provide some corrections. The experience of interviewing even a single real and unforgettable character, for instance, can be so vivid and compelling that staff members may come back from the field with very broad, entirely unwarranted conclusions about the questionnaire based on the infamous N of 1. A larger set of pretest interviews per person is desirable—5, for instance, would be much better. If this cannot be undertaken, quantitative data may help pretesters realize that their own experience was not entirely representative or general. And sometimes the live testimony of other interviewers who have just as vivid, entirely contrary views can help, too. In any case, both the colorful vignettes and some numbers can be useful. If interviewers' reports are often more instructive than the marginal frequencies (and in our experience, that has usually been the case), it is another indication of pretesting's qualitative hallmarks: small Ns, samples of convenience, hypothesis testing by hunch and judgment. Pretests would seem to be absolutely necessary even if almost never sufficient.

Just as most pretesting Ns are regrettably small, the number of pretest trials is often sharply limited—often to one. For a new study, to which investigators bring no previous hands-on experience, a minimum of *two* pretests is indispensable, in our view. For as we have already stressed, in a first trial the wording of the questions themselves is still uncertain enough—they are the focus of the testing—that the questionnaire does not yet have a very coherent shape. In the discussion that follows, we assume this minimum of two pretests. We will consider them in the framework of these three topics, developmental pretest I, evaluation, and polishing pretest II, and set forth some useful properties of each phase.

Developmental Pretest I

Most questions should be closed. Closed questions should generally be given the lion's share of the first pretest simply because they must generally be given the lion's share of the final interview schedule—and this is a pretest of it. To make that statement is to face one of the sternest limitations of survey research. Closed survey questions inevitably simplify and stylize the life and thought of individuals, even for the most routine of measures.

Try marital status, for instance, or number of times married. Reliably, the boxes (precoded responses) will not capture everyone's condition in a way that guides the selection of questions (skip patterns) in the rest of the questionnaire. For example, in most cases, this will be a straightforward sequence:

(A2) First, I would like to know your current marital status—are you now married, separated, divorced, or widowed, or have you not married?

(IF RESPONDENT IS DIVORCED, TURN TO PAGE 18)

But what of the man who is divorced from his first wife but lives with her and considers her his wife? He is certainly not Separated or Widowed, but is he Married, Divorced, or both? Legally, of course, he is divorced, but that does not solve our problem. Shall we ask him the questions to be asked of divorced people, or the questions to be asked of married people, or all of both?

Anyone who has conducted or coded a fair number of survey interviews knows that human experience is much too unruly in its diversity to be fully contained by the precoded responses of closed questions. When this richness thrusts out of the boxes, like so much jungle growth, we hastily set up another box, the residual "Other," and by relegating these wondrously oddball situations into this miscellaneous junk box, we lose entirely the vividness and "life" of individual character and unusual circumstance. There is little for it. Open-ended questions are far better for capturing those details and idiosyncrasies; entirely unstructured interviews conducted by master interviewers are better still; biographies and novels, of course, are probably best of all.

One repairs to closed questions for several good reasons. The first reason, and best, is that some boxes can be built to accommodate almost all cases. Our codes for marital status clearly did not cover everyone, but they covered *almost* everyone, which is not only good enough but absolutely splendid.

Another good reason is cost. To oversimplify the choices, one can pay interviewers to spend two hours with 250 respondents or less than one hour each with 500 persons. With the two-hour version, interviewers can ask and transcribe much more "in depth" detail, but an N of 250 will be too small to support any very compelling analysis. (The sampling error will be large for an N of 500, at that.) To undertake any statistical analysis at all, one will inevitably pare away much of the detail gathered in those two hours back to the bone of gross code categories. This risks a kind of triple squander of survey materials: one will pay to gather the detail (sacrificing a larger N in the process), then shear much of it away, paying for the time that takes too.

An even better reason for closed questions bears on validity. One may seek open-ended material in the very quest for greater validity, but the choice can sometimes work the other way around when the frame of reference for open questions is ambiguous. It is difficult to keep open questions free of the "tacit assumption" that Paul Lazarsfeld noted 50 years ago, with an example that remains one of our favorites. When school children in Austria were asked in an open-ended questionnaire item what they would most like to have in life, they wrote down economic and psychological goals such as big farms, good jobs, money, happiness. Nobody mentioned intelligence. When this alternative was included in a closed version of the question, it was a great favorite. The children had apparently assumed that the open question included only the goods that might be had for the striving, not the gifts of personal endowment (Jenkins, 1935: 355). There are other strengths and weaknesses about both open and closed questions that we have considered in Chapter Two. Suffice it here to say that one is well-advised to include many closed questions in Pretest I and probe their meaning in open ended follow-ups. Because open questions will usually constitute at most a small part of the interview schedule, they must be selected and trimmed with great care.

Rough codes for open questions should be designed in advance. In the press of field deadlines, it is usually difficult to find time to anticipate codes for open questions; but even if this preliminary code construction is done in a rather informal and approximate fashion, it enhances the realism of the first pretest and the particular value of any open questions used. It has the great value of helping investigators face up to what their objectives are in asking the question at all. And explaining the question objectives is essential for the interviewer, for without this information, the interviewer cannot know when a question has been answered.

The first pretest interview should be less than twice the final expected length. This is merely to say that the first pretest can be rather outsize, as long as one can also conduct a second pretest. A first pretest running as long as two hours can be useful, but this should be considered an absolute maximum. Beyond this length, the labor of cutting back to an hour or less will be formidable, and even if one can find respondents willing to spend two hours, the test of some questions may be doubtful if the length of the interview has tired them and dulled their attention and interest. Such a long trial may be testing personal endurance more than anything more cogent. If there is only one pretest in view, it should be much shorter: one should strive to make it an hour and a quarter as a maximum. Remember, too, that interviewers conducting a pretest may have to do most of their work in the evenings, and a long pretest may restrict them to one interview per evening; and in that case, the time scheduled for pretesting will have to be stretched.

Respondents should resemble the target population. A probability sample of the survey's target population would make an ideal pretest. But this is ordinarily much too expensive. One must nevertheless take a pretest out beyond the small worlds of colleagues, friends, or family, who offer much too thin a slice of life. Interviewers should not be left to their own devices. In a recent pretest conducted by DAS students, we found that almost half of our respondents were graduate students, hardly a cross section of the population.

There are two likely routes out of the small world. One way is to take advantage of group character or neighborhood stratification of importance to the study: One can go door-to-door in neighborhoods that are visibly ethnic, or elderly, or young and noisy with children, and so forth. A second is to interview strangers, by knocking on doors close to home or work. This seems an absolute minimum for pretesting. Going this route will ordinarily not yield as heterogeneous a collection of respondents as the first way, but it will certainly be more useful than interviewing one's own friends and relatives. (It seems fair to insist that interviewing in that inner circle should simply *not count* as a pretest.) If one is pretesting by telephone, one, of course, has no visual cues to heterogeneity, but one can achieve something of the same effect by selecting central office codes (the first three digits following the area code) that are known to span a range of neighborhoods, though one will unfortunately not be able to identify the neighborhoods themselves. One can also make a random selection of telephone numbers within those codes, staying within a close radius to save money and relaxing selection rules to save time.

A pretest N of 25-75 is reasonable. The Magic N for a pretest is of course as many as you can get. We see 25-75 as a valuable pretest range, which can vary first with the experience and talent of the interviewers. With student interviewers, one may have to settle for a yield of 2-3 interviews each. This is not an optimal number per individual but at least the task is manageable and each interviewer's share of the variance is appropriately small, both features of special value when the interviewers are inexperienced.

With experienced professional interviewers, the N usually has to be smaller because of costs, and in the best circumstances we think it safely can be. NORC's interviewing staff, for example, is ordinarily not augmented by student trainees, and the recommendation by Sheatsley (1983) that the N can range around 10-25 probably reflects that fact. SRC's practice is similar: Pretest Ns in recent years have averaged about 30, with a half dozen interviewers each conducting about 5 interviews. Even modest pretests of this order of magnitude have value for undergirding intuitive judgments with at least a jot of data and with the informed impressions of experienced pretest interviewers.

From the sizes we have been considering—an N of 25 with professional interviewers; an N of 50 or more with students—one might infer that professionals can be twice as effective as students for pretest work. That is not implausible, if the professional interviewers are selected for their pretesting skill and are an experienced, motivated elite of their group. A student group may well be the more highly educated, to be sure, but it is also likely to vary more in the interest, motivation, and talent for survey interviewing per se. Some students turn up in a survey practicum, after all, because they have to fulfill an academic requirement, not because they have any special interest, gift, or stamina for field work. Experienced professional interviewers who survive the winnowings are, to some extent at least, self-selected for just those qualities.

Two issues about who should conduct pretests: The first issue is whether or not pretest interviewers should represent the best of the professional staff, or the full range of talent that will ultimately work on the study. The DeMaio research group (1983), among others, favors using the full range. They feel that the most able interviewers can make even a poor schedule "work," and may not reveal the problems that a flawed schedule will present for some of the less able interviewers on the staff.

There are no data that we know to support one view or another, but our own experience argues for choosing the most talented pretesting interviewers. They tend to be strong advocates for their respondents' right to clear, sensible, interesting questions, and they spot questionnaire defects with a good deal of zest, yea, even dedicated nit-picking. The best professional interviewers are not loath to teach investigators, and in many instances their spirited counsel has been very valuable indeed. It should be noted that even among the most competent, experienced interviewers, pretesting is not everyone's cup of tea. Those with a special interest and flair for pretesting can not only catch poor designs, but also make extraordinarily good suggestions for revision (Flanagan, 1985). But this luxurious choice will be beyond the reach of many survey investigators, who will not have easy access or sufficient funds to hire professional interviewers for pretesting. In that case, everyone will be pressed into pretesting duty, whether especially talented for interviewing or not.

The second issue turns on whether or not investigators should be among them. Some writers feel that the research staff should not participate in pretesting unless they are skilled in standard interviewing techniques. Others feel that the field experience can be of value even without that training. We side with the latter. If investigators are poor interviewers, they do not need to conduct the questionnaire themselves; they can see how their questionnaire works in the field by going along with a better interviewer. Or at the very least, they can listen in on telephone interviews. Direct pretesting experience can make investigators more sensitive and sympathetic to the rigors of the interviewers' task, as well as knowledgeable (and humble) about the frailty of their questions. It is our impression that not enough researchers get their own feet wet and weary in the field.

Evaluating pretests

We have sketched out some design features for Pretest I, but these alone do not suggest how to make the best use of the pretest experience. The following six procedures all can offer something of value:

- marginal comments on the schedule
- oral debriefing
- written reports (section by section of questionnaire)
- written questionnaires (specific facets or problems)
- field observation of the questionnaire in action
- coding of answers and tallying of marginal frequencies

It is only the last two that do not depend directly on the observations of interviewers. The DeMaio group (1983: 119) has noted that:

> Interviewers are a key and often underrated element in the practice of survey research. They constitute the link between respondents and researchers, and in their direct contact with respondents, they can pick up valuable information which may be of interest to questionnaire designers.

As they say, "the systematic exploration of an interviewer's knowledge has been seriously neglected in the literature." In our own experience, that knowledge has been indispensable. Except where pretests are large in size and experimental in design, thereby making possible some statistical analysis, interviewers have a virtual monopoly on the prime information.

Copious comments written in the margins of the schedule should be encouraged. At this stage, the more the better. Interviewers can be asked to give a running account of their own impressions of the interview and of all respondent comments. Interviewers vary a good deal in their ability to do this—at the very least, it takes fast writing and the ability to seize instantly upon dialogue—so one cannot expect a rich running record from everyone. But from those who can do this kind of detailed transcription, investigators can mine evidence of problems and misinterpretations, and interviewers can go back to these marginal notes for the preparation of more systematic reports.

Oral debriefing, a group discussion with interviewers very soon after the pretest, has the advantage of immediacy: Interviewers can report while their memory of the experience is quick and their interest, usually, high. (The hazards of debriefing are those of any undisciplined discussion—if the best raconteurs or the more dominant personalities swamp the meeting and inhibit some of the less voluble interviewers from reporting their experiences at all; and the meeting should be structured accordingly.) It is not inexpensive to bring a set of professional interviewers together for what may well be a half-day's discussion, but we have found it money well spent.

Written comments may be fruitful, alone or in conjunction with a debriefing. When we have required written comments from student interviewers, we have sometimes collated the comments by topic, duplicated them, and given the entire set back to the students. The purpose has been to economize on academic class time; the schedule of the practicum was crowded enough, on occasion, that we had little time for debriefing; and given that constraint, it seemed important to provide feedback about *everyone's* experiences, so that individual students would not overgeneralize from their own. In any case, written reports have made for easy and systematic reference in revising the questionnaire.

We have also sometimes used both written reports and oral debriefing together. This has actually proved rather repetitive, for interviewers have tended to offer in discussion the same points that they make in writing. This may be a minor disadvantage, however, if the two reporting forms, in conjunction, enhance interviewers' interest and morale, while also providing useful pretest evaluation. And the combination has seemed to work that way.

A *questionnaire* can be a useful way to communicate with a far-flung interviewing staff. For example, questions such as these can serve as a useful focus for interviewer comments:

Questionnaire for Interviewers

Please make out a separate questionnaire for each pretest interview you conduct. For all "yes" answers, please specify the *question numbers* or section and *explain* what the situation or problem seemed to be.

(1) Did any of the questions seem to make R uncomfortable?

(2) Did you have to repeat any questions?

(3) Did R misinterpret any questions?

(4) Which questions were the most difficult or awkward for you to read? Have you come to dislike any specific questions? Why?

(5) Did any of the sections seem to drag?

(6) Were there any sections in which you felt that the respondent would have liked the opportunity to say more?

And so on. The specific questions of interest will depend, of course, on the survey and its particular problems.

Field observation of pretest interviewers, which comes highly recommended by the DeMaio group, allows an interviewer to give his or her entire attention to the conduct of the interview itself, while another person is free to listen to and observe how the questionnaire is working. Observation is sometimes practiced by field supervisors but it can be valuable for survey investigators (DeMaio, 1983: 101). Another variant is organizing pairs of interviewers (professionals or students) who work together during a pretest, taking turns as interviewer and observer. They can submit a joint report, concentrating their comments exclusively on properties of the questionnaire, without relaying any evaluation of each other as interviewers. Inexperienced interviewers may be more comfortable working this way in the beginning. They may learn more about the questionnaire and contribute more to its revision if they feel more confident interviewing in the presence of a peer observer than they would with a field supervisor or survey investigator. Berckmans (1985) reports some beneficial training experiences from the pairing of experienced and inexperienced interviewers.

Coding of responses, and preparation of marginal frequencies can provide a quick summary of variation. With a small pretest N, hand tallying of the closed question responses may be perfectly serviceable, and the open-ended answers can be quick coded for just a few gross categories, or even just an indication (yes/no) that the respondent interpreted the question as intended. With more substantial Ns, it may be more practical to edit the interviews quickly for direct data entry into a microcomputer.

Coding also can be used in a more ambitious way, as a part of interviewer training, to sensitize interviewers to the problems of coding and analysis that are created by poor interviewing. We usually have students code two or three pretest interviews just as a part of the practicum, to familiarize them with coding itself, and to get the work done. With the hope that the coding experience will sharpen sensitivity and skill in interviewing, we assign to student interviewers the coding of each other's pretest questionnaires. At least some then experience the plagues that poor interviewing visits upon coders, such as illegible handwriting, careless editing, poor probing; and we hope they take away the appropriate moral. For gathering data on occupation, familiarity with coding has come to seem essential. We suspect that many interviewers continue to ask occupation questions quite poorly until they have some experience or exercises in occupational coding. Experience reported by Hauser and Featherman (1977) supports that view.

Pretest II: the polishing pretest

The second pretest should be a "dress rehearsal" of the questionnaire as a whole. Pretest II is not a time to repair gross errors, or to make new exploration. It is rather a time for cutting, trimming, splicing, rearranging, and filling in new skip patterns, formatting for clarity—polishing.

As a dress rehearsal, the polishing pretest must necessarily be an undeclared one, which will be handled as a real interview. One *aspires* to produce a Pretest II schedule that is ready for the printer or final form on the computer (for Computer Assisted Telephone Interviewing). It has never worked quite that way in our experience—one always learns new information from a polishing pretest and revises accordingly—but one learns more from Pretest II by trying to make it as close as possible to the final questionnaire.

Because Pretest II is now a slimmer model, one can now ask outsiders to criticize a draft of it before it goes into the field, just as one asks colleagues to criticize academic papers in draft. The first pretest questionnaire is usually too fat to circulate (and may risk embarrassment, at that). It may be an imposition to ask colleagues to read it, and they probably cannot be much help at this point anyway, for the sheer bulk of the schedule may blur its main intellectual lines and certainly its formatting structure. (One can hardly expect to format completely a questionnaire that still has to be cut by some 50%.) But one can ask knowledgeable colleagues to read and criticize a draft of a polishing pretest, especially if one presents it along with the set of research objectives that are being operationalized. (Would that colleagues needed nothing more than the questions we present to deduce perfectly our research purposes.)

We have found our best critics to be colleagues interested in the subject matter who have, themselves, done some survey work in the area, and field or coding directors who have experience with a variety of survey questionnaires. The latter especially have shown a fine eye for the design properties of a questionnaire that affect production interviewing and production coding. The problem is time: finding a hole in the survey schedule that is big enough to get a draft out to colleagues and back with comments. When we have not found that time before Pretest II, we have asked colleagues to criticize a draft of the final questionnaire. Earlier is of course better when changes are less disruptive.

Collegial criticism is a new feature of preparing Pretest II. In other respects, the characteristics that were desirable for Pretest I are now almost mandatory: for example, most questions should be closed; code categories for the few open questions should be at least loosely sketched out in advance; respondents should be strangers who resemble the target population; the N should be around 25-75, and more if financially and humanly possible; study staff (including students, if any) should participate in conducting the pretest, along with the best and the brightest of a professional field staff.

To evaluate the second pretest and prepare the final interview schedule, we recommend only one additional procedure. It is to keep the barrier high to any new questions. This is hard discipline. Inevitably, after two pretests, study staff will have some new brainstorms. To fend off these last-minute inspirations, we have tried to stick by a rule that any new question must be given an independent test with some minimum number of respondents. This is not, finally, a thorough test of the question, because the trial is shorn of context. But at least the rule helps to discourage the less-serious people who are unwilling to find the requisite number of respondents. One may lose some splendid ideas by keeping this barrier in place but—given the problem of incorporating untried questions into an otherwise finished questionnaire—the risk seems acceptable.

The complex matter of how the final questionnaire is put into action in the field is beyond the scope of this book. We need only remind ourselves that a questionnaire is not writ in stone. It is *merely* a design, a plan for action and interaction; its execution depends on other directors and actors—able and motivated interviewers and field supervisors, effective procedures of quality control. This means that if investigators do not keep in touch with what is happening in the field, they can lose control of their questionnaire. But at that stage of a survey, responsibilities are always shared and sometimes diffuse, and how they are exercised will vary greatly by particular organizations. As Davis (1964: 231) has pointed out, if survey analysis is an art, it is more like architecture than sculpture or painting. The image seems apt for survey questionnaire design as well. Much painting and sculpture can finally be achieved by a single artist. Architects can make their drawings in solitary confinement, but their buildings take shape only as scores— sometimes hundreds—of other artists, craftsmen, technicians, take up the task. Survey questionnaire architects are no less dependent on all the others to carry their design into concrete form.

REFERENCES

ALEXANDER, C. S. and H. J. BECKER (1978) "The use of vignettes in survey research." Public Opinion Quarterly 42: 93-104.

ALWIN, D. F. and J. KROSNICK (1985) "The measurement of values in surveys: a comparison of ratings and rankings." Public Opinion Quarterly 49: 535-552.

BABBIE, E. R. (1973) Survey Research Methods. Belmont, CA: Wadsworth.

BELSON, W. R. (1981) The Design and Understanding of Survey Questions. Aldershot, England: Gower.

BELSON, W. R. and J. DUNCAN (1962) "A comparison of the checklist and the open response questioning systems." Applied Statistics: II: 120-132.

BERCKMANS, T. R. (1985) Personal communication.

BISHOP, G. F., R. W. OLDENDICK, and A. J. TUCHFARBER (1980a) "Experiments in filtering political opinions." Political Behavior 2: 339-369.

BISHOP, G. F., R. W. OLDENDICK, A. J. TUCHFARBER, and S. E. BENNETT (1980b) "Pseudo-opinions on public affairs." Public Opinion Quarterly 44: 198-209.

BRADBURN, N. (1983) "Response effects," in P. H. Rossi, J. D. Wright, and A. B. Anderson (eds.), Handbook of Survey Research. New York: Academic Press.

BRADBURN, N., S. SUDMAN, and Associates (1979) Improving Interview Method and Questionnaire Design. San Francisco: Jossey-Bass.

BRANNON, R. et al. (1973) "Attitude and action: a field experiment joined to a general population survey." American Sociological Review 38: 625-636.

CANNELL, C. F., L. OKSENBERG, and J. M. CONVERSE (1979) Experiments in Interviewing Techniques. Ann Arbor, MI: Institute for Social Research.

CARROLL, J. B., P. DAVIES, and B. RICHMAN (1973) The American Heritage Frequency Book. New York: American Heritage.

CONVERSE, P. E. (1970) "Attitudes and non-attitudes: continuation of a dialogue," in E. R. Tufte (ed.) The Quantitative Analysis of Social Problems. Reading, MA: Addison-Wesley.

———(1972) "Change in the American electorate," in A. Campbell and P. E. Converse (eds.) The Human Meaning of Social Change. New York: Russell Sage.

COWAN, C., L. MURPHY, and J. WIENER (1978) "Effects of supplemental questions on victimization estimates from the National Crime Survey." Proceedings of the Section on Survey Research Methods. Washington, DC: American Statistical Association.

DAHL, H. (1979) Word Frequencies of Spoken American English. Essex, CT: Verbatim.

DAVIS, J. A. (1964) "Great books and small groups: an informal history of a national survey," in P. E. Hammond (ed.) Sociologists at Work: Essays on the Craft of Social Research. New York: Basic Books.

DeMAIO, T. J. [ed.] (1983) Approaches to Developing Questionnaires, Statistical Policy Working Paper 10. Washington, DC: Office of Management and Budget.

Detroit Area Study (DAS) (1985) Questionnaire.

FINK, A. and J. KOSECOFF (1985) How to Conduct Surveys: A Step-by-Step Guide. Beverly Hills, CA: Sage.

FLANAGAN, H. (1985) Memos on pretesting. Detroit Area Study, University of Michigan. (unpublished)

FRANZEN, R. (1936) "Technical responsibilities involved in consumer research." Market Research 5: 3-7.

FREY, J. H. (1983) Survey Research by Telephone. Beverly Hills, CA: Sage.

GALLUP, G. H. (1935-1981) The Gallup Poll (9 vols). New York: Random House (1935-1971); Wilmington, DE: Scholarly Resources, Inc. (1972-1981).

GROVES, R. M. and R. L. KAHN (1979) Surveys by Telephone: A National Comparison with Personal Interviews. New York: Academic Press.

Louis Harris and Associates, Inc. (1970) The Harris Survey Yearbook of Public Opinion 1970: A Compendium of Current Attitudes. New York: Author.

———(1974) Family Finance Survey No. 2324 (Machine Readable Data File). Chapel Hill: Louis Harris Data Center, University of North Carolina.

HAUSER, R. M. and D. L. FEATHERMAN (1977) The Process of Stratification: Trends and Analysis. New York: Academic Press.

HENSON, R., C. F. CANNELL, and S. A. LAWSON (1979) "An experiment in interviewer style and questionnaire form," in Cannell et al. (eds.) Experiments in Interviewing Techniques. Ann Arbor, MI: Institute for Social Research.

HERZOG, A. R. and J. G. BACHMAN (1981) "Effects of questionnaire length on response quality." Public Opinion Quarterly 45: 549-559.

HITLIN, R. (1976) "On question wording and stability of response," Social Science Research 5: 39-41.

HOINVILLE, G., R. JOWELL, and Associates (1978) Survey Research Practice. London: Heinemann.

HUNT, S. D., R. D. SPARKMAN Jr., and J. B. WILCOX (1982) "The pretest in survey research: issues and preliminary findings." Journal of Marketing Research 19: 269-273.

HYMAN, H. and P. B. SHEATSLEY (1950) "The current status of American public opinion," in J. C. Payne (ed.) The Teaching of Contemporary Affairs. Twenty-first Yearbook of the National Council of Social Studies: 11-34.

JENKINS, J. G. (1935) Psychology in Business and Industry. New York: John Wiley.

KAHN, R. and C. F. CANNELL (1957) The Dynamics of Interviewing. New York: John Wiley.

KALTON, G., M. COLLINS, and L. BROOK (1978) "Experiments in wording opinion questions." Journal of the Royal Statistical Society Series C 27: 149-161.

KATZ, D. (1940) "Three criteria: knowledge, conviction, significance." Public Opinion Quarterly 4: 277-284.

KOHN, M. L. (1969) A Study of Values. Homewood, IL: Dorsey.

KORNHAUSER, A. and P. B. SHEATSLEY (1976) "Questionnaire construction and interview procedure," in C. Selltiz, L. S. Wrightsman, and S. W. Cook (eds.) Research Methods in Social Relations. New York: Holt, Rinehart.

160

KROSNICK, J. and D. F. ALWIN (forthcoming) "Response order effects in the measurement of values." Public Opinion Quarterly.

KUČERA, H. and W. N. FRANCIS (1967) Computational Analysis of Present-Day American English. Providence, RI: Brown University Press.

LADD, E. C. and S. M. LIPSET (1976) The Divided Academy: Professors and Politics. New York: Norton.

LAURENT, A. (1972) "Effects of question length on reporting behavior in the survey interview." Journal of the American Statistical Association 67: 298-305.

LENSKI, G. and J. LEGGETT (1960) "Caste, class, and deference in the research interview." American Journal of Sociology 65: 463-467.

LODGE, M. (1981) Magnitude Scaling: Quantitative Measurement of Opinions. Beverly Hills, CA: Sage

LOFTUS, E. F. and W. MARBURGER (1983) "Since the eruption of Mt. St. Helens did anyone beat you up? Improving the accuracy of retrospective reports with landmark events." Memory and Cognition 11: 114-120.

MACCOBY, E. E. and N. MACCOBY (1954) "The interview: a tool of social science," in G. Lindzey (ed.) Handbook of Social Psychology. Cambridge, MA: Addison-Wesley.

MARTIN, E. (1986) Report on the Development of Alternative Screening Procedures for the National Crime Survey. Washington, DC: Bureau of Social Science Research.

McKENNELL, A. (1974) Surveying Attitude Structures. Amsterdam: Elsevier.

MELLINGER, G. D., C. L. HUFFINE, and M. B. BALTER (1982) "Assessing comprehension in a survey of public reactions to complex issues." Public Opinion Quarterly 46: 97-109.

MILLER, W. E. and the National Election Studies (1982) Codebook, American National Election Study, 1980. Ann Arbor, MI: Inter-University Consortium for Political and Social Research.

MOSER, C. and G. KALTON (1972) Survey Methods in Social Investigation. London: Heinemann.

NETER, J. and J. WAKSBERG (1965) "Response errors in collection of expenditure data in household interviews: an experimental study." Technical Paper No. 11. Washington, DC: Bureau of Census.

NISBETT, R. E., E. BORGIDA, R. CRANDALL, and H. REED (1982) "Popular induction: information is not necessarily informative," in D. Kahneman, P. Slovic, and A. Tversky (eds.) Judgment under Uncertainty: Heuristics and Biases. Cambridge, England: Cambridge University Press.

NORPOTH, H. and M. LODGE (1985) "The difference between attitudes and nonattitudes in the mass public: just measurements?" American Journal of Political Science 29: 291-307.

PAYNE, S. L. (1951) The Art of Asking Questions. Princeton, NJ: Princeton University Press.

Public Opinion (1981) "An editors' report on the Yankelovich, Skelly and White 'mushiness index.'" 4 (April-May): 50-51.

RIESMAN, D. and N. GLAZER (1948) "The meaning of opinion." Public Opinion Quarterly 12: 633-648.

ROSSI, P. H. and A. ANDERSON (1982) "The factorial survey approach," in P. H. Rossi and S. L. Nock (eds.) Measuring Social Judgments. Beverly Hills, CA: Sage.

RUGG, D. and H. CANTRIL (1944) "The wording of questions," in H. Cantril (ed.) Gauging Public Opinion. Princeton, NJ: Princeton University Press.

SCHUMAN, H. (1966) "The random probe: a technique for evaluating the validity of closed questions." American Sociological Review 31: 218-222.

———(1983) "Review of Serge Lang, *The File* (New York: Springer-Verlag, 1981)." Public Opinion Quarterly 47: 601-607.

SCHUMAN, H. and S. HATCHETT (1974) Black Racial Attitudes. Ann Arbor, MI: Institute for Social Research.

SCHUMAN, H. and S. PRESSER (1981) Questions and Answers in Attitude Surveys: Experiments on Question Form, Wording, and Context. New York: Academic Press.

SCHUMAN, H., E. WALSH, C. OLSON, and B. ETHERIDGE (1985) "Effort and reward: the assumption that college grades are affected by quantity of study." Social Forces 63: 945-966.

SHARP, L. M. and J. FRAÑKEL (1983) "Respondent burden: a test of some common assumptions." Public Opinion Quarterly 47: 36-53.

SHEATSLEY, P. B. (1983) "Questionnaire construction and item writing," in P. H. Rossi, J. D. Wright, and A. B. Anderson (eds.) Handbook of Survey Research. New York: Academic Press.

SKOGAN, W. G. (1981) Issues in the Measurement of Victimization. Washington, DC: Department of Justice, Bureau of Justice Statistics.

SMITH, T. W. (1981) "Qualifications to generalized absolutes: 'approval of hitting' questions on the GSS." Public Opinion Quarterly 45: 224-230.

———(1983) "Attitude constraint as a function of non-affective dimensions," General Social Survey Working Paper. (unpublished)

———(1984a) "Nonattitudes: a review and evaluation," in C. F. Turner and E. Martin (eds.) Surveying Subjective Phenomena, vol. 2. New York: Russell Sage.

———(1984b) "The subjectivity of ethnicity," in C. F. Turner and E. Martin (eds.) Surveying Subjective Phenomena, vol. 2. New York: Russell Sage.

STARCH, D. (1923) Principles of Advertising. New York: McGraw-Hill.

SUDMAN, S. and N. BRADBURN (1982) Asking Questions: A Practical Guide to Questionnaire Design. San Francisco: Jossey-Bass.

SUDMAN, S., A. FINN, and L. LANNOM (1984) "The use of bounded recall procedures in single interviews." Public Opinion Quarterly 48: 520-524.

TURNER, C. F. (1984) "Why do surveys disagree? Some preliminary hypotheses and some disagreeable examples," in C. F. Turner and E. Martin (eds.) Surveying Subjective Phenomena, vol. 2. New York: Russell Sage.

TURNER, C. F. and E. KRAUSS (1978) "Fallible indicators of the subjective state of the nation." American Psychologist 33: 456-470.

TURNER, C. F. and E. MARTIN, [eds.] (1984) Surveying Subjective Phenomena (2 vols.). New York: Russell Sage.

WEBB, N. (1982) Comment, in G. Kalton and H. Schuman, "The effect of the question on survey responses." Journal of the Royal Statistical Society, Series A. Pt. 1: 42-73.

WEISBERG, H. (1980) "A multidimensional conceptualization of party identification." Political Behavior 2: 33-60.

WRIGHT, J. D. (1981) "Public opinion and gun control." Annals 455: 24-39.

COMPUTER-ASSISTED INTERVIEWING

PART III

WILLEM E. SARIS

PREFACE

Anyone who has been involved in survey research is aware that it requires a lot of people, effort, and money. Questionnaires must be designed, typed, printed, distributed by mail, filled in, returned, coded, entered into the computer, and validated. Only after all these steps have been taken can the analysis start.

The use of the computer in data collection can considerably reduce the amount of work. In computer-assisted data collection (CADAC), an interview program presents the questions on the screen and registers the answers, which are immediately entered into the computer. In this way one can skip the printing, mailing, coding, and data entry. If extra attention is paid to the construction of the interview, even the validation or editing phase can be reduced considerably. This reduction of work would suggest that computer-assisted data collection has the advantage of being faster and cheaper. Nicholls and Groves (1986), however, have mentioned that there is very little evidence for this general conclusion.

There is also another reason why CADAC has been recommended by many researchers. Nicholls (1978), Groves (1983), Fink (1983), Dekker and Dorn (1984), and many others have claimed that CADAC will lead to improvements in the data quality in survey and panel research. They have in mind data quality improvement by automatic branching and coding, consistency checks, and many other possibilities. There is very little empirical evidence (Groves and Nicholls, 1986), however, to suggest that these claims are justified.

Nevertheless, the use of CADAC is growing each year. It started in the 1970s with computer-assisted telephone interviewing (CATI), which is now widely used in commercial research, at universities, and by government agencies (Nicholls and Groves, 1986; Spaeth, 1990). The total number of

163

CATI installations is unknown, but is probably more than 1,000 over the whole world (Gonzalez, 1990). In 1988, the U.S. government alone already had more than 50 installations. The National Agricultural Statistical Service of the United States now is doing more than 125,000 CATI interviews each year.

More recently, computer-assisted personal interviewing (CAPI) has been introduced. Government agencies in the U.S. and Europe (Thornberry, Rowe, and Bigger, 1990; van Bastelaer, Kerssemakers, and Sikkel, 1988) and marketing research firms in Europe are among those using these facilities for data collection. In the Netherlands, the use of CAPI procedures by the Dutch Statistical Office alone has grown very rapidly, from nearly zero 5 years ago to more than 3,000 uses per month in 1990.

All large commercial firms now have CAPI facilities as well. A similar trend can be seen in most of the Western European countries and in the United States. There also have been experiments and commercial applications using computer-assisted interviewing procedures, in which no interviewers are used. All of them are designed for panel surveys. Some use videotex systems (Clemens, 1984); others use home computers (de Pijper and Saris, 1986a) or existing computer networks (Gonzalez, 1990; Kiesler and Sproull, 1986). There also have been experiments with the use of touchtone telephones (Clayton and Harrel, 1989) and voice recognition (Winter and Clayton, 1990). The last two procedures are used mainly on a small scale for obtaining business information. With the home-computer-based system, called *tele-interviewing*, 150,000 interviews per year are performed in the Netherlands.

This continuing growth of CADAC suggests that at least one of the three arguments should hold: increased speed, reduction in costs, or improvement in data quality. It is quite likely that all three arguments hold for different projects. On the one hand, simple research can be done very quickly and cheaply using CADAC if one is not trying to improve the data quality. On the other hand, complex research can be done better than before using the new tools of CADAC, but probably will not be cheaper or faster.

Many different topics would be interesting enough for discussion in this monograph. For example, we could discuss the following:

- The cost-effectiveness of the extra equipment and extra employees needed to maintain the computer systems
- The extra skills required of interviewers and respondents, and the consequences for training time and/or nonresponse
- The increased and decreased flexibility of the process

- The consequences of the introduction of CADAC systems for research organization

In this monograph, however, we do not want to discuss these topics. Instead, we want to concentrate on the improvement of data quality as the central issue. We have chosen this aspect because it is of concern to all social scientists who are collecting data. It already is possible to improve the quality of data using CADAC. One clear example of this is given by Tortora (1985), who has shown that 77% of the data errors in a standard survey, which were so serious they normally would require a second contact with the respondents, could be avoided by the use of CADAC with on-line edit facilities (allowing the program to check for inconsistencies and ask for corrections during the interview). This advantage, however, is not obtained for free: more must be done than "only" writing a questionnaire. To this task, the researcher must add the following (House and Nicholls, 1988):

- Branching and skipping instructions
- Specified "fills"
- On-line range and consistency checks
- Help screens
- Types of answers to the questions
- The way the answers must be registered

Some more tools will be added to this list of basic procedures in order to increase the possibilities. But one thing is clear: Computer-assisted interviewing requires not only the skill of writing normal questionnaires as taught in many books (e.g., Converse and Presser, 1986; Sudman and Bradburn, 1974), but also new skills related to the new possibilities. The purpose of this monograph is to give the reader an idea of these possibilities and the difficulties that will arise if one ventures down the road of computer-assisted interviewing.

We start in Chapter 1 with a general introduction to computer-assisted interviewing. In Chapter 2, we discuss the extra possibilities that computer-assisted interviewing has to offer to interviewer-administered interviewing, self-administered interviewing, and panel surveys. In Chapter 3, we discuss the design of questionnaires for CADAC. In Chapter 4, we give a brief overview of important features of programs for computer-assisted interviewing that must be considered if one wants to purchase a CADAC program.

A number of examples of questionnaires from research are given. These examples are not limited to a specific interview program. We concentrate on the logical structure rather than on the language used. In this monograph, examples are presented as annotated versions of normal questionnaires (Baker and Lefes, 1988). In such questionnaires, their relation to the usual paper questionnaires remains visible, and the extra statements needed for computer-assisted interviewing become very clear. There are programs that use quite different procedures, as we discuss later, but for my purposes the procedure used here is sufficient to illustrate the task of the interview designer.

1. COMPUTER-ASSISTED INTERVIEWING

Personal and telephone interviews consist of a specific type of dialogue between an interviewer and a respondent. In such a dialogue, the task of the interviewer is rather complex. She or he must do the following.

- Obtain cooperation
- Present information, questions, answer categories, and instructions
- Motivate the respondent to answer
- Build up sufficient confidentiality for honest answers to be given
- Stop the respondent from recounting irrelevant stories
- Check if the answers are appropriate
- Help the respondent if the question is not correctly understood
- Code the answers in prespecified categories, or write the answers down
- Look for the next question

Compared with the task of the interviewer, the respondent has a simpler task. He or she must only do the following.

- Interpret the question
- Examine his or her memory (or papers) for the information
- Answer the question orally or write it down
- Possibly code the answer using a specific code book

Given the list of tasks the interviewer must perform in an interview, one might wonder whether anyone can perform all of them in one interview. Surprisingly, the process normally leads to satisfactory results. That does not mean that the interview has not been criticized in the past. Some critics have shown that respondents provide biased answers as a result of misunderstanding the questions (Belson, 1981; Molenaar, 1986; Schuman and Presser,

1981), social desirability (Bradburn, Sudman, Blair, and Stocking, 1978; Kalton and Schuman, 1982; Phillips and Clancy, 1970), or response set (Converse and Presser, 1986; Schuman and Presser, 1981). Others have concentrated on the problems of interviewer effects (e.g., Dijkstra and van der Zouwen, 1982; Groves, 1989). Bruinsma, Saris, and Gallhofer (1980), Andrews (1984), van Doorn, Saris, and Lodge (1983), and Saris (1988) have shown that the choice of response scale has a considerable effect on the results of a study. There also has been a lot of discussion in the literature about failure to recall information (Sikkel, 1985; Sudman and Bradburn, 1973, 1974) in interviews that ask questions about past behavior. Such studies, which often use diaries, are notorious for their high nonresponse (Thornton, Freedman, and Camburn, 1982), mainly due to the amount of effort asked of the respondent. Recently, there has been an increasing tendency to use electronic equipment instead of diaries. Modern techniques allow the registration of some kinds of behavior, such as watching TV, using the telephone, buying consumer goods, and so on, without putting any questions to the subjects. Such systems can be seen as a promising effort to design unobtrusive measurement instruments (Webb, Campbell, Schwartz, and Sechrest, 1981) that could replace the notoriously unreliable diaries. (See Saris, 1989, for an overview article on this development.) If these procedures turn out to be efficient, they will certainly lead to a complete change in data collection with respect to behavioral data. However, this monograph does not deal with that development, but instead concentrates on data collection by questionnaires.

Besides the above-mentioned methodological problems, there is a practical problem with interviews: namely, the costs of interviewing. In the United States, the costs of face-to-face interviewing are already so high that most research is done by telephone or mail.

Other problems are nonresponse in the form of complete refusals, especially in large cities, and partial nonresponse as a consequence of complex routings in the questionnaires.

The recently developed computer-based procedures for data collection can solve at least some of these problems. Below, we will discuss in historical order computer-assisted interviewing procedures that are efficiently replacing the paper-and-pencil procedures of the past, but first, we consider the requirements for an interview program if it is to replace a paper questionnaire or an interviewer.

CADAC as a Substitute for Paper Questionnaires

At a minimum, an interview program should be able to replace a paper questionnaire. A more ambitious goal would be for the program to replace the interviewer, or at least to reduce the task of the interviewer to minimal proportions. One could imagine the computer program doing all the administrative work, which it can do better than the interviewer, leaving for the interviewer the task of motivating and explaining, which the interviewer probably can do better than the computer.

The requirements for an interview program to replace a paper questionnaire are as follows.

- The presentation of information, questions, answer categories, and instructions
- The registration of the answers etc.
- Branching to the next question

These requirements are minimal and all interview programs can perform these tasks. Nevertheless, they are more complex than they may appear. One reason is that any type of question must be possible, and the computer should know the type of response (i.e., numeric or alphanumeric) and the size of the response. In order to present a question on a screen, the interview program must have the following information (Nicholls and House, 1987).

- What type of question is asked
- What the size of the answer is
- Where the data must be stored
- Where the text starts
- Where the text ends

Any interview program must deal with these tasks and each of them does it in a different way. Some programs provide a computer programming language, and are therefore very flexible but difficult to use; others are interpreters and try to stay as close as possible to the form of normal interviews (de Bie, Stoop, and de Vries, 1989). Some are question-based, and others are screen- or form-based (Nicholls, 1988). No matter what program is used, some extra information must always be provided, as we have indicated above. In these examples, we use a language derived from the program INTERV (de Pijper and Saris, 1986b), because by using that program (an interpreter) it becomes very clear what part of the questionnaire is added to instruct the computer.

Type = Num range=[10   120] var=Age
How old are you ?
(type the answer below)
END

Figure 1.1. Example 1

Let us see how a normal question can be formulated for an interview program. As an example, take the question, "How old are you?" In order to specify the task for an interview program to present this question on the screen, the instruction must be written like the one presented in Example 1 (Figure 1.1). A program requires that the lines containing instructions to the computer are distinguished from the lines of text that should appear on the screens. Therefore, all instructions to the program are printed in bold letters, and screen text is printed in plain letters in all figures.

The following information is indicated in the first line of Example 1 (Figure 1.1): the type of question (numeric), the acceptable range of answers (10 to 120), and where the question must be stored (in the variable *age*). After this instruction line, the question itself follows with the instruction to the respondent. Because these lines are not in bold, the program automatically assumes that these lines are to be presented on the screen. The researcher has complete control over the layout of the screens by placing the text wherever she or he wants. The interview screen will look exactly as specified. The text is followed by a last instruction. This line is necessary to indicate where the text of the screen stops. Normally, the specification of the next instruction is automatically the end of the previous one. If there is no next question, the end of the questionnaire is indicated by "END."

If this small interview were tried on a computer, the result should be as indicated in Figure 1.2. This example demonstrates how the program interprets the instructions and presents on the screen exactly what has been written down for the screen text.

If the interviewer types in the answer (for example, "25") this number is automatically stored in the variable *age* and can be used at any moment later in the interview.

In this simple example with only one question there is no need to indicate where to go after the first question. Example 2 (Figure 1.3) is an illustration of a longer questionnaire, with several different questions and indications for branching.

```
How old are you ?
(type the answer below)
```

Figure 1.2. Screen of Example 1

This more realistic example demonstrates more clearly the different characteristics that an interview program should have if it is to be used for the presentation of questions during an interview. These basic characteristics are as follows.

- Instructions and screens should be distinguished (bold or not)
- The type of response should be indicated (by type=)
- The size of the response should be indicated (by a range= [a b])
- The registration of answers should be organized (in the data file and in variables)
- The beginning and end of a screen should be indicated
- The branching should be indicated (condition)

Example 2 (Figure 1.3) shows how these different requirements are satisfied for the program used here. The interview starts with an information screen, and, therefore, the first instruction is **Information** so the program does not expect an answer. After the information screen, it is indicated that seven questions will be asked. Several types of questions are possible. Here are illustrated questions that require numeric answers (type=num), self-made category scales (type=cat), a prestructured 5-point rating scale (type=rating), a time scale (type=time), and an open question (type=open). A program can provide many more types. For example, the program INTERV has 16 different types of questions, including line-production scales, prestructured-category scales, multiple-answer scales, money scales, and an automatic-coding scale.

Branching is done automatically by the computer program. The branching can be arranged in different ways. Branching is indicated here by conditional statements (lines starting with the instruction **Condition**). This is very similar to how instructions to interviewers commonly are done (e.g., "Only for people with work"). In this case, these instructions are interpreted by the program, which presents only the appropriate questions to the interviewer

---

Information
In this interview, we would like to
ask you about your activities.
# of Questions=7
Type=cat range= [0   1] var=work
Do you have a job ?
  0 No
  1 Yes
Type=open var=job
Condition Work=1
What is your occupation ?
(describe the occupation as fully as possible)
Type=num range=[0   20] var=hours
Condition Work=1
How many hours did you work yesterday ?
Type=time var=time
Condition Work=1
At what time did you start your work ?
Type=cat range =[1   6] var=other
Condition Work=0
What is your situation ?
  1 housewife
  2 pensioner
  3 student
  4 unemployed
  5 disabled
  6 other
Type=code var=act
Condition Work=0
What was your main activity yesterday ?
Type=rating text=var
Did you enjoy your day or not yesterday ?
terrible   very pleasant
day   day
END

Figure 1.3. Example 2

or respondent depending on the answers given. Other procedures will be discussed later. The resulting screens for Example 2 are shown in Figure 1.4.

Figure 1.4 shows that there are two routes specified to this questionnaire. The route chosen depends on the response to the question "Do you have a job?" and thus the value of the variable *work*.

173

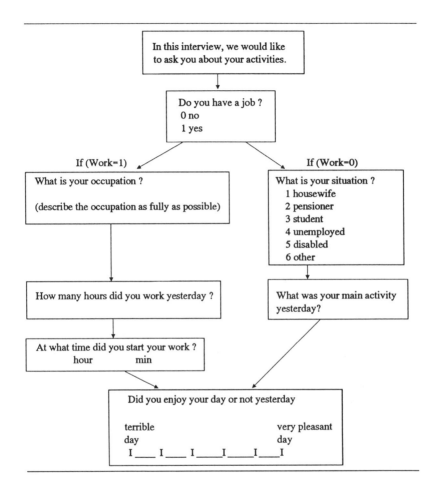

Figure 1.4. Screens of Example 2

This extended example illustrates that it is not too difficult to write questionnaires for interview programs that can replace paper questionnaires; in fact, the difference between the two is not so large. The computer questionnaire simply requires a few more instructions for the computer.

CADAC as a Partial Substitute for Interviewers

Let us now look at the requirements for an interview program to replace completely the paper questionnaire *and* interviewer. In this case, there are a number of extra requirements. Looking again at the list of tasks required of the interviewer, the following tasks have not yet been fulfilled by the interview program.

- Obtain cooperation
- Motivate the respondent to answer
- Build up sufficient confidentiality for honest answers to be given
- Stop the respondent from recounting irrelevant stories
- Check if the answers are appropriate
- Help the respondent if the question is not correctly understood
- Code the answers in predetermined categories
- Write the answer down

It is clear that an interview program cannot perform the social tasks as well as the interviewer. This, however, does not necessarily mean that the programs are worse on all counts. For example, respondents do not tell irrelevant stories to computers, and they are often more willing to report undesirable behavior to a computer than to an interviewer. However, here we concentrate on those technical tasks that can be performed as well or even better by the computer than by the interviewer. These tasks are as follows.

- Check if the answers are appropriate
- Help the respondent if the question is not correctly understood
- Code the answers in predetermined categories
- Write the answer down

The interviewer has only very limited possibilities for checking the correctness of the answers (range checks). A computer program not only can carry out range checks, but also can check the answer against any kind of existing knowledge that may validate or invalidate the answer.

The interviewer can certainly help people if necessary, but if a research project is well designed, one can build help options into an interview program as well.

Coding during an interview is a very time-consuming and difficult task for the interviewer. While concentrating on the coding, she or he also must keep up the contact with the respondents, which can lead to problems. Two computer procedures that can be substituted for coding by the interviewer or respondent are shown below.

Finally, it is not difficult to provide a simple editor that allows people to write short remarks. Experience shows that the respondents are very reluctant to do so in the beginning, but after some experience they like it and even ask for it.

Example 3 (Figure 1.5) illustrates how these possibilities can be realized using an interview program. The example is a typical marketing research questionnaire about cigarette smoking. The questionnaire starts with a general question, but it quickly becomes clear that the researcher is only interested in the type and brand of cigarettes the respondent may have bought. The line in the questionnaire is easy to follow by looking at the questions. If one also takes into account the branching, it is even clearer. In this case, for each categorical answer to a question, the instructions indicate in sequence which question should be asked next. For example, if the answer to the first question is "yes," the next question is "what?" whereas if the answer is "no," the next question is "end." This means that the program jumps to the end of the questionnaire. Therefore the routing indicates that only respondents who bought something to smoke should answer further questions. These respondents are asked to characterize in three questions the type of smoking articles they bought. On the basis of the category values used, the interview can distinguish seven types of smokers from the three questions of the "tree" type:

1	cigars
211	cigarettes, filter, low tar
212	cigarettes, filter, high tar
221	cigarettes, no filter, low tar
222	cigarettes, no filter, high tar
3	cigarette-rolling tobacco
4	pipe tobacco

The tree-type questions automatically produce the above specified codes on the basis of the category codes of the different questions. For example, if one bought cigars, a "1" is coded on the first question and nothing more. If one bought low-tar, filter cigarettes, the answers on the tree questions are, respectively, 2, 1, and 1, and the code is 211. This has been called *tree-structured coding*, because it is a procedure by which the

176

Information
   In this interview, we would like to
   ask you about your shopping.
# of questions=7
Type=cat range=[1   2] var=shop
   Did you buy anything to smoke yesterday ?
   1 yes -----→ what
   2 no -----→ end
Type=tree range=[1   4] var=what
   What did you buy ?
   1 cigars   ------→ end
   2 cigarettes   ------→ filt
   3 cigarette-rolling tobacco ------→ end
   4 pipe tobacco   ------→ end
Type=tree range=[1   2] var=filt
   Did they have a filter or not ?
   1 filter
   2 without filter
Type=tree range= [1   2] var=tar
   Was it a high-or low-tar cigarette ?
   1 low
   2 high
Type=code var=brand
   What brand of cigarettes did you buy ?
   Codes: 1 "pall mal" "pal mal " "pal mall" "pall mall"
             2 "marboro" "mar_" "marlboro"
             3 "lucky_" "_ strike" "lucky strike"
             4 "camal" "cammel" "camell" "camel"
Type=price range=[0   2000] var=costs
   How much did you pay ?
Type=price   Help var=corr
Condition (costs > 300 or costs < 200)
Help screen
   Most packs of cigarettes cost between
   200 and 300 cents.
Question Screen
   The price you mentioned is very unlikely.
   For further information press F3.
   If you made a mistake press F1.
   If the answer was correct specify the reasons
   below. You can use the rest of this
   screen for your comments.
End

Figure 1.5. Example 3

interviewer or the respondent can code products or activities by answering simple tree-structured questions.

Of course, this is a very simple example, but the same has been done for the coding of occupations (150 different categories) and companies (100 categories) for labor-force surveys, activities (350 different categories) for time-budget research (Verweij, Kalfs, and Saris, 1986), and consumer products (3,000 different categories) for consumer expenditure surveys (Hartman and Saris, 1991). This procedure avoids the need for an elaborate code book to be used by the respondent (or interviewer or coder). It is hypothesized that this reduction of effort will lead to more precise and valid results, but there has not yet been any detailed research on this point.

In the third part of the interview in Example 3 (Figure 1.5), the brand of the product is asked for in an open question. The codes that have been mentioned after the questions are the categories of the code book that are used for "string matching" in order to classify the answers. These codes are not presented on the respondent's screen. Because many different errors can be expected in the writing of the respondents, the code book is made in such a way that it allows the respondents to make errors. This can be done in two ways. First of all, all expected errors can be specified (see Pall Mall and Camel). Secondly, one can ask the computer to match only a characteristic part of the word; the rest is indicated by a line (see Marlboro and Lucky Strike).

Both coding procedures, by tree-structured questions and string matching, serve one purpose, the classification of answers to questions that normally need coding, without putting the full burden of the coding on the respondents or interviewers. Which of the two procedures is used depends on the topic and the taste of the researcher, but one should be warned that both procedures require a lot of research in advance.

The last two questions of Example 3 (Figure 1.5) illustrate the help, checking, and writing possibilities of interview programs. The first question asks for the price. The second question starts by instructing the program that it is an open question, that there is a help screen, and gives the name of the question (var=corr), after which a check on the range of the answer to the previous question is specified. If the answer to the previous question is outside the expected range, the last question is asked. In this question, help is provided on a screen and this can be requested by pressing "F3." In this case, the question consists of two parts, a help screen and a question screen. The program should be told that there are two screens, so the help is mentioned in the instruction line. Of course, this grammar is program specific, but a similar facility has been created in most advanced programs.

This question suggests that the last answer might be wrong; further information is given on the help screen, and the previous question can be corrected by pressing "F1," which will present the previous question again. It is also possible that the answer is correct, but that (for example) more than one pack of cigarettes was purchased. This answer can be given on the rest of the screen by writing a remark down. Of course, the editor provided should be very simple so people can handle it without help. In INTERV, the editor allows writing without returns at the end of the line (word wrap) and corrections can be made using the backspace key, but no other possibilities are provided.

Now that we have discussed the questionnaire as it is specified in this particular case, I will illustrate the sequence of screens that result from this questionnaire (Figure 1.6). Because the reader probably knows by now what the screens look like, we only illustrate the structure of the interview with a flow chart indicating the names of the screens and variables.

This example illustrates that writing a questionnaire that takes over certain tasks of the interviewer is not very complicated. We illustrated procedures for automatic branching, two automatic coding procedures, help options, checks, and possibilities for open-ended questions. In the next section, we hope to show that there are several tasks that the computer can do even better than the interviewer.

CADAC Can Be Better Than Normal Interviewing

Although we would not say that interview programs are better than interviewers in all aspects of the task, there certainly are a number of aspects in which the interview programs are better. Let us look at the following technical skills.

- Calculations
- Substitutions of previous answers
- Randomization of questions and answer categories
- Validation of responses
- Complex branching
- Complex coding
- Exact formulation of questions and information
- Provision of comparable help

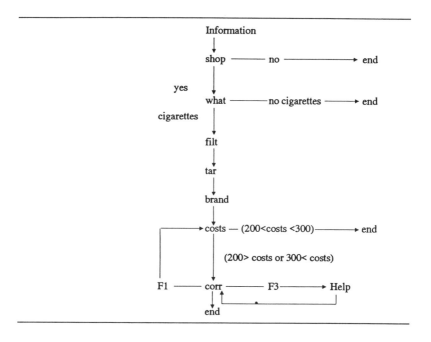

Figure 1.6. Flow Chart for Example 3

In the case of the last two skills, the advantage of using an interview program is obvious. It is well known (Brenner, 1982; Dijkstra, 1983) that interviewers do not read the questions exactly as they have been formulated. Also, help, when needed, does not always take the same form. As a consequence, it is unclear whether the responses to the questions are comparable. In computer-assisted interviewing where self-administration is used, this problem no longer exists, because the interviewer does not read the questions and therefore the questions on the screen are the same for all respondents.

The discussion of complex coding and routing also can be kept very brief, as these possibilities have already been discussed in the previous section. The only further remark needed is that the possibilities an interviewer has during an interview with respect to coding and branching are very limited, as the interviewer's task is already difficult enough. It is impractical to take longer than 30 seconds between questions to determine the code or the routing. For complex coding or branching more time is needed, and the interviewer will have trouble with the different tasks that must be performed. For a computer, such tasks are no problem; it can easily determine a routing on the basis of the answers to 10 or more questions within a second, and the complex codings also can be performed very quickly. String matching with 256 categories does not lead to a noticeable time delay in INTERV. Given these qualities of the interview programs, it is better to assign these tasks to an interview program than to an interviewer. Let us now turn to an example that illustrates the possibilities of programs with respect to calculation, substitution, and branching.

It is clear that one cannot ask an interviewer to make calculations during the interview. Nevertheless, sometimes it is useful to make calculations to determine the branching to the next question or to substitute the result of the calculations in the text of the interview. Example 4 (Figure 1.7) illustrates this point in a simple questionnaire that is nevertheless too complex for interviewers.

This example again concerns the purchase of cigarettes, using two questions from the previous example. The new aspect in this example is that a more complex situation is discussed. The possibility that more than one pack of cigarettes could have been purchased is explicitly taken into account. We expect the price of a pack of cigarettes to be between 200 and 300 cents, and so the lower and upper bound of the price paid for cigarettes are, respectively, "number * 200" and "number * 300," where "number" is the number of packs bought. A computer can calculate these costs simply, but it would be too much for an interviewer to do calculations like this in the course of an interview. The computer also can calculate how many packs most likely have been bought, assuming that the total amount paid is correct. This number is estimated to be "costs divided by 250." If all these numbers have been calculated, more detailed help can be given to the respondents during the interview. Example 4 (Figure 1.7) shows that after the two basic questions, calculations are made (grouped in what is called a *calculation block*). The calculated values of the variables then are used in the condition for the next question and the help screen. This is done by substituting these numbers for different variables in the text (for this purpose quotation marks are used before the variable to be substituted). Clearly, this information cannot be provided by interviewers, who do not have time to make such calculations. In computer-assisted interviews, such calculations do not cause any delay.

This example illustrates the extra possibilities offered by computer-assisted interviewing as a result of the facility to make calculations. Calculations

---

# of Questions=2
Type=num range=[0   25] var=number
How many packs of cigarettes did you buy yesterday ?
type=price range=[100   1000] var=costs
How much did you pay for the cigarettes ?
Calculations
V2= number*200
V3= number*300
V4=costs/250
# of Questions=1
type=price Help var=corr
Condition ((costs > v2) Or (costs > v3))
Help Screen
Most packs of cigarettes cost between 200 and 300 cents.
Thus the costs for "number packs would be between "number*200="v2
and "number * 300="v3.
The price you mentioned of "costs is very unlikely. It would mean that you have bought
approximately "costs/250="V4 packs of cigarettes and not "V1 as you mentioned.
Question screen
The price you mentioned is very unlikely.
For further information press F3.
If your answer was correct type 0.
If you made a mistake specify the proper costs :
END

Figure 1.7. Example 4

can play an important role in substitution and branching, which can be considerably more complex in computer-assisted interviewing than in paper-and-pencil interviews.

Example 4 (Figure 1.7) also illustrates another, very important, new feature of computer-assisted interviewing, the improved facilities for validation. Normally, the interviewers do not have the time or skill to carry out the validation during the interview. In computer-assisted interviewing, validation can be done immediately. As soon as the answer to a question is given, it can be checked against other information to check the quality of the answer. In case of doubt, the program can immediately ask the respondent for clarification and corrections (see Figure 1.7). This is a very important advantage of computer-assisted interviewing. It means that one can clean the data while the respondent is still available. Normally, these checks are done later, and if errors are detected, one can only change the incorrect answer into a missing value to avoid returning to the respondents for additional information. In computer-assisted interviewing, these checks are made during the interview, and if the questionnaire is constructed with care, the data from the research can be considered optimal immediately after the interview is finished; later validation will not be necessary. We will illustrate this point elsewhere in this monograph, as it is one of the most important advantages of computer-assisted interviewing.

The last two points to be mentioned in this section are randomization of questions and randomization of response categories. Because of the "order effect" in interviews (Billiet, Loosveldt, and Waterplas, 1984; Schuman and Presser, 1981), it has been suggested that the sequence of questions and response categories be randomized. In normal paper-and-pencil interviews this is not very easy. It requires different versions of the questionnaire, which is very costly, and only a few variants can be created.

In CADAC, randomization can be realized in a simple way, because a random-number generator can easily be created and used during the interview to determine the order of the questions. The researcher must decide only in which way to tell the program which questions have to be randomized. This requires a statement specifying the names of the questions to be randomized. If the questions already are brought together in a block (as in a stimulus block; see de Pijper and Saris, 1986b), the questions can be randomized by default, or only one sign has to be used to specify that randomization is requested. The same holds for category randomization, but in that case the categories already belong together, and only a sign in the instructions for the program is necessary.

Disadvantages of CADAC

There are also some disadvantages associated with CADAC. Groves and Nicholls (1986) mention the following points.

- The size of the screen is smaller than a questionnaire page, which might lead to a lack of overview when using CADAC
- Corrections are more easily made on a form
- Coordination of hand and eye is lost

Because a screen is smaller than a questionnaire page, a screen cannot contain as much information. In the earlier CADAC programs, each question was presented on a separate screen in order to have enough space for the questions. The disadvantage of this approach is that people can lose track of the purpose of the questions, especially if automatic branching is used extensively. The problem has been recognized in the literature and has been referred to as the "segmentation" problem (House and Nicholls, 1988). One solution to this problem is to use programs that present more questions on one screen (Nicholls, 1988). Another solution is to use screens that summarize information. We will return to these options later.

The second problem is that paper questionnaires give a continuous overview of the questions and answers, so that one can easily see where errors have been made and correct them. In a computer-assisted procedure these corrections are not so easily made if an "item-based" program is used. The CADAC user must return to the error in the questionnaire by moving backwards through the questionnaire, or the researcher must provide correction possibilities at any place where problems can occur. The first option might lead to errors if the program or questionnaire is not protected against such errors (Nicholls and House, 1987). The second option requires a lot of effort on the part of the researcher.

The last problem—the lack of coordination of hand and eye in CADAC—is a very interesting problem. In paper questionnaires, people write where they look. In CADAC procedures, people type on a keyboard, but they have to look at a screen for the result. If they look at their fingers and not at the screen while they are typing, there is a possibility of making an error in the response. Such an error is very unlikely in paper questionnaires. Although this problem has not been very closely studied, it is probably the experience of many users of CADAC systems that typing errors do occur in CADAC procedures and that they can have a negative influence on the data quality. The solution to this problem is to use summary screens, which we will discuss later.

All three problems indicate that CADAC procedures are not the same as paper-and-pencil interviews. Simple translations of paper-and-pencil interviews to computer-assisted procedures will not necessarily lead to better quality data. More effort in the design is required in order to make the CADAC questionnaires better than paper-and-pencil questionnaires. Facilities that can be used for this purpose are the topic of Chapter 2, but first, let us summarize the results so far.

Summary

We have shown in this chapter that interview programs combined with good questionnaires not only can replace paper questionnaires, but also can replace the interviewer, at least partially. We also have demonstrated that computer-assisted interviewing can even be superior to personal interviewing, because of the possibility of calculations, complex fills, complex branching, coding, randomization of questions and answers, and, most important, the possibility of validating the answers during the interview while the respondent is still present. During the interviews, checks can be done and the respondents can introduce the necessary corrections or can indicate why their case is different from the normal case.

On the other hand, we also have mentioned that there are some problems with CADAC procedures that require extra attention. Therefore, it should be clear that there is a price to pay for improving data quality with the use of CADAC. The price is not the cost of the computer itself, which is quickly covered as a result of the efficiency of the procedures. The higher costs result from the time one must spend on the development of good questionnaires that take full advantage of the facilities of computer-assisted interviewing to improve the data quality. Such a time investment makes more sense for questionnaires that are very frequently used.

Because the procedures for improving the data quality differ according to the data-collection techniques used, we will discuss the possibilities of each of the different data-collection techniques in Chapter 2.

2. DIFFERENT CADAC APPLICATIONS

Having dealt with the general possibilities and difficulties of computer-assisted interviewing in Chapter 1, this chapter now discusses different possible applications of these techniques and their potential.

The oldest application of CADAC is computer-assisted telephone interviewing (CATI). Commercial applications of CATI began in the 1970s (Fink, 1983), and it is now widely used in commercial research, at universities, and by government agencies (Nicholls and Groves, 1986). The most recent figures for the universities given by Spaeth (1990) show that 69% of those university research institutions in the United States who replied to a questionnaire were using a CATI system, and that 22% more were planning to start CATI applications in the near future.

The first systems used as hardware were mainframes or minicomputers with connected terminals. Examples of such systems still existing are the Cases system (See Appendix) in the United States, and the Research Machine (Pulse Train Technology, 1984) in Europe. In recent years, more and more personal-computer- (PC-) based systems, stand-alones, and networked systems have become available (Carpenter, 1988).

Typical of all CATI systems is that the interviewer sits behind the terminal or PC and calls a respondent. Once contact is made, all necessary information and questions appear on the screen and the interviewer immediately types in the answers on the keyboard of the computer or terminal. This description shows that as far as the respondent is concerned, there is no difference between a CATI interview and a paper-and-pencil telephone interview. The difference for the interviewer is that part of the work is done by the computer (branching and skipping, fills, consistency checks, etc.). This is partially an advantage, but there are also disadvantages associated with this approach if the questionnaire is not well designed. The extra facilities offered by CATI systems are sample management by the CATI system, call management by the CATI system, and on-line monitoring of the interviewers.

The first two facilities will not be discussed further here, because they affect the quality of the sample rather than the quality of the responses. For further information on these points, see Nicholls and Groves (1986) and Weeks (1988), and other articles referenced in those texts. The third facility offered by CATI will be given some attention below.

The second CADAC system to be developed and tested was the computer-assisted personal interview (CAPI). As far as we are aware, the first tests were carried out in 1980. Although at that time computers still were not really practical for this purpose, a Dutch research group was experimenting with these procedures using Apple IIc computers and, later, transportable Kaypro computers, in order to test the possibilities of more efficient measurement procedures for attitudes, evaluations, and preferences (Saris, de Pijper, and Neijens, 1982). The first experiments with portable computers by a statistical office were reported by the Swedish Census Bureau (Danielsson and Maarstad, 1982). More recently, the Dutch Statistical Office has done several experiments (Bemelmans-Spork and Sikkel, 1985, 1986). Similar reports are now coming out of the United States (e.g., Couper and Groves, 1989; Couper, Groves, and Jacobs, 1989; Thornberry et al., 1990).

Since 1980, portable computers, or "laptops," have become much cheaper, lighter, and better. Therefore, it comes as no surprise that several statistical offices have decided to do at least a large part of their routine face-to-face interviewing with CAPI systems. As far as we are aware, this decision has been made in the Netherlands, Sweden, the United Kingdom, and the United States. Commercial firms also have started to use CAPI systems recently (Boerema, Baden, and Bon, 1987).

In CAPI, the interviewer takes the computer to the respondent's residence. Normally, the computer is used in the same way as in CATI applications: The questions appear on the screen, and the interviewer reads the questions for the respondents and types the answers into the computer. However, from the very start there has been another way of working, in which the interviewer leaves the reading of the questions and the entering of the answers completely to the respondent. This is sometimes called a "computerized self-administered questionnaire," or CSAQ.

From a respondent's point of view, the interviewer-administered CAPI interview is not very different from the paper-and-pencil interview, although it has been suggested that the mere presence of the computer might change the situation (Couper and Groves, 1989). The studies of the Dutch statistical office (Bemelmans-Spork and Sikkel, 1985), however, do not indicate any difference with respect to refusals or partial nonresponse, even for sensitive questions such as income. Nevertheless, there are differences: The CAPI interviews take longer than paper-and-pencil interviews, and the notes made by the interviewer on the computer are shorter (Couper and Groves, 1989).

Whatever the conclusion on this point in the future, may be it is safe to say that the interview situation changes quite dramatically in the self-administered approach. A much more active role is required of the respondent, as well as more skills than in interviewer-administered interviewing. (The latter does not apply if the program is sufficiently user friendly.) Saris et al. (1982), who used this approach in the Netherlands, did not report any problems, nor did Gavrilov (1988), even though his study was done with farmers in the Soviet Union who had very limited schooling.

Another important difference between the two CAPI systems is that in the self-administered procedure, the interviewer no longer has anything to do during the interview. It is for this reason that alternatives have been developed. One possibility is to create a situation where one researcher can help a number of respondents at the same time. For example, this can be done by placing a number of computers on a bus that then is driven to a place where the respondents are asked to come to answer the questions. In the bus, many interviews can be done simultaneously under the supervision of one researcher. This was the system used by Gavrilov in the farmlands of the Soviet Union. Another possibility, which will be discussed below, is to organize completely automatic interview procedures.

In order to make the CAPI procedure truly efficient, one must provide the interviewer with a modem by which the interviews can be sent from the central computer to the computer of the interviewer and the data returned to the central computer. This can be done during the night or in the morning when no other activities take place. As a result, mailing costs are considerably reduced, the speed of research is increased, and one has better control of the sample.

The latest developments in the field of CADAC have taken place in panel-survey research (repeated observations of the same cases of the population). Panel-survey research normally is done by a mixture of face-to-face interviewing, telephone interviewing, and write-in procedures (diaries). The development of computer-assisted interviewing also has created new possibilities for panel research. One possibility is the collection of the data by CATI or CAPI, or by a mixture of both procedures. In these procedures, interviewers play an important role. The role of the interviewer is considerably reduced if self-administered interviews are used.

There also have been developments toward completely automatic panel-survey research. This has been done in several ways. Clemens (1984) has reported experiments with the Prestel videotex system in the United Kingdom, where respondents answer on-line, in self-administered mode, questions that appear on the screen of the terminals in their homes. Kiesler and Sproull (1986) have reported on an experimental research project where an ad-hoc sample of computer users, connected to a computer network, answered questions on the computer available to them. De Pijper and Saris (1986a) have developed one of the more successful systems in this class, the "tele-interviewing." In this system, a random sample of the population is provided with a home computer and modem. With this hardware and a normal telephone, it is possible to send an interview from a central computer to the home computer or PC of the respondent. The respondent answers the questions on the computer, and afterward the answers automatically are returned. The advantage of this procedure is that interviewers are required only to ask the subjects for their cooperation and to explain the procedure. After that first contact, the respondents can answer all questions on the home computer, and the interviewer is no longer needed. This system has been tested successfully by the Sociometric Research Foundation (de Pijper and Saris, 1986b) and has been applied in commercial research by the Dutch Gallup Organization since 1986 with a sample of 1,000 households (van Doorn, 1987-1988). At the moment, a similar panel with a sample of 2,400 households has been set up by the University of Amsterdam.

TABLE 2.1
A Classification of CADAC Procedures

Name	Description	Role of Interviewer	Observation
CATI	computer- assisted telephone interviewing	interviewer - administered	ad hoc and repeated
CAPI	computer-assisted personal interviewing	interviewer or self-administered	ad hoc and repeated
TI	tele-interview using PCs and modems	self-administered	repeated
PDE	prepared data entry	self-administered	repeated
TDE	touchtone data entry	self administered	repeated
VRE	voice recognition entry	self-administered	repeated

An alternative procedure for tele-interviewing has been developed in the United States and is known as *prepared data entry* (PDE). Since 1988, the Energy Information Administration in the United States has asked firms to provide information via a PC interview. In some cases, the information is sent to the central computer by mail. In other cases, the transport of data is done electronically.

There are two further procedures that were developed for business research and are completely automatized. These two systems are called *touchtone data entry* (TDE) and *voice recognition entry* (VRE). In both systems, the computer reads questions from a record and the respondent has to answer by use of the telephone. The first system requires a touchtone telephone that allows numeric answers to be typed. The second system allows the respondents to speak into the telephone directly, and the computer at the other side tries to recognize the numeric answers (Clayton and Harrel, 1989; Winter and Clayton, 1990). Although both systems are operational and have great potential, especially the VRE, it is still too early to predict their future. At the moment, they can only be used for very short interviews with respondents who are familiar with the system.

In Table 2.1, the information about the most important systems has been summarized. This table also indicates whether or not interviewers are needed for data collection, and whether the system can be used for ad hoc research or only for repeated observations of the same cases. These two features of the systems are mentioned because they are much more important in describing different CADAC systems than the technology that has been used in the different systems.

As can be seen from this overview, computer-assisted panel research (CAPAR) can be interviewer-administered in the case of CATI or CAPI, and also self-administered in the form of CAPI, tele-interview (TI), PDE, TDE and VRE. Cross-sectional surveys can be done by CATI and CAPI, but systems that can collect data from a fixed panel repeatedly also can be used for description of a situation at a specific moment. So the technology does not differentiate between the different possible applications.

On the other hand, we will argue that interviewer-administered and self-administered interviews require very different approaches by the interview designer in order to get good quality interviews. We also will show that repeated observations allow much more quality control in the interviews, but require much more effort. Given that we want to discuss procedures to improve data quality, we will distinguish between procedures for cross-sectional surveys and panel surveys, and between procedures for interviewer-administered and self-administered CADAC, and will not concentrate so much on the technology required. (A few words on this point will be said in the last chapter.)

Interviewer-Administered Survey Research

As we already have mentioned, we will discuss two different procedures in this monograph: CATI, which is by necessity an interviewer-administered procedure; and CAPI, as far as the interviewer plays an active role. Because both procedures are CADAC procedures, they have all the advantages and disadvantages of these procedures mentioned in the first chapter. However, these two procedures have several characteristics in common due to their use of interviewer-administered questionnaires. We concentrate on these characteristics in the next section.

Complex Questions and Answer Categories. One of these characteristics, a very general one not necessarily connected with the computer aspect of the procedure, concerns the fact that it is very difficult for respondents to memorize a large series of possible alternative answers or a very long instruction read to them by the interviewer. This problem is mentioned here because it is one of the differences between this procedure and those discussed later.

Two examples can illustrate this point. The first example is a common question about the political agenda:

What is, according to you, the most important political issue at the moment?

1. Unemployment
2. Pollution
3. Danger of a nuclear war
4. Poverty in the Third World
5. AIDS
6. Crime in the cities
7. Homeless people
8. Drugs
9. Danger of catastrophes
10. Terrorism

If one tries such a question in an interviewer-administered questionnaire, two reactions occur very frequently. First, many respondents ask the interviewer to repeat the question again. Second, the respondent often says "the first" or "the last" issue. The first reaction clearly indicates that the respondent could not remember all the options that had just been read to him or her. The second reaction leaves this interpretation open. It is possible that this is a serious answer, but it is more likely that the respondent has given this answer in order to avoid repetition of the question, which would take more time, and which could also give the bad impression that he or she is not able to remember all the options.

One might think that in such a situation it is probably better not to read the possible answers to the respondent, making it an open question instead. However, research by Schuman and Presser (1981) and Billiet et al. (1984) has indicated that quite different results are obtained if such an open question is used. A better alternative, if one is interested in the differences in the relative importance of the different issues and not in the individual responses, is to randomize the order in which the options are read to the respondent.

This option exists in CADAC procedures, but not in normal interviews. In this way, at least on an aggregate level, reasonable results are obtained.

A similar problem exists if the instruction is very long. The next example illustrates this point:

> Political parties differ in their political orientation. Some are more right-wing oriented and others more left-wing. We would like to ask you to evaluate the political orientation of the different parties. An extreme left-wing position is indicated by zero and an extreme right-wing position by 100. We ask you to express your opinion about the parties' positions with a number. So, how would you then evaluate the position of the . . . ?

Again, a common reaction to this question is that the respondents ask: "Can you say it again?" or "what did you say: right-wing is zero and left-wing is 100?" Or they start to answer the question and reverse the direction of the scale. In this case, there is little one can do except repeat the reference points once more just before they start to answer.

These problems are typical of all interviews where the interviewer reads the questions to the respondent. Such questions must not be long or complex; otherwise the respondents cannot remember the necessary information. In self-administered questionnaires this problem is less severe, because the respondents are able to look back in the text. An alternative is the use of show cards during the interview, but this is possible only in CAPI applications; also, it would mean that the interviewer would have to carry a computer *and* a pack of cards, which would increase considerably the weight he or she must carry. Thornberry et al. (1990) found that this is still a problem. The introduction of the notebook computers in the near future will considerably reduce this problem. In the long run, it is not impossible that this situation also will improve for CATI systems, if drastically different telephone networks (ISDN) are introduced that will allow pictures to be transmitted from the interviewer to the respondent at a speed of 64 KB per second. There is even a possibility of a system (broadband-ISDN) that is 10,000 times faster (Gonzalez, 1990). These developments suggest that in the future, the problem of the visual aids will be solved for CAPI as well as CATI; however, at the moment one has to recognize that the problem of complex questions and instructions exists in interviewer-administered interviews.

Due to the recent changes in Eastern Europe, a suggestion has been made that the NATO and Warsaw Pact countries should draw up new treaties governing the first use of nuclear weapons.

What do you think of a proposal whereby both parties would agree never to use nuclear weapons as a first-strike weapon ?

(A first strike is intended to destroy the other country, so that it cannot attack so easily any more. For an explaination of NATO and WARSAW PACT press F3.)

   1 agree
   2 disagree
   9 don't know

Figure 2.1. Example 5

Help by the Interviewer. A positive feature of the procedures where the interviewer plays an important role is that the interviewer can help the respondent to understand the questions correctly and give the appropriate answer. In CADAC procedures these possibilities also exist, but it is more difficult for the interviewer to be of much help: The questionnaires can be so structured with respect to branching and skipping in the questionnaire that each interview looks very different to the interviewer. In this case, the interviewer is hardly more likely than the respondent to be able to understand the questions, unless intensive training has been given to the interviewers.

Nevertheless, no matter how much training is given to the interviewers, it is always very wise in designing CADAC interviewer-administered questionnaires to provide the interviewer with as much information as possible to give him or her a better understanding of the meaning of the question. This extra information can be given on the screen where the question is presented, or on a separate help screen that is only called up if necessary. We will illustrate this point with an example.

There are situations where it makes sense to provide help information on the screen for all interviewers, because it is likely that only a few of them will know that information. An example is the military use of the *first-strike* concept. If an opinion about the first-strike capabilities of NATO (North Atlantic Treaty Organization) is requested, it is probably wise to explain the concept of first strike to all interviewers and respondents.

There are also situations in which the interviewer and the respondent usually will know what is meant by the terms used, but occasionally will need further information. For example, if the questionnaire asks people for their opinions about NATO, many people will know what this organization is, but some people might need help. In a case like this, help should be given on a separate help screen in order to avoid overcrowded screens. Example 5 (Figure 2.1) illustrates this possibility.

This example illustrates how in CADAC procedures extra information can be supplied that interviewers need in order to be helpful to the respondent. The information can be given directly on the screens to all interviewers, or it can be given only to those people who need the information. In the latter case, help screens that only appear on request are used. In order to obtain this extra information, the interviewer must press some key (i.e., the function key F3).

Example 5 (Figure 2.1), however, also illustrates that help could be given directly to the respondent without being presented by the interviewer. Only occasionally will the interviewer play an important role, namely when the questionnaire is not very suitable for the respondent and all kinds of problems arise. However, even in these situations, the interviewer cannot do very much because of the relatively rigid structure of CADAC procedures. We will return to this point later.

Keeping Up the Pace of the Interview. A very important aspect of inter-viewing, especially of telephone interviewing, is that there should only be a very short time between questions. If the delay is more than a few seconds, respondents can get annoyed and withdraw their cooperation or reduce it to the minimum (House, 1985). This can have very negative effects on the quality of the data. The speed with which the interviewer can move from one screen to the next depends on (a) the quality of the hardware and software, (b) the activities that are organized between two questions, (c) the layout of the screens, (d) the difficulty the interviewer has with corrections, and (e) the flexibility of the questionnaire or program in the event of serious problems arising. A similar list of points has been given by House (1985) for CATI interviewing, but many of the arguments given for CATI can be generalized to other applications as well. Let us look at these different points more closely.

First of all, *the replacement of one screen by another* is dependent on the quality of the hardware and the software. If the interviews are done on a terminal connected to a central computer, the response time can be rather slow when other users are making use of the same computer. But even if a personal computer is used, the response time can be slow due to the way the software is operating. Delays are mostly due to reading from and writing to the diskettes, or to very complex codings or calculations. If a program is reading or writing all the time, the process is slowed down. Such delays can be considerably reduced by writing to and reading from a RAM (random-access memory) disk instead of a diskette or hard disk. On the other hand, the tasks need to be very complex indeed to slow down a computer due to coding and calculations.

Also, the *design of the questionnaire* can affect the speed of the program. The designer of a questionnaire can increase the pace of the interview considerably by avoiding situations where the computer has to do many different tasks at the same moment between two questions (i.e., coding a complex response, writing the answers to a disk, reading a new part of the interview, making some calculations, and evaluating a complex branching statement). All of these tasks can be designed to happen between two questions, but with a little bit of effort, it often is possible to spread them over several questions, so although some moves may take a little longer, a very long delay is avoided.

A second way in which the questionnaire designer can influence the pace of the interview is by designing *screen layout* procedures that are immediately clear to the interviewer. If the screen is not immediately clear to the interviewer, she or he will need some time to study it before the question can be formulated. House (1985) suggests some important rules to follow:

1. Standard procedures should be used to indicate questions and instructions. For example, questions can be given in normal letters and instructions in inverse video (reverse screen). Words that should be stressed could be underlined or bold; extra information can be given in a different color. Of course, these suggestions are arbitrary; more important is that the interviews should always look the same to the interviewer so that quick orientation is possible.

2. The different parts of the screen should always be used in the same way (e.g., first some short instructions to the interviewer, then, below that, the questions and the response categories, and to the right of the categories extra information if available).

3. The screen should not be too full of text. It is my experience that lines with important information should be separated by blank lines to make them immediately recognizable to the interviewer. If there are many answer categories that need not be read by the interviewer, they can be closer together.

The time between questions certainly will be too long if the answers of the respondents do not fit in the specified categories and there are no facilities for the interviewer to solve these problems. It goes without saying that CADAC questionnaires should be tested thoroughly. But even if this is done, it is unavoidable that once in a while a respondent will give answers that do not fit into the system of the questionnaire. This is one of the major problems with CADAC procedures. The one thing that can be said about it is that one should do the necessary tests (We will come back to this later) and that one should allow for a way out if "impossible" events occur. One way is always to allow an "other" category, with some suggestion of what this other possibility may be. This option requires choices with respect to branching and skipping, which might be complicated. Another possibility is to allow the interviewer to comment at any time (or at frequent intervals) on the responses and possible errors that may have occurred. The disadvantage of this option is that one still has to edit the data after the data collection is done.

Another aspect of the design that can speed up the interview concerns the *procedures to correct inconsistencies*. If these procedures are too complex, the time between the question that led to the contradictory answer and the next question becomes too long. Because this concerns the more general issue of how the interviewer must deal with inconsistencies, this point is discussed further in the next section.

Clearing Up Inconsistencies. As the final point in this section, the general problem of clearing up inconsistencies is discussed. In Chapter 1, we mentioned that this facility of CADAC procedures is one of its major attractions. Nevertheless, these procedures are not without dangers. One has already been mentioned: If the procedure for correcting inconsistencies is not clear to the interviewer, it might take too much time before the next question can be asked.

There are different procedures in use to make these corrections. The start, however, is always the same: The program compares the answers to different questions and detects inconsistencies that cannot be tolerated or finds combinations of answers that are extremely unlikely. But what the program does not and cannot tell is which of the answers is incorrect.

One way to proceed in such a situation is to provide the interviewer with all the available information, point out that there is an inconsistency, and ask him or her to sort it out. If only two questions are involved, this is not very difficult. For example, the program can say:

Question	Answer
Age father	35
Age son (John)	36
Not possible!	

In this case, when the names of the questions are available, it should be clear to the interviewer what must be done.

1. Mention that there is something wrong.
2. Ask for clarification.
3. Go back to the question that has been wrongly answered and correct the answer there.
4. If other questions depend on this answer, these questions also should be asked so that complete and correct data are obtained.
5. Finally, the program should return to the point where the inconsistency was found.

What is not specified in this procedure is how the interviewer should approach this task. Should she or he say:

"You made an error because . . ."
"I am sorry, but there is a difficulty . . ."
"I am sorry, but the computer detected that . . . ," or
"I may have recorded something incorrectly here . . ."

Although the first formulation is correct, one cannot use it too frequently if one wants the respondent to remain motivated.

An additional complication is that it may be not only the age information that is wrong, but also the information about the relationship with the respondent. The name of this question is not on the screen, and the interviewer will have to look for it in order to make the necessary corrections. This can be a complicated matter that takes some time if the question is far away in the questionnaire and there is no easy way to find its name. This is a typical situation in which the time between two questions can become too long, as previously mentioned.

Of course, it would have been better if the designer of the questionnaire had foreseen this possibility and given the name of this question on the screen. In this case, all necessary corrections could be made. If this procedure is used, the sequence of questions and the formulation of them is no longer under the control of the researcher. The interviewers have to decide for themselves which question to correct. Previous research has indicated that they do not necessarily correct the proper questions. Some interviewers chose to correct the question that is simplest to correct, which is often the last one. However, that is not necessarily the appropriate question to correct (van Bastelaer, Kersssemakers, and Sikkel, 1988).

An alternative approach that allows the researcher to maintain complete control is to specify extra questions to deal with all possible inconsistencies. In this case, the interviewer does not have to make decisions about which direction to take. The interview always goes forward, never backward. Of course, the specification of the extra questions is not an easy task, but if one can specify a consistency check one also can specify extra questions. For the problem mentioned above, the designer could present a question next to the given information:

> I am sorry, but the computer has detected that in one question you mentioned that your age is 35 and in another that the age of your son John is 36.
> Of course, this is very unlikely.
> Is your age wrong, is the age of your son wrong, are both wrong, or is there another error (more than one answer is possible)?
>
> 1. My age
> 2. Age of my son John
> 3. John is not my son
> 4. Other problem

If one (or both) of the given ages is wrong extra questions about it will follow, and then the normal questioning continues. If John is not his son, a question follows about their relationship.

It will be clear that both procedures have their advantages. The first procedure gives some freedom, but this can be dangerous in the sense that wrong questions are asked or wrong corrections are made for simplicity, or the interview cannot be continued because the name of the question that should be corrected is missing.

The second procedure is more controlled, but also is more rigid. The designer must analyze the problems well in advance. On the other hand, if the designer is not doing this, the first procedure also runs into problems because question names that are needed to jump to the question with the wrong answer are missing.

Monitoring the Behavior of Interviewers. It is inherent in the role of the interviewer in these procedures that the interviewers can do things that the researcher does not wish them to do. At worst, they talk to the wrong person, or falsify interviews or parts of interviews. It is not known how frequently this occurs (Groves and Nicholls, 1986), but all research institutes at some time are confronted with such occurrences.

Less extreme, but also very unpleasant, is the fact that the interviewers have a tendency to change the wording of the questions, partly in anticipation of the answers expected of the respondents (Brenner, 1982; Dijkstra, 1983). In CAPI applications, not much can be done to stop these activities, because it is not easy to control the interviewers except by calling the respondents to verify information. However, although doing so allows the researcher to check whether the interview was or was not completely falsified, it cannot change the way the interview was performed. In the next section, we will discuss various radical solutions to this problem in CAPI applications. In CATI, it is possible to check up on the interviewers. Technically, it is possible not only to monitor their behavior on the phone, but also to copy the text of their screen to the screen of a control computer. In this way, the research management has complete audio- and video-monitoring possibilities. Only samples of the whole process can be monitored, but given that the interviewers are aware of the possibility that their behavior may be observed, they will take more care and not engage in the devastating activities mentioned above, and may even reduce the amount of reformulation of questions. These monitoring facilities are certainly of great value in the CATI applications, even though the monitoring can lead to some stress on the part of the interviewers.

It will have become clear from the discussion in this section that the interviewer-administered CADAC procedures CATI and CAPI have many possibilities, but that good results are not obtained without costs. One must make a considerable investment of time in good questionnaire design. This is especially true for consistency checks and on-line editing. If one wants to use these facilities, a lot of effort and time is required. Whether this is worthwhile for ad-hoc survey research remains to be seen.

Self-Administered Survey Research

The most important difference between the self-administered procedures and the interviewer-administered procedures is the role of the interviewer. In the self-administered surveys, there is no interviewer reading the questions and typing in the answers. If there is an interviewer present during the interview, his or her role is only to clarify general points.

The major advantage of this approach, of course, is that there is no interviewer to change the questions. As a result, all respondents are presented with the same questions and the same answer categories. This does not mean that all respondents will read the text equally carefully, but (at least from a researcher's point of view) the presentation is optimal, because one can completely determine which information, questions, instructions, and answer categories are presented to the respondents.

Although this is a very attractive situation, it also requires a lot of effort on the part of the questionnaire designer, who cannot rely on an interviewer for clarification. The whole process needs to be spelled out well in advance. Also, given that some people have only limited reading and writing abilities, and even less computer experience, the procedures must be very simple so that anybody can do the interviews. The requirements for such an approach will be the topic of this section. We also will discuss other aspects specific to the self-administered questionnaire that can help the respondents in their work. The tools that can be provided may be so efficient that they more than compensate for the absence of an interviewer: visual aids, calendars, summary and correction (SC) screens, more complex category scales, the use of psychophysical scales, and complex instructions.

User-Friendliness. Self-administered questionnaires require much more user-friendliness from the interview program and questionnaire than interviewer-administered procedures. Although programs that can be done by the respondents themselves also can be done by interviewers, the opposite is not always true. In particular, the instructions and consistency checks are quite different in self-administered questionnaires.

Let us first discuss the instructions. Clearly, one cannot give instructions like "Do not read the categories" if one would like to ask an "unaided recall" question. Such a question should be presented as an open question in these procedures. But if it were a real open question, routing would be impossible. Therefore, the answers have to be coded immediately, using a dictionary specified by the researcher. After coding in several categories, further branching is possible.

A typical example of such a question would be a question asking respondents to mention names of cigarette brands to see which are the best known. Next, the people are asked if they know those brand names that they did not mention. An illustration of such a questionnaire is presented in Example 6 (Figure 2.2).

This example is a little bit complicated using the language of the INTERV program, because the program does not provide a standard procedure for this type of questionnaire. But the result is the same as that achieved automatically in other programs.

# of questions=1
Type=code Var=V1
    Please give the name of the first
    brand of cigarettes that comes
    to your mind ?
    Codes: 1 "pall mal" "pal mal" "pal mall" "pall mall"
           2 "marboro" "mar_" "marlboro"
           3 "luck_" "_strike" "lucky strike"
           4 "camal" "cammel" "camell" "camel"
Calculation
V20=1
Repeat 5
Calculation
V20=V20+1
# of questions 1
Type=code var=V[V20]
    If you know more names
    type another name below.
    Otherwise type: NO
    Codes: 1 "pall mal" "pal mal" "pal mall" "pall mall"
           2 "marboro" "mar_" "marlboro"
           3 "lucky _" "_strike" "lucky strike"
           4 "camal" "cammel" "camell" "camel"
           5 "NO"
Until (V[V20]=5)
Calculation
V11=0   V12=0   V13=0   V14=0
[v1=1 or v2=1 or v3=1 or v4=1 or v5=1] V11=1
[v1=2 or v2=2 or v3=2 or v4=2 or v5=2] V12=1
[v1=3 or v2=3 or v3=3 or v4=3 or v5=3] V13=1
[v1=4 or v2=4 or v3=4 or v4=4 or v5=4] V14=1
# of questions=1
Type=multi range=[1 4] var=aided
    Which of the following brands have you also heard of ?
Condition V11=0
    { 1. Pal Mall}
Condition V12=0
    {2. Marlboro}
Condition V13=0
    {3. Lucky Strike}
Condition V14=0
    {4. Camel}
    You can mention more than one brand.
    Type a number after each number
    and press F5 at the end.
END

Figure 2.2. Example 6

```
Please give the name of the first
brand of cigarettes that comes
to your mind ?
```

Figure 2.3. Screen 1 of Example 6

The first question presented on the screen will be the question in Screen 1 of Example 6 (Figure 2.3). Notice that the dictionary from the question text is not presented. After the first question, a second question is repeated maximally five times. This second question asks for other brand names. This is also an unaided recall question, because the names of the brands are not mentioned on the screen, only in the dictionary. This "repeat until" procedure stops before the fifth round if the respondent answers "no" on the second question, meaning that she or he knows no other names.

Now imagine that the respondent mentioned the names *Pall Mall* and *Lucky Strike*. Then the next step is that in a calculation block the variables $V11$ and $V13$ obtain the value 1, and the variables $V12$ and $V14$ will have the value 0.

After that calculation, the last question is presented. Only the names of those brands that were not mentioned by the respondent are presented, as shown in Screen 2 of Example 6 (Figure 2.4). The last question is a multiple-response question by means of which the respondents can indicate which names of brands they can remember in aided recall.

```
Which of the following brands
have you also heard of ?

2. Marlboro
4. Camel
```

Figure 2.4. Screen 2 of Example 6

This is a typical example of how instructions and procedures are changed to make up for the fact that there is no interviewer present. On the one hand, the procedure becomes more difficult for the researcher to write, whereas on the other hand, the procedure for the respondents becomes simpler.

Example 6 (Figure 2.2) also illustrates the point that this procedure can be used in self-administered and interviewer-administered interviews, but the interviewer-administered version with the instruction to the interviewer not to read the specified categories cannot be used in the self-administered procedures.

The same complications occur with respect to the consistency checks. The previous section showed two procedures to deal with inconsistencies. One was interviewer-dependent, as the interviewer just got a message that inconsistencies had occurred, and the names of the questions involved were presented. It was then up to the interviewer to decide how to solve these inconsistencies. This procedure cannot be used in self-administered interviews.

The second procedure took into account all possible errors and proposed several specific questions to solve the inconsistency. It is this procedure that should be used for self-administered interviews. Again, procedures for self-administered interviewing, being more explicit, can be used in inter-viewer-administered procedures, but not vice versa.

Use of Visual Aids. One of the procedures frequently used to improve data quality is the use of visual aids. As seen above, the use of these tools is not possible in the CATI application and is difficult in CAPI applications that are interviewer-administered, but in self-administered procedures they can be used.

An example would be the use of pictures to help respondents remember whether they have seen or read a newspaper or magazine, whether they know a certain person, and so forth. In media research, such aids play an important role. For example, if one would like to know if people have seen the latest edition of a magazine, it is often very difficult without visual aids for them to remember whether they have seen it. They may not know whether the last issue they have seen was from this week or last week. If, however, the front page of the magazine is shown and they are asked to say whether they have seen it, it is easier for the respondent to answer the question correctly.

Technically, the application of these procedures in self-administered questionnaires is not difficult. The pictures can be scanned and stored on the interview diskette. In the question text, an instruction can be given that the picture can be obtained by pressing a function key (Sociometric Research Foundation, 1988). When the key is pressed, the picture appears on the screen, and when the respondent wants to return to the questionnaire, the same function key is pressed again. If the picture does not cover the whole screen, it also can be integrated into the questionnaire text, with the question text around the picture. With modern text processors, these procedures are not too difficult, but they do take time.

The fact that the pictures require a lot of space in memory and on the diskettes can cause problems. A full-sized picture requires 64 KB. One solution is to combine several pictures on one screen, which would still require 64 KB but now for, say, four pictures instead of one. Another possibility would be to use pictures that are smaller than a full screen. A third possibility is to use the larger storage capacities of hard disks, although this would be much more expensive.

Use of a Calendar. Another application of visual aids is the use of calendars in interviews. In the literature, the problems of memory effect, complete loss of memory, and telescoping have been mentioned frequently (e.g., Sikkel, 1985; Sudman and Bradburn, 1974). The solution to this problem suggested in the literature is to offer reference points in time by providing a calendar. In interviewer-administered interviews this is too difficult, but in self-administered interviews it is no problem; the procedure can be organized in the same way as for the pictures in the previous example. If the respondent presses a function key, the calendar is shown, and if he or she presses it again, the calendar disappears, and the program returns to the appropriate question in the questionnaire (Kersten, 1988). Various well-known events can be noted in the calendar, such as national holidays (e.g., Memorial Day) and religious feasts (e.g., Christmas); the birthdays of the respondent and other members of the household also can be included if this information is available. With these dates fixed in the calendar, it has been suggested that other activities, such as visits to the doctor, purchases, or other behavior, can be located more precisely in time (Loftus and Marburger, 1983).

Summary and Correction Screens. A similar tool to improve the quality of the data in self-administered interviews is the *summary and correction screen,* or SC screen. In Chapter 1, we mentioned that CADAC has the disadvantage that respondents and interviewers face the problem that the answers are typed on the keyboard but the questions are presented on the screen, which might lead to errors in the responses. Also, for other reasons, errors can occur in the data. These errors might remain undetected by range checks and consistency checks because they represent plausible answers, but these answers may be incorrect nevertheless. If branching and skipping depend on these answers, this might lead to problems later in the interview. Therefore, SC screens have been developed (Kersten, Verweij, Hartman, and Gallhofer, 1990). These screens summarize important responses and allow the respondent to make corrections. These procedures are especially useful before important branching decisions are made.

A typical example of such a situation is information on the household. If this information about the members of the household and their ages is to be used later on in the interview, (e.g., to select the persons who should be asked for further information about their work hours in the past week), it is very important that the basic household information is correct, or problems will arise.

These problems can be twofold. The less difficult problem is that for one person the information is not requested, when it should have been. The second, more serious problem that can arise is that information is requested about a certain person when this person is, for example, too young to work. In such a situation, the respondent will have problems if no easy way out is provided. However, if the information was requested far back in the questionnaire, returning to the question is very difficult. In this case, the respondent has serious problems.

In order to avoid such problems, the vital information used for later branching should be summarized in an SC screen, and the respondent should be asked to check the information once more very carefully. It would take too much space to show the whole procedure here, but a typical SC screen for a household with four people (two parents and two children) is presented in Figure 2.5.

For the lines that are incorrect, questions about the name and age follow again. Then the SC screen is given again, and this procedure is repeated until the respondent is satisfied with the result. This procedure does not give a complete guarantee of the correctness of the data, but it certainly ensures the quality of the data better than procedures that do not use SC screens.

Psychophysical Scaling. The previous section showed that interviewer-administered interviews cannot make use of scales with many categories unless show cards are used, because respondents cannot remember all the categories that have been read to them. In self-administered procedures this is not a problem, because the respondents can always look back. They have the time and all the information in front of them. This means that this limitation does not apply to the procedures discussed here. However, not only can questions with many categories be used, but also there are possibilities that are completely out of the question in interviewer-administered

```
┌─────────────────────────────────────┐
│  Person            Age              │
│  (1)  John          40              │
│  (2)  Mary          39              │
│  (3)  Harry         17              │
│  (4)  Lucy          12              │
│                                     │
│  Please check carefully whether the names │
│  and ages of the people in the table are correct │
│  because other questions depend on this │
│  information being correct.         │
│                                     │
│   If all information is correct, type 0 │
│   and press F5                      │
│                                     │
│   If lines are incorrect type their numbers │
│   with a return in between          │
│   and press F5.                     │
└─────────────────────────────────────┘
```

Figure 2.5. Typical SC Screen for Household of Four People

interviews. These possibilities include the use of all kinds of scales that make use of some kind of response manipulations by the respondent. Some examples of such scales are analogue-rating scales, line-production scales, sound-production scales, and other psychophysical scales (Lodge, 1981; Saris, 1982; Stevens, 1975; Wegener, 1982).

These scales have an advantage over the commonly used categorical scales in that they allow the respondents to express their opinions on continuous scales. This allows more precision in expressing their opinions (Lodge, 1981). This is an important point, because van Doorn, Saris, and Lodge, (1983) and Költringer (1991) have shown that the categorization of theoretically continuous variables can lead to considerable bias in the estimates of the strength of relations between variables.

The attraction of the CADAC procedures for these scaling purposes is that one can ask the respondents to express their opinions through the length of lines that are automatically measured by the computer. This way, one does not have to rely on manual measurement, as was done in early experiments with psychophysical scales (see Lodge, Cross, Tursky, and Tanenhaus, 1975).

206

Furthermore, the availability of different modalities for the expression of opinions makes it easier to ask respondents to express their opinion twice, in different modalities. These repeated observations make it easier to correct for unavoidable measurement errors without reducing the validity of the measures. For detailed discussion of these points, see the psychometric literature (e.g., Lord and Novick, 1968) and sociometric literature (e.g., Andrews, 1984; Saris, 1982; Saris and Andrews, in press).

These procedures are not without problems, however, due to the variability in the way people answer questions. Each respondent can use his or her own scale to express his or her opinions, but due to this variation in the response scales (or as Saris, 1988, has called it, the variation in the response functions), the scores obtained for the different respondents are not comparable. In order to remedy this point, more complex instructions to the respondents are necessary. A previous section showed that complex instructions can lead to problems in interviewer-administered interviews, but not as much as in self-administered interviews. The following section will deal with complex instructions, and so also will illustrate the psychophysical scales.

Complex Instructions. Psychophysical scaling (and other questions) requires a complex instruction, which could lead to problems in interviewer-administered interviews, but not in self-administered questionnaires. The reason is the same as before: respondents can look back and find very quickly what they have forgotten. We will illustrate this point with an example of psychophysical scaling, taking into account the problem of variation in response functions across respondents. Bon (1988) has shown that it is impossible to correct for the variation in the response functions. Therefore, if one wishes to use individual data or the study of relationships between variables, the only possible solution is to prevent the variation in response functions as far as possible. Experiments by Saris, van de Putte, Maas, and Seip (1988), Batista and Saris (1988), and Saris and de Rooy (1988) have made it clear that providing respondents with not one reference point, as is commonly done, but two reference points with a fixed meaning will improve the data considerably. In other words, these authors suggest that instructions like the one below should be used:

We are now going to ask your opinion about a number of issues. If you are in complete agreement with the expressed opinion, draw a line of the following length:

_____

If you completely disagree with an opinion, draw a line like this:

‾‾‾

The more you agree, the longer the line you should draw.

Although clearly such a scale is not possible in an interviewer-administered interview because of the use of line production, the instruction is still too complicated even if magnitude estimation is used instead of line production.

The above scale has been used for many years with very good results, frequently leading to reliabilities of 0.90 to 0.95, which is very high compared with other scales (Saris, 1989). One of the reasons for these good results is the extra precision of the 38-point scale. Another reason is that the scale is fixed by two reference points.

This overview has shown that the self-administered questionnaire has quite a number of advantages over the interviewer-administered interview. In the previous section, we described some procedures that can help keep the quality high. In this section, we pointed to several procedures that can improve the quality. But, again, these advantages are not obtained for free. They require extra effort from the designer of the questionnaire. The formulation demands more effort and time. And it is not only the writing of the questionnaire that requires extra time, but the testing of the questionnaire as well.

One of the reasons why testing is necessary is that help screens are essential components of these questionnaires, and the best place for these help screens can only be found through tests. How the tests are carried out will be discussed later.

Computer-Assisted Panel Research

As mentioned previously, computer-assisted panel research can be done by CATI, CAPI, computer-assisted mail interviewing (CAMI), tele-interviewing, or videotext systems. The rest of this chapter will concentrate on the continuous character of panel research and on the possibilities it offers to improve the quality of the data collection if any type of CADAC is used. In this section, we will return to several topics already mentioned, but with the difference that we now will be making use of a continuous stream of information about the same persons. This means that not only information about background variables, but also information about several important variables at different points in time will be available. A typical example of research where such a situation occurs is the ongoing family expenditure studies that are carried out in many countries and that normally are done by a combination of personal interviews and self-administered diaries.

In order to refine these procedures, some new facilities have been developed, which can be classified into two groups: procedures with the aim of directly reducing the number of errors, and procedures designed to reduce the amount of effort on the part of the respondent. The second type of procedure also may lead to a reduction in the number of errors, but only indirectly. We will discuss both types of procedures.

New Procedures for Data Validation. The most common procedures for data validation or editing are range checks and consistency checks across time. In paper-and-pencil interviews, these checks are performed after the data have been collected. At that moment, when the respondent is no longer available, errors are difficult to correct, but at least one can clean the data and eventually assign some values for erroneous answers on the basis of some more or less plausible assumptions.

A fundamental difference with computer-assisted interviewing is that the checks are all performed during the interview while the respondent is still present. This means that the respondent can immediately correct any errors. If all the possible and necessary checks are done during the interview, the validation phase after the data collection can be eliminated, or at least considerably reduced.

All the procedures discussed so far use data from one interview. In panel research, one gets an extra source of information to check the quality of the data, namely, the information from the previous interview(s). Validation procedures that use this information are dynamic range and consistency checks, dynamic SC screens, and dynamic calendars. We will discuss these different procedures in sequence.

Dynamic Range and Consistency Checks. *Range checks* are checks that are based on prior knowledge of the possible answers. For example, if the question is about the prices of different products, it is easy to type in "200" instead of "20"; such errors can lead to values that are too high by a factor of 10 or more. Most interview programs have the facility to specify range checks on the answers. For example, the program INTERV can specify a lower and an upper bound for continuous responses. If the program detects an answer outside the acceptable range, it automatically mentions at the bottom of the screen that the answer should be within the specified range and the response is ignored, which means that the respondent has to answer again.

These range checks are "hard checks" in the sense that one cannot continue with the next question until an answer is given that falls within the acceptable range. It will be clear that one should be very careful with these hard checks in order to avoid problems. This means that they are normally only used for checks on obvious typing errors, where it is certain that the answer is wrong.

A second type of check that can be performed and that is also available in most interview programs is to specify the conditions under which a question is presented. This procedure can be used for consistency checks, because these checks are used as conditions for questions that ask for clarification. We have discussed these possibilities before, but will give another example. If we are interested in people's income, we might ask those who work the following question:

Type=price range=[1   200,000] var=income
How much did you earn last month?

In the Netherlands, we would expect an answer between 1,000 and, say, 10,000 gulden (one U.S. dollar equals approximately two guldens). All answers outside this range are very unlikely, but not impossible. This means that we cannot do a range check using these values. A range check can only be done with the values 1 and perhaps 200,000.

But in order to have a more sensitive check, we can use a "soft check," which consists of a conditional question only asked if the answer to the first question is below 1,000 gulden and above, for example, 5,000 gulden. The extra question would be

Type=price var=check
Condition (1000>income or income>5000)
You gave a very unlikely income of "income "
If you made a mistake, press F1 and answer the question again. If the answer is correct go on to the next question by pressing ENTER.

This example shows that this is not a hard check. The answer may be correct even though it is very deviant, and in that case the respondent can go on; but in 99% of cases the answers will be wrong, and the respondent is given a chance to correct the error.

The latter checking procedure is already much more flexible than the range check, but it is still very rough and can be annoying for people with a very deviant income, because in a panel study they will get the correction question each time their income is requested. This is neither necessary nor desirable, and should be avoided so as not to annoy the respondent.

Therefore, a dynamic range check should be used that adapts to the information given through time, on the basis that the information about a person at time t is often the same as at time t - 1. Thus, if the information about income at t can be saved and used the next time, this would be the most efficient check on the answers in an interview. The above specified procedure could then be adjusted as follows:

Type=price var=check
Condition {$(.9*$income$(t-1)>$income$)$ or $(1.1*$income$(t-1)<$income$)$}
You gave a very unlikely income of "income
whereas, last time your income was "income$(t-1)$"
If you made a mistake, press F1 and answer the question again. If the answer is correct, go on to the next question.

Now, the check question is asked whenever the income has been changed by more than 10%, but not if the income is deviant but stable. We consider this to be the most efficient way of making checks, for the following reasons: (a) The range specified can be as narrow as one wishes, (b) it uses as much information as possible from the respondent, (c) people with a constant but deviant position are not bothered all the time by check questions, and (d) the check adjusts itself automatically to a changing situation. If someone's income changes, the check will be adjusted the next time, too.

Here we have given the example of an income question, but the same procedures can be used for many more variables, such as expenditure components (Hartman and Saris, 1991).

Dynamic SC screens. A second general procedure that has been developed to provide possibilities for error correction is the use of SC screens. In panel research, these procedures differ from the SC screens in cross-sectional research in that information from a previous wave can be used.

Let us continue with the example of the income question to illustrate this possibility. If we ask a household for the first time about their incomes, and three out of five people in the household have an income, a typical answer

Person	Income Last Month
(1) John	2,000
(2) Mary	9,000
(3) Harry	1,200
(4) Anna	0
(5) Elizabeth	0

If there is anything wrong in this summary, type the numbers of the lines that are incorrect with a return in between: press F5 if your answer is finished.

If nothing is wrong, press 0 and F5 to continue.

Figure 2.6. An Example of a SC Screen

could be like the one shown in Figure 2.6. This example illustrates a situation where it is possible that all information is correct, but where it is also possible that Mary's income is 10 times too high due to a typing error. The respondent who is filling in the questionnaire will spot this error immediately and correct it, whereas there is no way a program can detect the error if it is the first interview. Furthermore, the next time the question of Mary's income arises, the dynamic range check will assume that her income is 9,000 gulden and will start to complain if the answer given is 900. As this could lead to confusion, the information should be checked before it is used in the next interview. The SC screen provides an easy way to make these corrections.

In panel research, SC screens can be used very efficiently if they are slightly adjusted. Providing the respondents immediately with information about the previous wave and asking them for corrections may prevent errors. The previous example would be adjusted in the manner indicated in Figure 2.7.

The purpose of this procedure is to prevent typing errors as much as possible and to reduce the effort for the respondent. Both purposes are realized by prespecifying, on the basis of the existing information, the most likely answer. If no change has occurred the respondent has only to type a "0" and to press RETURN to answer for all household members the questions about their incomes. If one of the incomes has changed only that income needs to be corrected, and not all incomes must be specified again.

```
According to our information the members
of your household had the following incomes:

Person                  Income in
                        September

(1) John                2,000
(2) Mary                  900
(3) Harry               1,200
(4) Anna                    0
(5) Elizabeth               0


If the incomes have changed in October, press the
numbers of the lines that are incorrect with
a return in between; press F5 if your
answer is finished.

If all the incomes remain the same, press 0 and F5 to continue.
```

Figure 2.7. An Example of a Dynamic SC Screen

In this way the respondent's task is made easier, as discussed below, but more important, one can avoid many typing errors without reducing the possibility of specifying changes. The procedure also is designed in such a way that changes through time automatically are taken into account. For this reason, it is called a *dynamic* SC screen.

A Dynamic Calendar. In a previous section, the possibility of preventing errors due to memory failure by using a calendar was mentioned, including public holidays and personal information that could be found in the background variables. However, in panel research, one is getting much more information through time. For example, it is possible to mention in the calendar specific events like visits to the hospital by a family member, a change of job, a special party, or any other event that has been mentioned by the respondents as important. The introduction of these events into the calendar gives the respondents many more reference points to determine when other specific events occurred. The information about these events can be collected during the panel study in other surveys. It is also possible to build up this information from questionnaires on different topics, such as school career, working career, and so forth.

Such procedures might be especially attractive for collecting information about life histories, which is a very popular topic in sociology nowadays.

Life histories are very difficult to specify without memory aids. A calendar full of information about events in the life of the respondent might be a very useful tool for improving the data quality in these studies.

Procedures to Reduce the Work for Respondents. Having discussed several procedures for the detection and correction of errors in the data, we now present some procedures to reduce the workload of the respondents. These procedures do not prevent or correct errors directly, but it can be expected that reducing the workload of the respondents will improve the data they provide and reduce their reluctance to cooperate in unattractive questionnaires. Here, we discuss three different approaches: the use of dynamic SC screens, scheduling, and grouping in SC screens.

The Use of Dynamic SC Screens. In paper-and-pencil questionnaires the possibilities for branching are very limited. Therefore, a large number of questions are printed and asked that do no apply to a specific person. For example, if a person has a pension and is not working anymore, all questions with respect to income from work, holiday money, overtime, and so on, do not apply. Nevertheless, in paper-and-pencil interviews these questions still exist, and it is up to the interviewer to determine which to skip and which to ask. If the conditions for skipping are very simple, an interviewer can do the job, but the interviewer does not have the time or the capability to evaluate complex conditions.

In computer-assisted interviewing, any level of complex branching is possible as long as the researcher understands what she or he is doing. The advantages of automatic branching in the questionnaire are that no errors occur in the branching, thus avoiding partial nonresponse, and that the amount of text the respondent has to read is reduced.

For the pensioner mentioned above, all questions about work as a source of income are automatically skipped, reducing the number of questions considerably. The same kind of approach can be used for information about the household, work, the home, the children's school, and so forth.

However, in panel research one has to take into account that the composition of the household can change, that people may change jobs, move to another house, and so on. This means that it is not enough to request this information once. The information has to be updated in order to prevent errors when it is used for branching in other questionnaires. For this purpose, SC screens are very useful because they allow a very brief summary of the information and allow quick updates. For example, the household information can be summarized in a screen such as the one shown in Figure 2.8.

214

According to our records, your situation was as follows in the last interview. Please check if the situation is still the same.

Person	Work/School	#hours	Where
(1) John	work	38	university
(2) Anna	work	22	school
(3) Harry	work	38	Philips
(4) Mary	school	—	secondary
(5) Elizabeth	school	—	primary

If there is anything wrong in this summary, press the numbers of the lines that are incorrect with a return in between; press F5 if your answer is finished.

If nothing is wrong, press 0 and F5 to continue.

Figure 2.8. An SC Screen of the Household Box Information

In this way, this information does not have to be requested again. The information from the last interview is presented and the respondents can immediately see whether or not there has been any change in their situation since the last interview; if so, they can give their new situation by replying to a few follow-up questions. After this check, which normally takes less than a minute, the updated information can be used for the rest of the interview.

Clearly, this procedure is very efficient, especially in panel research, and will save the respondents a lot of effort, leaving them to concentrate on the new questions and, most likely, to answer them with more precision and care.

Scheduling. Background information can be used not only to reduce the number of questions asked, but also to evaluate the regularity of information that is collected. For example, in the Netherlands, family allowance money comes only once every 3 months, and the telephone bill must be paid only once every 3 months. The same might be true for mortgages, energy bills, and so forth, and often insurance is paid only once a year. Membership fees for different organizations will fall due at different times, but in general there will be a fixed sequence of months in which payment is required. If detailed information is requested once, so that not only the amount is known, but also when the last payment was made and how many months it covered, then an intelligent interview program can calculate the next time that the same payment has to be made. If the amount to be paid is stored, the program can even mention something such as the following:

According to our calculations, last month you had to pay your mortgages, and the amount you had to pay was ___ gulden.
Did you indeed pay this amount last month?
1 = yes.
0 = no.

If the answer is "no," extra questions are asked about the reasons for the change, but normally the amounts and timing will be correct. This way, the amount of effort required of the respondent is much less than when all the different regular expenditures have to be evaluated in the traditional way.

In the months when there is no payment to be made, the work is reduced even further, because in those months the question can be skipped completely, or one can use the same procedure to suggest that the people had nothing to pay this month and ask for a confirmation or correction.

This procedure, which we have called *scheduling,* has been used for all regular income sources and expenditures (Kersten et al., 1990). It considerably reduces the amount of work required of the respondents, especially when combined with the procedure described below.

Grouping in SC Screens. A very simple but efficient way to reduce the amount of work for the respondents is the use of *natural grouping* of items in SC screens. This is especially efficient for regular sources of income and expenditure. By natural grouping, we mean an ordering of the items in such a way that it is immediately clear to the respondents what the researcher wants to know.

If this procedure is combined with scheduling (allowing the respondent to type "0" and press RETURN if nothing has changed), then a long list of boring questions can be answered by one answer and in less than 30 seconds, and the procedure does not reduce the possibilities for indicating changes, because the respondent can correct any number on the screen.

Natural groupings of items can be used for many different topics (e.g., the household-box information, the income of the household, the costs of the house, insurance, membership fees, etc.). When the amounts obtained or spent do not change much through time, these procedures are very efficient and time-saving. If there are considerable changes in these amounts, there is no great advantage to be obtained using these methods, but they will certainly not increase the amount of work.

Some General Comments. Summarizing the above-specified options, panel research allows all the possibilities for improving data quality mentioned before.

The amount of possibilities depends on whether the procedure is interviewer-administered or self-administered. In this section, to the possibilities discussed earlier have been added procedures that are only possible in panel research. We have mentioned several procedures that prevent or detect errors in data and allow for corrections in panel research. These procedures directly improve the data collection: In this connection, we discussed dynamic range checks, dynamic SC screens, and the use of a dynamic calendar. Besides that, we discussed several procedures for reducing the amount of work required of the respondents. These procedures do not directly lead to improvements in the data, but we would nevertheless expect a positive effect on the data quality due to the lesser burden on the respondents.

One point we have not yet mentioned is that the scheduling procedures also have the advantage of reminding the respondent very explicitly of a number of items that have to be mentioned. In this way, scheduling is a very attractive way of aiding the memory of the respondents. In this respect, these procedures are similar to what is known in the literature as *bounded recall,* where people are reminded of what they said last time in order to get better data this time (Neter and Waksberg, 1963, 1964, 1965). In our approach, this possibility is extended to offer memory support over much longer periods, because it is not necessarily the last answer that is mentioned, but the most appropriate answer for a particular point in time.

Of course, there are also disadvantages connected with these procedures. There is the danger of panel effects, but that is not a specific problem for the procedures mentioned here. This is a feature these procedures have in common with all others for panel research. More specific problems are the following: Respondents may have a tendency to indicate no change if this option is made too easy. If scheduling is used, small changes in time, an earlier payment, or a later payment than expected could lead to errors. These errors, however, can be solved relatively easily.

The tendency to indicate no change could be solved in two ways. One is to ask the respondents explicitly to confirm each separate item on the screen, which requires more effort and is not so different from changing a number. A second possibility is to introduce extra questions for those who indicate that no changes have occurred. These questions could appear to be checking why no changes have occurred. If the questions are complex enough and time-consuming enough to balance the two options, the respondents will not make unjustified use of the no-change option in the future. Further research on this point is necessary.

The second problem, of deviations from the expected schedule in periodic activities, can be counteracted by asking extra questions. For example, in a questionnaire asking about different periodic expenditures using a scheduling system, deviations from the scheduling can be counteracted by producing a screen specifying all relevant items where no payment is made, as follows:

Is it correct that you did not make any payment for the following items last month?
—
—

The lines refer to the different expenditures that were expected to be zero according to the scheduling system. The advantage of this procedure is that one can be more sure about the correctness of the data. On the other hand, it is more work for the respondents. Further research is required on this point as well.

For a delay in payment, the solution is much simpler. In that case the information that no payment was made or received is stored to be used in the next interview. In the next month's interview, the same question is asked again. This procedure is used for a number of income sources in questionnaires designed for income and expenditure by Kersten et al. (1990).

This section has shown that computer-assisted panel research has even more possibilities for improving data than the same procedures in cross-sectional research, but one has to check the questionnaires very carefully. Without good questionnaire-checking procedures, there is a serious danger that the complex questionnaires themselves are going to produce errors, due to errors in the programs. Besides this, the programs can become so complex that one will be very reluctant to ever change the questionnaire, because any change would be very difficult to incorporate. As a consequence, the data collection procedures can become inflexible. Researchers will have to decide in the future which characteristic of the data collection instruments they will give priority to: research flexibility or the quality of the collected data. This point and other points connected with the technical aspects of designing CADAC questionnaires are the topic of Chapter 3.

3. WRITING QUESTIONNAIRES

In the first two chapters, we have tried to impress on the reader that designing CADAC questionnaires requires not only the commonly recognized skills for writing questionnaires, as discussed in many textbooks, but also some new skills related to the new possibilities of CADAC. In the past, many designers of programs for CADAC, myself included, have tried to make the point that for their program the questionnaire designer only needs the skills needed to design paper-and-pencil questionnaires. This is indeed true for certain programs, if one does not design complex questionnaires and if one does not use all the possibilities of the systems.

House (1985), Nicholls and House (1987), and House and Nicholls (1988) have argued very convincingly that CATI instruments should be treated not only as survey questionnaires but also as computer programs. Their arguments should be extended to any type of CADAC instrument. Therefore, it is also necessary in this monograph to discuss the programming aspects of these procedures. Because House and Nicholls have made a considerable effort to clarify this point, we will rely in this chapter very much on their contribution, but will generalize their arguments to any type of computer-assisted data collection system.

Looking at the design of questionnaires from a programming point of view, it seems reasonable that the instruments should satisfy the following requirements:

The first and most obvious requirement is that the questionnaire should be able to collect the information for which it has been designed, under all circumstances. Nicholls and House have paid a lot of attention in their papers to the fact that questionnaires should produce correct results not only under normal circumstances, going forward in the questionnaire, but also if one goes back in the questionnaire to change some answers, or if one takes any other action that the system permits. It requires a lot of effort to check whether a program is correct under normal conditions, let alone to check whether programs work correctly under all circumstances.

Second, the instruments should be designed in such a way that it is not too difficult to change the questionnaire for future use. This requirement is not automatically satisfied. Questionnaires can be so complex, as we have mentioned before, that researchers will be very reluctant to change them for fear that the first requirement of correctness will not be satisfied anymore. If the use of CADAC instruments were to result in inflexible questionnaire design, this would be a very bad consequence. Therefore, extra attention should be paid to this point in the design stage.

The third requirement House and Nicholls (1988) have drawn attention to is the *portability* of questionnaires. By portability, they mean that it should be easy to use the same questionnaire or parts of a questionnaire in different studies without the risk of getting a lot of errors. It is, of course, always possible to adjust a new questionnaire till it satisfies the first criterion mentioned above, but it is better to take portability into account during the actual design of the questionnaire, so that one does not need so much time for testing.

The last point we would like to mention is the requirement for questionnaires to be designed in such a way that not only the first author but also other people can change the questionnaire and use it in different contexts. If this requirement is not satisfied, the effort put into the design of a complex questionnaire cannot be fully exploited. Given the mobility of highly qualified people, even the best questionnaires will have a short life if this requirement is not taken very seriously.

In order to satisfy these requirements, one has to take them into account in the process of designing questionnaires. We will make some general remarks about what this means for the design of instruments first, and then in the rest of this chapter we will try to make some suggestions for structuring the design process so that these rules are taken into account.

Starting with the first requirement, it will be clear that a lot of testing is needed before one can be sure that the questionnaire program satisfies this requirement. These tests can be divided into three subtests. The first is the test of the syntax of the questionnaire, the second is the test of the branching and skipping procedures, and the third is the test of correct interpretation by respondents. The first two types of tests evaluate quite different aspects of the questionnaire. Even if the syntax of a questionnaire is correct, this does not guarantee at all that the appropriate information will be collected.

These two types of tests are only sufficient for testing the correctness of the code. They do not guarantee that the questions will be correctly interpreted by respondents. This aspect of the correctness requires field tests in small pilot studies.

However, syntactic and semantic correctness and validity do not guarantee correctness under all circumstances (e.g., under conditions of backing up and making corrections). Nicholls and House (1987) have correctly stressed this point, arguing that programs should be designed in such a way that no errors result from such moves. We will return to this important point in the next chapter. In this chapter, we will concentrate on the other tests to satisfy the requirement of correctness of the questionnaire.

The second important requirement mentioned was flexibility, so that the questionnaires can be changed. This requirement can be satisfied if the questionnaire is designed in such a way that the effects of changes in the questionnaire are limited in scope. In other words, it should be easy to determine what part of the program will be affected by any change. In computer programming, modular design is used for this purpose. This means that one "decomposes" the total task of the program into subtasks and then

220

subdivides these further, until one reaches a very elementary level of sub-routines that can exist independently of each other, and therefore can be designed and tested independently of the other parts of the program. These independent parts, which we call *modules,* can be changed without affecting the other parts of the program as long as the input and output remain the same. From a CADAC point of view, groups of questions concerned with a similar topic should be grouped in such modules. By doing so, changes can be introduced into modules without affecting other parts of the questionnaire. In this way, future changes in the questionnaire are already taken into account in the design.

The use of modules also can be very helpful in making the questionnaire, or parts of it, portable. Given that the modules are clearly defined with respect to their input, output and function, they can be easily implemented in other questionnaires as well. So the modular design also satisfies the third require-ment. It is then possible to make a kind of "library" of modules that can be combined to formulate questionnaires for different studies.

Finally, the use of a clear design using modules helps to make it possible for different people to understand the same questionnaire. But normally this is not enough. Often the designs still can be so difficult that a second researcher will be afraid to look into somebody else's program. In order to avoid this as far as possible, one should add to the modular design a good documentation of each module. This should be done both on paper and in the questionnaire, if the CADAC program allows such comments.

Often the documentation is left till last, and it is common practice not to do it at all. This common practice has a devastating effect on the life span of questionnaires. Therefore, the documentation should be taken up during the design of the questionnaire. This has the further advantage that it also simpli-fies communication. We will come back to this point later.

These considerations have led to the formulation of the following impor-tant steps, which should be taken into consideration during the design of a questionnaire:

1. Start by decomposing the research problem into smaller tasks that can be studied independently of all other parts. If these smaller tasks, or modules, are con-nected to each other, indicate the order in which they should be performed.
2. Design the procedure to be used for each module, using flow charts to document the program.
3. Specify the questionnaire, the input and output variables needed in the module, the criterion values used for checks and branchings that might be variable through time, and the responses that will be produced.

4. Test the syntax and semantics of each module and the combination of modules.
5. Do a field test with the questionnaire in the presence of an interviewer in order to establish whether the respondents understand the questions in the way they are supposed to be understood.
6. Check if the program generates the data that are needed, for the statistical analysis.

Only after all these steps have been carried out successfully can one have some assurance that the questionnaire satisfies the above specified criteria with respect to quality, flexibility, portability, and understandability. It also means that one can be reasonably sure that the instrument will work without too many problems and that the data will satisfy the data requirements.

In the next section, we will say a few more words about each of these steps in the design process and illustrate the procedure with an example. The example that will be used is a questionnaire designed by Kersten et al. (1990) for family income and expenditure surveys, designed for a completely automatic panel study.

The Modularization of the Questionnaire

Most of the time, questionnaires are too complex to be designed as a whole. It is better to divide the questionnaire into parts that perform different tasks. In order to arrive at the level of manageable modules, one sometimes has to decompose the different parts several times.

In the income and expenditure survey mentioned above, four different parts were distinguished, and then the expenditure questionnaire was again split into two parts: one part for regular expenditure and one for incidental expenditure. This decomposition process led to the following five quite independent modules.

- The household box
- The special-events box
- The income box
- Regular-expenditure box
- The incidental-expenditure box

The first two questionnaires were planned to provide the background information needed in the other three questionnaires to reduce the size of the questionnaires for the respondents.

The household box asks for all necessary information about the household composition. This information plays a role in the questions about income; for example, children under 12 will not be asked about their work. Note that the household box provides information for the income box but not vice versa; the questionnaires need to be presented in a specific order, but they can be developed independently.

In the special-events box, information about the house and any illnesses in the last month is asked for. This information is needed from all household members, so the household box must be filled in before the special-events questionnaire. The information from the latter questionnaire then is used in the questionnaire about expenditure.

The use of information from one questionnaire in another determines the sequence of the questionnaires, as indicated in Figure 3.1. The sequence is indicated by the direction of the arrows. The figure shows that the question-naires have to be done in sequence, going from the top (the household box) to the bottom (the regular expenditure box).

Figure 3.1 also indicates that each questionnaire has its own information source that is used after the first interview, called a *matrix*. These matrices are intended to be used for presentation in the dynamic SC screens in order to update the information on the specific topic. This example shows quite clearly how the decomposition of the questionnaire into modules can be represented. A rather complex questionnaire is presented here in a very simple way. Once this picture is understood, each individual module can be considered without worrying about the other modules in the questionnaire. This is precisely the reason for decomposing the questionnaire.

Design of the Modules

Before the questionnaire is written in detail, it always makes sense to make a flow chart of the questionnaire to be developed. In doing so, the problems of the questionnaire will become clear and one can look for solutions by improving the flow chart. Different rules for the formulation of flow charts are used in practice (Jabine, 1985). The rules we have used are indicated in the flow chart of the household box, presented in Figure 3.2.

In Figure 3.2, the following rules have been applied:

1. Procedures that indicate decisions by the program have been indicated by diamonds; for example, if it is the first interview, the program follows the scheme on the right, and if it is a subsequent interview the program starts on the left.

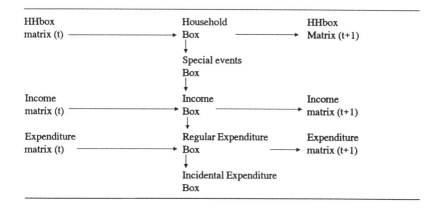

Figure 3.1. The Structure of an Income and Expenditure Questionnaire

2. Questions to which the responses determine the further procedures are presented in screens with the question text. For example, the question "How many people are living in the household?" determines later on how many questions have to be asked about names, birthdays, and so on.

3. Elaborate procedures containing sets of questions concerning factual information are presented in boxes, and the topics are indicated with bold letters. We call these procedures *question procedures*.

4. SC screens are presented by a combination of a screen and a question. For example, there is an SC screen with the text:

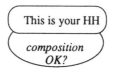

The top part indicates that an SC screen is presented and the bottom part shows the question presented on the screen.

5. Arrows indicate the direction in which the process goes. A double headed arrow indicates that the process can go back and forth. For example, if the names are incorrect, the program goes to the procedure "correct names." There the correct names are requested. Then the result is again presented and checked by the respondent. If there is still an error, further corrections can be made, and so on.

224

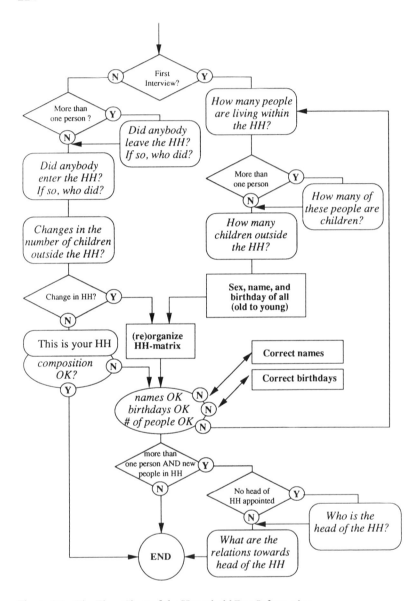

Figure 3.2. The Flow Chart of the Household Box Information

It should be mentioned that range checks and consistency checks are not indicated in this figure. For most of the questions, checks could be specified: Loops and question procedures should be indicated for all questions, but this would take too much space and would be more confusing than clarifying. Therefore, the checks are not indicated in the flow chart.

Having described the form of presentation used in the flow charts, we can now describe the basic characteristics of the household-box questionnaire as presented here.

First of all, a distinction is made as to whether it is the first interview or not. If it is the first interview, all the basic information has to be collected as indicated on the right-hand side of Figure 3.2. Once all the necessary information has been collected, an SC screen is presented to ask the respondent to check the correctness of the information. If errors are present, corrections can be made until all information is correct according to the respondent. Finally a "head of the household" is chosen. When this choice has been made, the questionnaire asks the relationship of all persons in the household to the head of this household. After these questions the process is finished and the next interview can start.

If the respondent has to fill in this questionnaire again, the procedure is normally much simpler because most of the information concerning names, gender, ages, and so forth remains the same. The only possible changes are that someone has left the household or has come into the household.

If nothing has changed, the respondent goes immediately to the SC screen that provides all the information about the household and asks whether the composition is still the same. If that is the case, this questionnaire is finished and new interviews can be carried out. If changes have occurred, minor corrections have to be specified, the SC screen is again shown, and then the questionnaire is finished. The use of the SC screen in this case is clearly very efficient and saves a lot of time and effort.

This illustration indicates very well the usefulness of the flow charts. It is a handy tool for the design of questionnaires. It also facilitates discussions with clients and other designers of questionnaires about the structure of the questionnaire.

On the other hand, the design is still not complete with the design of the flow chart. Often, the final formulation of the questionnaire is a creative process that can change the flow chart. The design of a flow chart, however, is a useful tool not only for communication between researchers but also as documentation for later use.

Specification of the Questionnaire

The next step is the specification of the questionnaire itself. Although the flow chart specifies in considerable detail what should be written in the questionnaire, the flow chart is still program independent and easily understood. The text written for different CADAC programs starting with the same flow chart can be very different. Also, the way the text will be produced is very different: Some remarks on this point will be made in the next chapter. Here we will concentrate on the more general aspect of the specification of the questionnaire. Having specified the flow chart, the following steps still must be taken.

- Edit the questions in sequence and in the appropriate syntax
- Specify the branching and skipping
- Specify any procedures not yet specified
- Specify consistency checks and the extra questions necessary for this purpose
- Specify the information saved and stored for later use
- Specify the responses to be stored in the data file

In this process, so many new components will be added to the questionnaire that it is necessary for documentation purposes to provide additional information (besides the flow chart) in order to make the questionnaire understandable to other people. One way to do this is to provide a paper version of the questionnaire text as well as the computer version of it. In itself, however, this is not enough. It is very useful to do the following.

- Place comments in the questionnaire text, if possible
- Provide an overview of the different variables that are used in the module

An illustration of the first recommendation would be to write in the questionnaire text "The procedure CORRECT NAMES starts here" or "Variable V1 contains the age of the respondent" or "Consistency check of the age and relationship with the head of the household." The structure of the questionnaire is much easier to understand with the help of such comments.

The second point mentioned concerns the specification of variables. The specification of the variables has two purposes. The first purpose is to indicate what values have been chosen for the constants used in the questionnaire. Criteria for consistency checks are relatively arbitrary. For example, a clarifying question can be asked when the father is 50 years older than his presumed daughter or when the age difference is only 13 years. However, these criteria are arbitrary. In order to indicate which criteria are used and to be able to correct them in all places where they are used simultaneously, one can start the interview with a specification of the values of these constants by writing (for example)

V60=50 \ the upper limit for a father-daughter age difference\
V61=13 \ the lower limit for a father-daughter age difference\

In the questionnaire, the check now is written as

If (age>v60) or (age<v61) then . . .

If in a later study these limits need to be changed, they can be changed on the first page of the questionnaire, and this change automatically will be taken into account at all places in the questionnaire where V60 or V61 is used. This procedure will prevent programming errors that occur when a correction is forgotten.

The second purpose of the specification of the variables is to indicate explicitly the relationship between the module and other parts of the questionnaire. The other parts can only communicate with the module in question by providing information about values of input variables or by using the values of the output variables obtained from the relevant module. In the case of the household box, the input and output variables are the same. These variables, for all members of the household, are membership number, gender, year of birth, day of birth, relationship with the head of the household, membership number of last month, and the name of the respondent. This information is summarized in Table 3.1. The household box module uses this information for specification of the SC screens of the next month (input); the same variables also are produced by this module as output variables each month, and these values will be used in other modules to reduce the number of questions in them.

Finally, it is useful to make a list for each module of the responses that are returned to the researcher for further analysis. It is possible that not all answers will be of interest to the researcher; for example, if consistency checks are made, the incorrect answers do not have to be returned. In this case it should be clear which answers are to be returned and which are not. This information is important if one has to check whether the appropriate information is provided by the questionnaire.

TABLE 3.1

The Variables Used in the Household Box

Member	1	2	3	4	5	6	7	8	9
Member # last month	V11	V12	V13	V14	V15	V16	V17	V18	V19
Gender	V21	V22	V23	V24	V25	V26	V27	V28	V29
Year of birth	V31	V32	V33	V34	V35	V36	V37	V38	V39
Month of birth	V41	V42	V43	V44	V45	V46	V47	V48	V49
Day of birth	V51	V52	V53	V54	V55	V56	V57	V58	V59
Relationship with head	V61	V62	V63	V64	V65	V66	V67	V68	V69
Name	X11	X12	X13	X14	X15	X16	X17	X18	X19

The writing of the questionnaire is only a part of the task that must be performed. It should be kept in mind that the documentation is at least as important if one would like to use a specific questionnaire more than once.

Testing the Syntax and Branching

Any new questionnaire will contain some errors. These errors can be of different natures. One of the most difficult type of errors to avoid is the syntax error. By a syntax error, we mean that text is made that is not in agreement with the grammar used in the CADAC program. Such errors can lead to many problems if the program does not provide tools to detect them. The errors could appear very minor to the questionnaire constructor, but an omitted bracket or a comma instead of a period can interrupt the program, and the error can be very hard to detect.

In order to prevent such errors, some CADAC programs provide menu-driven questionnaire writing facilities. This makes it impossible to make syntactical errors. On the other hand, such programs often are not very sophisticated in their possible applications.

Other programs provide what amounts to a computer language to write questionnaires. The written code is compiled to make a questionnaire pro-gram. These programs normally have a facility in the compilation stage to indicate where a syntactical error has been found in the program.

Finally, there are CADAC programs that require the designer of the questionnaire to add some instructions for the program to a normal questionnaire. The INTERV program used in this monograph is an example of this type. Programs of this kind interpret the written text and present the different pieces of information on the screen. They normally do not have syntax-checking facilities. If there is an error, one will discover it while doing the interview, when the program ends in an error or does not present the correct questions and answer categories on the screen. Although these programs have the advantage that they do not require compilation, which means that the questionnaire can be used immediately, their disadvantage is that they do not indicate syntax errors. In the case of the INTERV program, this problem has been solved by developing another program (SYSFILE) that checks the syntax, among other things.

We cannot generalize much about these specific checking procedures, because they are very program-dependent. There is one general remark, however, that should be made on this point. Above, we have stressed the importance of modular design, partly with the testing problems in mind. It is of the utmost importance in the construction of complex questionnaires that they be tested at the modular level first. This makes the detection and correction of errors more simple and manageable. If one is testing large questionnaires, a diagnostic often is not very helpful, because it might be due to an error at a different point in the text. Also, the effect of changes at the modular level is very limited for the whole program, so the changes are also of restricted magnitude.

Only after all modules have been tested and shown to be correct, can one start testing the combination of modules. If an error is detected in a combination of modules that already have been tested, the error must lie in the connection between the modules. Thus, the modular construction also helps in the diagnostics.

Concerning the testing of the branching and skipping patterns in a questionnaire, the same argument holds: It is better to start by testing the modules before testing the whole questionnaire. In fact, it is even more necessary in this case, because there are as yet no formal tools available to check the validity of the branching and skipping specifications, although some theoretical work has begun in this field (Willenborg, 1989). Obvious errors that can be spotted very easily are (a) questions that cannot be reached from any other question, due to incorrect specification of a question name; and (b) branching that leads to the end of the questionnaire.

Such problems can even be indicated by a program; for example, the above mentioned program SYSFILE has these possibilities for questionnaires written for INTERV. But even in these cases, the programs cannot indicate where errors have been made in the branching and skipping specifications. This can only be determined by the researchers.

There are also many branchings that are correct from a syntactical point of view, but wrong from a theoretical point of view. In trying out a questionnaire, these errors will be detected if the order of the questions leads to very strange combinations. But the questionnaire also can look normal and nevertheless be wrong. If one does not have special tools, it can take a lot of time to detect these errors in a complex questionnaire, and one needs to have a very clear idea of what should happen in the questionnaire.

Programs could provide interpretations of the branching and skipping specifications in tree structures or other forms. If such presentations are compact and clear, they can provide a lot of help in the detection of errors. The development of such programs should be a top priority of survey-research programmers, because they would be very useful tools. Without these programs, one has to rely on manual checking of the questionnaires. This is a very time-consuming but nevertheless necessary task in all CADAC studies.

Testing Questionnaires in Pilot Studies

As we have already mentioned, the syntactical correctness and the validity of the branching and skipping specifications do not mean that the questionnaire will work properly. It is our experience, and the experience of many survey researchers, that carefully chosen text can be misinterpreted by respondents in many different ways.

For this reason, it is absolutely essential to test any CADAC instrument in the field in small pilot projects before it is used in a large survey. It is common practice to carry these tests out in two stages. The first test is done in the institute by other survey researchers, on the basis that a group always knows more than an individual. This is certainly a necessary step, but it is not sufficient to be sure of the correct interpretation. A second test then is done in a small field study, and should be carried out by interviewers even if the questionnaire is a self-administered questionnaire. In the latter case, the interviewer should not read the questions but only listen to the remarks the respondents are making or the clarifying questions they ask. Our department (University of Amsterdam, Methodology Department) normally uses 30 to 50 interviews to test questionnaires. The amount depends on whether new errors still are being reported by the interviewers.

The problems that are reported will lead to the reformulation of questions and to the introduction of help screens where necessary, or even to complete changes in the questionnaire design. If there are many problems reported, it might be necessary to do a second pilot study. This was the case in the design of a CADAC questionnaire for time-budget research that led to many problems in a first pilot study (Kalfs, 1986).

If one has several alternative formulations for the same questions and one does not know which to chose, CADAC has the attractive feature that split-ballot experiments can be designed very easily if one has the facility of a random generator in the program. In that case, one can randomly determine which respondent gets which form of the questionnaire and determine afterwards which form was more successful. This experimental work within a questionnaire has been discussed recently in the literature (Shanks, 1989), but these possibilities have been available for a long time.

Recently, the discussion between cognitive psychologists and survey researchers has led to cognitive analyses of the tasks that survey researchers set their respondents. These studies now are providing new suggestions for experiments with different formulations of tasks that should be experimented with (see, e.g., Blair and Burton, 1986; Silberstein, 1989). CADAC provides good facilities for these purposes.

The work of Belson (1981) has made it very clear that this kind of testing should be done. He even recommends in-depth interviews to find out how the questions are interpreted. Although his point is clear, one does not usually have the time or money for such experiments. But in the case of a long-term study that uses the same questionnaire over and over again, it is certainly recommended to consider this possibility before the definite questionnaire is chosen.

As a weak substitute for Belson's recommendation, we provide the respondents in our self-administered CADAC questionnaires with one page for comments on our questions after each module. Most of the time, the respondents report errors they have made, which provides us with valuable information about problems that occur in the questionnaire, but sometimes they clearly indicate problems they have had with the questions. In this way, information is obtained that can help us to improve data collection instruments.

Our general impression is that this phase does not get enough attention in practical research. Researchers normally assume too quickly that their interpretation of questions is the same as the interpretation by the respondents. For a more elaborate discussion of the design of field tests, see Nelson (1985).

Testing the Data

The last test to be performed before the instrument can be used in practice is a test of the data produced by the CADAC instrument. As we mentioned earlier, it is possible that some answers (later on corrected) are not stored in the data file. But if such an option is provided by a program, it is also possible to make errors. If the specification for the deletion of an answer is given for the wrong question, one will not get the data one needs in the statistical analysis. Such errors, if they are not detected, can completely ruin a study, as the necessary data can never be recovered (unlike in paper questionnaires), because the data are omitted during the data collection and not stored. One suggestion would be to store all information, but sometimes the number of variables is so large that one has to reduce this quantity to be able to analyze the data efficiently.

Many CADAC programs are able to generate a system file for different statistical packages. Such programs use the specified questionnaire to generate an input for the job to make a system file. In such a job, all the information about the variable names and variable labels is mentioned, and such a text can be used to check the correctness and completeness of the data file generated by the questionnaire. If errors exist in this structure, one can still make the changes; if one has finished the data collection it is too late.

This is also a good place to mention that the above specified programs or subroutines are a very attractive component of the CADAC procedures. Not having to make the system files manually saves the researcher a lot of time. In the past, this job could easily take 3 days or more. Using these programs, this task can be done in a few minutes, so it is possible to start the data analysis within a few minutes after the data collection has been finished.

Nevertheless, with respect to the testing of the data structure, we would recommend that such a check on the correctness and completeness of the data file is always done before the data collection. Only when this last test has been done can one start the data collection with some confidence in the whole process.

4. CADAC HARDWARE AND SOFTWARE

It would be impossible here to give an overview of all existing hardware and software for computer-assisted data collection, nor is that the purpose of this chapter. What we can do in this chapter is provide the reader with the information that will help to make the important choices when choosing a system. On this point, there is very little systematic information, and there are many different systems available. The information that is available is mainly directed at the evaluation of CATI systems. In this chapter, we will put forward a more general approach that takes into account the various possible applications discussed above. Perhaps we can provide some insight into this jungle of computer programs by discussing some of the hardware and software choices that are relevant for the user. Let us start with the hardware.

CADAC Hardware

With CADAC hardware, there are two major issues at stake. The first concerns the choice of a computer system, the second has to do with the choice of a communication system. The issues are connected, but they can be discussed separately. Of course, the major issue is the choice of computer system, so we will start with this point.

From Mini- to PC-Based Systems. Computer-assisted data collection started with CATI systems that were designed for mainframe or minicomputers connected by direct lines with terminals (Dutka and Frankel, 1980; Fink, 1983). All the processing is done on the central computer; the terminals present only the results of this processing and receive the keyed answers. Such a system is efficient for CATI systems if all the interviewers are working in a room close to the computer, but it is not suitable for other applications discussed in this text like CAPI and CAPAR.

Although terminals connected through modems to central computers could have been used in other applications, this has not in fact happened. Experiments with computer-assisted interviewing on PCs have been going on since 1980 (Danielsson and Maarstad, 1982; Palit and Sharp, 1983; Saris, de Pijper and Neijens, 1982). PCs are more flexible, because they can function independently of a central computer. Given their improved portability, PCs can be used for personal interviewing as well as for CATI and CAPAR. Because many special interest groups among respondents, such as doctors or business people, have a PC at home, these systems can also be used for compuer assisted mail interviews or CAMI.

The major advantage of using a PC- (especially an MS.DOS) based system for CADAC, besides reduction of costs, is that the same interview program can be used for all the different applications mentioned. This means that the research staff need only become familiar with one program for data collection, and the data collection can be done in many different ways. In the previous chapter, we mentioned that programs that can be used for self-administered CADAC interviews can be used for all other applications. This is not the case for the older mini-based systems. Some of these older systems are now also available in PC-based versions, because of the wider range of applications of PC-based systems.

Some organizations claim that this wide range of applications is a special feature of their system. We hope that we have made it clear here that this is nothing special for a PC-based system, because all PC-based systems have this potential. The versatility of a PC-based system depends on the amount of effort put into developing a good communication and management system for the different applications.

Having expressed a preference for PC-based systems for their wide range of possible applications, and for MS.DOS systems because of their widespread use, we now come to the next choice: the communication system. (First, however, we should stress that this preference for PC-based systems does not mean that mini-based systems do not have their value for CATI applications. There are some very sophisticated mini-based CATI systems that certainly can compete with PC-based systems for the same application. If one chooses such a system, however, one should be aware that it will probably be necessary to learn a different program if one also would like to use CADAC for other applications.)

Communication Systems for CADAC. Choosing a PC-based system does not limit the choice of communication system or the choice of central computer. In principle, four different procedures can be used.

- A stand-alone or mail-based system
- A wide area modem-based system
- A local area network (LAN)
- Direct lines between the PC and the central computer

The most elementary use of a PC-based system is as a "stand-alone" computer, to collect the data with no need for contact with a central computer. In that case, the program, administration, and interviews can simply be mailed, or handed over to the interviewer if the data collection occurs close to the research center. When the interviews are finished, the diskette is returned, and the results are stored in a central computer for analysis. In this way, no communication system is needed. Such a system is very cheap, but it can be used only on a very small scale. Above approximately 10 stand-alone computers, such a system becomes unreliable, because one easily can make mistakes when handling the data on the diskettes. On the other hand, it is definitely the cheapest form in which CADAC systems can be used.

The second system, the wide area modem-based system, is especially useful for CAPI and CAPAR applications. Information can be exchanged through modems and telephone lines with computers at a distance via the RS232 connector on the PC. This kind of system allows interviews and administration to be sent over the telephone line from a central computer to the remote PC of an interviewer or household. The interview then can be carried out on the remote PC because the computer can function on its own. In this way, interviews can be carried out independent of and very far from the central computer. This system is efficient for CAPI and CAPAR, especially tele-interviewing, but also can be used for decentralized CATI applications. For centralized CATI applications such a system is not recommended, because over small distances it is better to use local area networks. If long distance telephone calls are very expensive in a particular country, however, it would make sense to consider a decentralized modem-based CATI system.

In the future these systems will no longer require modems, when the new ISDN standard is introduced for telephone and datalines. Communication then will also be much faster. This is especially attractive for transmitting pictures over long distances, which now takes a long time and is therefore rather expensive. For more details on these developments and their consequences, see Gonzalez (1990).

The third possibility, the local area network (LAN), has been developed for centralized CATI systems. In this system, the computers are connected to a server (a stronger PC) by special cards and coaxial cables, allowing fast communication between computers over small distances. In a LANs, the PCs can work alone, but still obtain and provide information fairly frequently from or to a server through the network. The very fact that this system is called a "local area network" indicates that this system is especially useful for CATI applications, although because LAN can be used to connect remote PCs nowadays, it can also be used for CAPI, CAPAR, or CAMI. The information exchanged in the system between the PCs and the server can vary. The frequency of contact and the amount of information transmitted each time depends on the management program used. For example, one may give an interviewer a set of names and numbers of people to be called and return all information only after the whole list has been done. It is also possible for the server to keep complete control over the whole process, so that contact with the server is made by the PC each time a task has been completed. Depending on the management system used, the PCs can work more or less independent of the server.

Finally, the old mini-based system can be simulated by using the PCs as terminals connected to a central computer. This kind of system, where the PCs do not function on their own but are only used as screens to convey messages between the PCs and the central computer, only makes sense for centralized CATI applications and cannot be used for any other application. This system would appear outdated nowadays, because it ignores one of the important advantages of the PC, namely, that it can function on its own as a data collection system. To use a different data collection system one has to rewrite the whole interview program.

It should be clear from this discussion that systems that can use PCs as stand-alone computers are very attractive, because they can be used for many different applications. This is especially true for the first three options, although the first option is only reasonable if one wishes to test the possibilities of such systems. The most serious candidates for practical research are the wide area modem-based system and the LAN-based system. These also can be used next to each other. They have different applications that require different management systems, but the interview program can remain the same. Whether the different programs provide the facilities for the different applications depends on the company and the amount of effort put into developing the management systems. Therefore, there is no reason to prefer one over the other as far as the scale of possible applications is concerned. The choice should be based on the planned application and the potential of the software under consideration.

CADAC Software

Besides the choice of hardware, the choice of software must be made. These two choices are not independent of each other. Most of the time the software is provided for a specific hardware system (i.e., stand-alone computers, a LAN-based system, or a modem-based system, or combinations of these systems). Therefore, the next question is "What are the requirements for the software?" This question has been answered unanimously for CATI systems (Baker and Lefes, 1988; Nicholls, 1988; Nicholls and Groves, 1986). The functional requirements can be generalized to other CADAC applications quite easily. In doing so, the following requirements for the software can be specified:

1. The sample management should be done by the system and not by the researcher.
2. The contacts between interviewers and respondents or the selection of interviews for the household members should be scheduled by the program.
3. On-line interviewing should be arranged by the program.
4. The quality and quantity of the work of the interviewers should be controlled by the system.
5. The system should produce more or less automatically the data files for statistical analysis.

We would like to add to this list a sixth requirement:

6. The questionnaire authoring system should not be too difficult to use and should provide sufficient flexibility and testing facilities.

We will now make some brief comments on each of these requirements.

Sample Management. Even when the population from which the sample is drawn is the same, the sample frame used for different CADAC applications can be quite different. For CATI, one could use telephone directories or random-digit dialing methods, whereas for CAPI, lists of addresses are the most obvious source of information. But whatever the sample frame, a program should be able to draw a sample from a list of cases provided to the program. Furthermore, the program should be able to keep track of the results of the data collection: whether a household has been contacted; if so, what the result of this contact was, or why the household refuses to cooperate, and so forth. All this information should be organized by the program. If it has to be done on paper by the researcher, it requires a lot of work and this can lead to errors and arbitrary decisions. This has been shown convincingly by Palit and Sharp (1983). Imagine that one wishes to interview people with a specific characteristic that occurs in only 10% of households, and one would like to talk to 1,000 people with this characteristic. Then 10,000 calls are needed to find these 1,000 people. If random dialing is used, with a success rate of 30% one must manipulate 30,000 records to realize these 1,000 interviews. This example illustrates the necessity of a computer-based management system in the central computer.

Scheduling of Contacts. In each application, different procedures are used to select, administer, and schedule contacts. In CATI systems, the combination of interviewer and telephone number has to be selected, and a schedule for the calls has to be designed. In CAPI applications, interviewers and addresses have to be selected, and a sequence of visits has to be determined. But in tele-interviewing, the computer only has to make a combination of interviews and household members if not all members get the same interviews.

In all applications, the status of the work has to be administered, and decisions have to be made about what the next step in the process should be. All these tasks can be done better by the computer than by human beings, if the program works well. This does not mean that the computer program can do all the work. There are still a large number of decisions that researchers have to make.

Although these management programs are similar with respect to their tasks, they will be sufficiently different to require different modules depending on the application used. Often, not all modules are available in all programs: The programs are often specialized to one application.

Programs also will be different in the way they organize these tasks. Some programs (CATI-oriented systems) will organize these tasks mainly on the central computer. Programs more oriented toward CAPI and CAPAR will organize these tasks mainly on the PCs, which has the advantage that the systems can continue to function if the network fails. This is not the case with the other systems, which are more dependent on the central computer.

On-Line Interviewing. In earlier texts on CATI procedures, the following necessary characteristics of CATI systems have been mentioned (Nicholls, 1988; Nicholls and Groves, 1986):

1. The system displays instructions, survey questions, and response categories on the computer screen.
2. Screens may contain "fills" or alterations of the display text based on prior answers or batch input from case records.
3. Answers to closed questions may be numeric or alphanumeric codes; and these codes and other numeric entries may be edited by sets of permissible values, by ranges, or by logical or arithmetic operations.
4 Edit failures may result either in an unaccepted entry (requiring another attempt) or in the display of additional probes or questions to be asked.
5. Extended text answers may be entered for open questions.
6. Branching or skipping to the next item is automatic and may be based on logical or arithmetic tests of any prior entries or input data.

7. Interviewers and respondents may interrupt and resume interviews in mid-course; review, back up to, and (if permitted) change prior entries; and enter interviewing notes at appropriate points.

These characteristics can be generalized quite easily to any kind of CADAC system, but they give only the minimum requirements for these programs. There are two very elaborate evaluations of computer programs for CADAC of which we are aware. These evaluations (Carpenter, 1988; de Bie et al., 1989) provide many more criteria and an evaluation of programs on the basis of these criteria. They evaluate criteria such as the number of question types, randomization of questions and response categories, and facilities for high-lighting. They also mention more detailed criteria, such as the procedures for skipping and branching (*if, then, else*), and many other possibilities. However, this is not the place to discuss all these criteria; besides, these programs change rather quickly and the state of the art has changed considerably in the last 2 years. Nevertheless, these evaluations also show that the most elaborate systems have most of the important features mentioned. These reports are mainly interesting (we feel) to make readers sensitive to the criteria that they might consider when they have to decide on the purchase of CADAC software. A good example of such a study is that of Connett et al. (1990), who had to make the decision with respect to a new CATI system for the Survey Research Center.

There also are two specialized papers on evaluation research of CAPI systems by Couper and Groves (1989). These papers are especially interesting because they compare the performance of different interfaces between the computer and interviewers. Most common for MS.DOS computers in survey research are menu-driven systems, where the respondent has to type the number of the response category. There are many alternatives, however, that can be considered. The GridPad provides facilities to write answers in uppercase letters in the box provided on the screen. The coding is done by handwriting recognition. The Datellite provides a touch screen, whereby one answers a question by touching the part of the screen where the answer is presented.

In addition to the interfaces studied by Couper and Groves, there is another quite common interface that is also menu driven, but where the answer is chosen by moving the cursor with the cursor keys or a mouse to the appropriate answer. A completely different possibility is the use of bar codes for categories and a bar-code reader for the coding.

Couper and Groves (1989) have made a start with research on the consequences of the choice of the interface for data quality. On the basis of their most recent study, they conclude:

> Both the handwriting recognition and touchscreen machines performed worse than "traditional" laptop computers in terms of speed and certain types of errors. However, such differences could well disappear given sufficient familiarity with and training on these machines. Furthermore, these technologies are still in their relative infancy. It is expected that hardware and software developments (some of which have already been announced) will make these systems easier to use and less error-prone.

Although their results are very interesting, much more research on this point has to be done before it becomes clear which data-entry system is the best for survey research. The conclusion of these studies could well be that the choice should depend on the type and amount of data that is to be collected.

Recently, a distinction was made between different software packages on the basis of another aspect of the use of the screen. It has been suggested that there are item-based, screen-based, and form-based CADAC systems (Nicholls, 1988). *Item-based systems* display one survey question and answer space at a time, perform edits after each entry, and typically erase the screen before the next item appears. *Screen-based systems* present more questions on the screen, but the branching and skipping is still under control of the program. The more recent *form-based systems* provide many questions on the screen, but the interviewer or respondents can move in any direction on the screen and answer the questions in the order they prefer. The edits are done after all questions have been answered.

Although the distinction is very interesting, CADAC systems cannot be characterized so simply on this basis. The systems are adapting so quickly to new demands that systems that were originally item-based now provide facilities that are comparable to those of screen-based and form-based systems. Thus, the systems can not be simply characterized in this way, and the choice should not be based on this feature.

There are other criteria, however, that have not been mentioned yet that deserve more attention. We would like to mention the following criteria.

- The maximum length of the interview
- The facilities to put together complex questionnaires tailor-made for the purpose
- The flexibility of the program for introducing changes into the questionnaire

Some programs limit the length of the questionnaire by the number of questions or by the size of the program that has to be compiled from the interview text. As personalized questionnaires can become very long, this is an important criterion.

The second point stresses an obvious requirement, namely, that one should be able to make the questionnaires one would like to make. Some CADAC programs are very simple to use, but do not provide much flexibility for the design of questionnaires.

The third point relates to a previous discussion, where we argued in favor of programs that allow flexibility in the design and in adjustment of questionnaires. One generally recognized problem in this field concerns the use of numbers for the questions or screens used. If one would like to change a questionnaire, the branching of which is based on numbers, one has to change all the numbers in the questionnaire, and the likelihood of errors in such systems is clearly very high. We will come back to this discussion later. These three points should certainly be taken into account when evaluating good quality CADAC systems.

Quality and Quantity Control. In CATI systems, a distinction is made between quality control by monitoring and control of the quantity of work done by interviewers. The latter task is done by collecting information on the number of calls, outcome of the calls, amount of time spent, productivity, response rate, and so on. In the other applications this distinction cannot be made, but quality controls can still be made by counting the correct codings, the length of the verbal responses, the number of alternatives mentioned in multiple response questions, and so forth.

It is a useful facility if a program can report this information automatically, as some programs do. On the other hand, it is already quite attractive if the information is available and can be evaluated by statistical analysis of the data, which is the case for most programs. Therefore this point does not lead to a very different evaluation of the different programs.

Production of System Files. The production of system files for statistical analysis of the data with one of the commonly used statistical packages, such as SAS, BMDP, SPSS, or any other package, should be a standard facility in any CADAC system. Some packages provide their own statistical package for the CADAC data, but it is difficult to see this as an added attraction, because such a package can never be as complete as the well-known statistical packages. Most of the better CADAC programs, therefore, provide procedures, which on the basis of the information available in the questionnaire, generate system files for different statistical packages.

Although we do not consider this feature of CADAC systems to be an important criterion in the choice of a CADAC system, because all elaborate systems have the facility, we also do not want to underestimate its importance. In the past, the development of a correct input file for constructing a system file could take up to a week. With the automatic procedures available in the CADAC systems, this job is done in a few minutes. This is a very important advantage of CADAC systems.

The Questionnaire-Authoring System. Last but not least, we would like to draw the attention of the reader to the different aspects that are important in the evaluation of the authoring system connected with the CADAC systems.

Some systems seem very attractive because of their simple authoring system, mostly menu-driven. However, these systems are often the least flexible when it comes to designing questionnaires. At the other extreme, there are authoring systems that more or less provide a computer language for writing questionnaires. These systems are certainly very flexible in terms of their possibilities for designing any kind of questionnaire, but one has to be a computer programmer to design such questionnaires, or at least have programmer-like capabilities.

A middle-of-the-road option has been chosen in systems that work on the basis of a program that requires a questionnaire text with extra symbols for the computer. In such systems, like INTERV used in this monograph for illustrative purposes, simple questionnaires can be written very quickly, whereas the possibility to write complex questionnaires depends on the facilities provided by the program. In my experience, the possibilities are as unlimited as in the program-based systems.

A related point is that it should be relatively easy to change a questionnaire if necessary. A typical problem arises when numbers are used for questions or screens, as we have already mentioned. Another point is that it should be possible to develop separate modules that can be combined together in different questionnaires. This facility is provided by most programs. It depends mainly on the author of the questionnaire whether these facilities are properly used (as described in Chapter 3).

One feature that tends to vary quite a lot from one program to another is the very important facility of checking the syntax of a questionnaire and getting some insight into the structure of the branching and skipping patterns specified in the questionnaire. The first facility is very important in helping to avoid wasting a lot of time on very small errors. The programs that provide a kind of computer language to specify questionnaires and that require a compilation stage to produce an interview program from a questionnaire have the advantage of automatically providing an error-detection facility.

Menu-driven authoring programs prevent errors by leaving the authors only limited freedom. But the programs based on interpreters do not normally have error detection facilities. If these facilities do exist in a program, they are developed separately from the interview program. One should take care that such a program is available if one is buying a CADAC system, because it will save the questionnaire authors a lot of time.

An equally attractive feature of a system would be providing tools for representing the branching and skipping in a questionnaire. These specifications can contain many errors, which can cause a lot of problems if not detected by syntax-checking programs. Although these facilities are very important, it will be some time before they will be available on a large scale.

Having discussed the different characteristics that we consider important in the choice of a CADAC system, we also provide a list of CADAC programs in the Appendix for those who are interested in using such a system. It is not possible in this context to offer an evaluation of the different programs (see the evaluations of Carpenter, 1988; Connett et al., 1990; de Bie et al., 1989), but we also should warn the reader that such evaluations are out of date the moment they appear, because the design of CADAC programs is one of the most dynamic fields in computer programming. It is also my conviction that knowledge of the possibilities of these systems is still very limited. We expect that in the near future many new ways will be found to improve computer-assisted data collection. This is one of the reasons why this is such an interesting field of research.

APPENDIX: COMPUTER PROGRAMS FOR CADAC

We provide a list of computer programs for CADAC on PCs without the pretention of completeness and without an evaluation of the quality of the programs. For more information about these programs, see Carpenter (1988), de Bie et al. (1989), and Connett et al. (1990).

ACS Query
Analytical Computer Service, Inc.
640 North Lasalle Drive
Chicago, IL 60610
USA
(312)751-2915

Athena
CRC Information Systems, Inc.
435 Hudson St.
New York, NY 10014
USA
(212) 620-5678

Autoquest
Microtab Systems Pty Ltd.
2 Tanya Way
Eltham, Victoria
3095 Australia
(03)439-6235

Blaise
Central Bureau of Statistics
Hoofdafdeling M3
P. O. Box 959
2270 AZ Voorburg
The Netherlands
(70)694341

CAPPA
The Scientific Press
540 University Ave.
Palo Alto, CA 94301
USA
(415)322-5221

Cases
Computer Assisted Survey Methods
University of California
2538 Channing Way
Berkeley, CA 94720
USA
(415)642-6592

Cass
Survey Research Laboratory
University of Wisconsin
610 Langdon St.
Madison, WI 53703
USA
(608)262-3122

Ci2
Sawtooth Software, Inc.
208 Spruce N.
Ketchum, ID 83340
USA
(208)726-7772

INTERV
Sociometric Research Foundation
Van Boshuizen Str 225
1083 AW Amsterdam
The Netherlands
(020)-6610961

ITS
Information Transfer Systems
2451 S. Industrial Hwy.
Ann Arbor, MI 46104
USA
(313)994-0003

245

MATI
Social and Economic Sciences
Research Center
Washington State University
Pullman, WA 99164
USA
(509)335-1511

PCRS/ACRS
M/A/R/C Inc.
7850 North Belt Line Rd.
Irving, TX 75063
USA
(214)506-3400

PC-Survent
CfMC, Computers for Marketing
547 Howard St.
San Francisco, CA 94105
USA
(415)777-0470

Quancept
Quantime Limited
17 Bedford Square
London WC1B 3JA
England
(1)6377061

Q-Fast
Statsoft, Inc.
2325 East 13th St.
Tulsa, OK 74104
USA
(918)583-4149

Quester Writer
Orchard Products
205 State Rd.
Princeton, NJ 08540
USA
(609)683-7702

Quiz Whiz
Quiz Whiz Enterprises, Inc.
790 Timberline Dr.
Akron, OH 44304
USA
(216)922-1825

Reach
World Research
P. O. Box 1009
Palatine, IL 60078
USA
(312)911-1122

REFERENCES

ANDREWS, F. M. (1984) "Construct validity and error components of survey measures: A structural modeling approach." *Public Opinion Quarterly* 48: 409-442.
BAKER, R. P., and LEFES, W. L. (1988) "The design of CATI systems: A review of current practice," in R. M. Groves, P. P. Biemer, L. E. Lyberg, J. T. Massey, W. L. Nicholls II, and J. Waksberg (eds.) *Telephone Survey Methodology* (pp. 387-403). New York: John Wiley.
BATISTA, J. M., and SARIS, W. E. (1988) "The comparability of scales for job satisfaction," in W. E. Saris (ed.) *Variation in Response Function: A Source of Measurement Error* (pp. 178-199). Amsterdam, The Netherlands: Sociometric Research Foundation.
BELSON, W. A. (1981) *The Design and Understanding of Survey Questions.* London: Gower.
BEMELMANS-SPORK, M., and SIKKEL, D. (1985) "Observation of prices with hand-held computers." *Statistical Journal of the United Nations Economic Commission for Europe* 3(2). Geneva, Switzerland: United Nations Economic Commission for Europe.

246

BEMELMANS-SPORK, M., and SIKKEL, D. (1986) "Data collection with handheld computers." *Proceedings of the International Statistical Institute, 45th Session* (Vol. 3, Topic 18.3).
Voorberg, The Netherlands: International Statistical Institute.

BILLIET, J., LOOSVELDT, G., and WATERPLAS, L. (1984) *Het Survey-Interview
Onderzocht* [*The Survey Interview Evaluated*]. Leuven, Belgium: Department Sociologie.

BLAIR, E., and BURTON, S. (1986) "Processes used in the formulation of behavioral frequency
reports in surveys," in *American Statistical Association Proceedings* (pp. 481-487). Alexandria, VA: American Statistical Association.

BOEREMA, E., BADEN, R. D., and BON, E. (1987) "Computer assisted face-to-face interviewing," in *ESOMAR Marketing Research Congress, 40th Session* (pp. 829-849). Amsterdam, The Netherlands: European Society for Opinion and Market Research.

BON, E. (1988) "Correction for variation in response behavior," in W. E. Saris (ed.) *Variation
in Response Function: A Source of Measurement Error* (pp. 147-165). Amsterdam, The
Netherlands: Sociometric Research Foundation.

BRADBURN, N. M., SUDMAN, S., BLAIR, E., and STOCKING, C. (1978) "Question threat
and response bias." *Public Opinion Quarterly* 42: 221-234.

BRENNER, M. (1982) "Response effects of role-restricted characteristics of the interviewer,"
in W. Dijkstra and J. van der Zouwen (eds.) *Response Behaviour in the Survey Interview* (pp.
131-165). London: Academic Press.

BRUINSMA, C., SARIS, W. E., and GALLHOFER, I. N. (1980) "A study of systematic errors
in survey research: The effect of the perception of other people's opinions," in C. P.
Middendorp (ed.) *Proceedings of the Dutch Sociometric Society Congress* (pp. 117-135).
Amsterdam, The Netherlands: Sociometric Research Foundation.

CARPENTER, E. H. (1988) "Software tools for data collection: Microcomputer-assisted
interviewing." *Social Science Computer Review* 6: 353-368.

CLAYTON, R., and HARREL, L. J. (1989) "Developing a cost model for alternative data
collection methods: Mail, CATI and TDE," in *American Statistical Association Proceedings*
(pp. 264-269). Alexandria, VA: American Statistical Association.

CLEMENS, J. (1984) "The use of viewdata panels for data," in *Are Interviewers Obsolete?
Drastic Changes in Data Collection and Data Presentation* (pp. 47-65). Amsterdam, The
Netherlands: European Society for Opinion and Market Research.

CONNETT, W. E., BLACKBURN, Z., GEBLER, N., GREENWELL, M., HANSEN, S. E., and
PRICE, P. (1990) *A Report on the Evaluation of Three CATI Systems*. Ann Arbor, MI: Survey
Research Center.

CONVERSE, J. M., and PRESSER, S. (1986) *Survey Questions: Handcrafting the Standardized
Questionnaire*. Beverly Hills, CA: Sage.

COUPER, M., and GROVES, R. (1989) *Interviewer Expectations Regarding CAPI: Results of
Laboratory Tests II*. Washington, DC: Bureau of Labor Statistics.

COUPER, M., GROVES, R., and JACOBS, C. A. (1989) *Building Predictive Models of CAPI
Acceptance in a Field Interviewing Staff*. Paper presented at the Annual Research Conference
of the Bureau of the Census.

DANIELSSON, L., and MAARSTAD, P. A. (1982) *Statistical Data Collection with Hand-Held
Computers: A Consumer Price Index*. Orebo, Sweden: Statistics Sweden.

de BIE, S. E., STOOP, I. A. L., and de VRIES, K. L. M. (1989) *CAI Software: An Evaluation
of Software for Computer-Assisted Interviewing*. Amsterdam, The Netherlands: Stichting
Interuniversitair Institut voor Sociaal Wetenschappelijk Onderzoek.

de PIJPER, W. M., and SARIS, W. E. (1986a) "Computer assisted interviewing using home
computers." *European Research* 14: 144-152.

de PIJPER, W. M., and SARIS, W. E. (1986b) *The Formulation of Interviews Using the Program
INTERV*. Amsterdam, The Netherlands: Sociometric Research Foundation.

247

DEKKER, F., and DORN, P. (1984) *Computer-Assisted Telephonic Interviewing: A Research Project in the Netherlands*. Paper presented at the Conference of the Institute of British Geographers, Durham, United Kingdom.

DIJKSTRA, W. (1983) *Beinvloeding van Antwoorden in Survey-Interviews* [*Influence on Answers in Survey Research*]. Unpublished doctoral dissertation, Vrije Univeristeit, Amsterdam, The Netherlands.

DIJKSTRA, W., and van der ZOUWEN, J. (eds.) (1982) *Response Behaviour in the Survey Interview*. London: Academic Press.

DUTKA, S., and FRANKEL, L. R. (1980) "Sequential survey design through the use of computer assisted telephone interviewing," in *American Statistical Association Proceedings* (pp. 73-76). Alexandria, VA: American Statistical Association.

FINK, J. C. (1983) "CATI's first decade: The Chilton experience." *Sociological Methods and Research* 12: 153-168.

GAVRILOV, A. J. (1988, November) *Computer Assisted Interviewing in the USSR*. Paper presented at the International Methodology Conference, Moscow.

GONZALEZ, M. E. (1990) *Computer Assisted Survey Information Collection* (Working Paper No. 19). Washington, DC: Statistical Policy Office.

GROVES, R. M. (1983) "Implications of CATI: Costs, errors, and organization of telephone survey research." *Sociological Methods and Research* 12: 199-215.

GROVES, R. M. (1989) *Survey Errors and Survey Costs*. New York: John Wiley.

GROVES, R. M., and NICHOLLS, W. L., II. (1986) "The status of computer-assisted telephone interviewing: Part II. Data quality issues." *Journal of Official Statistics* 2: 117-134.

HARTMAN, H., and SARIS, W. E. (1991, February) *Data Collection on Expenditures*. Paper presented at the Workshop on Diary Surveys, Stockholm, Sweden.

HOUSE, C. C. (1985) "Questionnaire design with computer assisted interviewing." *Journal of Official Statistics* 1: 209-219.

HOUSE, C. C., and NICHOLLS, W. L., II. (1988) "Questionnaire design for CATI: Design objectives and methods," in R. M. Groves, P. P. Biemer, L. E. Lyberg, J. T. Massey, W. L. Nicholls II, and J. Waksberg (eds.) *Telephone Survey Methodology* (pp. 421-437). New York: John Wiley.

JABINE, T. B. (1985) "A tool for developing and understanding survey questionnaires." *Journal of Official Statistics* 1: 189-207.

KALFS, N. (1986) *Het Construeren van Meetinstrumenten voor Quasi Collectieve Voorzieningen en Huishoudelijke Productie* [The Construction of Measurement Instruments for Quasi Collective Goods and Household Products] (Research Memorandum No. 861117). Amsterdam, The Netherlands: Sociometric Research Foundation.

KALTON, G., and SCHUMAN, H. (1982) "The effect of the question on survey response answers: A review." *Journal of the Royal Statistical Society* 145: 42-57.

KERSTEN, A. (1988) *Computer Gestuurd Interviewen* [*Computer Assisted Interviewing*]. Unpublished master's thesis, University of Amsterdam, The Netherlands.

KERSTEN, A., VERWEIJ, M., HARTMAN, H., and GALLHOFER, I. N. (1990) *Reduction of Measurement Errors by Computer Assisted Interviewing*. Amsterdam, The Netherlands: Sociometric Research Foundation.

KIESLER, S., and SPROULL, L. S. (1986) "Response effects in the electronic survey." *Public Opinion Quarterly* 50: 402-413.

KÖLTRINGER, R. (1991, April) *Design Effect in MTMM Studies*. Paper presented at the meeting of the International Research Group on Evaluation of Measurement Instruments, Ludwigshafen, Germany.

LODGE, M. (1981) *Magnitude Scaling*. Beverly Hills, CA: Sage.

248

LODGE, M., CROSS, D., TURSKY, B., and TANENHAUS, J. (1975) "The psychophysical scaling and validation of a political support scale." *American Journal of Political Science* 19: 611-649.

LOFTUS, E. F., and MARBURGER, W. (1983) "Since the eruption of Mt. St. Helen did anyone beat you up? Improving the accuracy of retrospective reports with landmark events." *Memory and Cognition* 11: 114-120.

LORD, F. M., and NOVICK, M. R. (1968) *Statistical Theories of Mental Test Scores.* London: Addison-Wesley.

MOLENAAR, N. J. (1986) *Formuleringseffecten in Survey-Interviews: Een Nonexperimenteel Onderzoek [Question Wording Effects in Survey Interviews].* Amsterdam, The Netherlands: Vrije Univeristeit Uitgeverij.

NELSON, D. D. (1985) "Informal testing as a means of questionnaire development." *Journal of Official Statistics* 1: 179-188.

NETER, J., and WAKSBERG, J. (1963) "Effect of interviewing designated respondent in household surveys of home owner's expenditures on alterations and repairs." *Applied Statistics* 12: 46-60.

NETER, J., and WAKSBERG, J. (1964) "A study of response errors in expenditures data from household interviews." *Journal of American Statistical Association* 59: 18-55.

NETER, J., and WAKSBERG, J. (1965) *Response Errors in Collection of Expenditures Data by Household Interviews* (Technical Report No. 11J). Washington, DC: Bureau of the Census.

NICHOLLS, W. L., II. (1978) "Experiences with CATI in a large-scale survey." *American Statistical Association Proceedings* (pp. 9-17). Alexandria, VA: American Statistical Association.

NICHOLLS, W. L., II. (1988) "Computer-assisted telephone interviewing: A general introduction," in R. M. Groves, P. P. Biemer, L. E. Lyberg, J. T. Massey, W. L. Nicholls II, and J. Waksberg (eds.) *Telephone Survey Methodology* (pp. 377-387). New York: John Wiley.

NICHOLLS, W. L., II, and GROVES, R. M. (1986) "The status of computer-assisted telephone interviewing." *Journal of Official Statistics* 2: 93-115.

NICHOLLS, W. L., II, and HOUSE, C. C. (1987) "Designing questionnaires for computer assisted interviewing: A focus on program correctness," in *Proceedings of the Third Annual Research Conference of the U.S. Bureau of the Census* (pp. 95-111). Washington, DC: Government Printing Office.

PALIT, C., and SHARP, H. (1983) "Microcomputer-assisted telephone interviewing." *Sociological Methods and Research* 12: 169-191.

PHILLIPS, D. L., and CLANCY, K. J. (1970) "Response bias in field studies of mental illness." *American Sociological Review* 35: 503-515.

PULSE TRAIN TECHNOLOGY. (1984) *Limited Questionnaire Specification Language.* Esher, United Kingdom: Author.

SARIS, W. E. (1982) "Different questions, different variables," in C. Fornell (ed.) *Second Generation of Multivariate Analysis* (pp. 78-96). New York: Praeger.

SARIS, W. E. (1988) *Variation in Response Functions: A Source of Measurement Error.* Amsterdam, The Netherlands: Sociometric Research Foundation.

SARIS, W. E. (1989) "A technological revolution in data collection." *Quality and Quantity* 23: 333-348.

SARIS, W. E., and ANDREWS, F. M. (in press) "Evaluation of measurement instruments using a structural modeling approach," in P. P. Biemer, R. M. Groves, L. E. Lyberg, N. Mathiowetz, and S. Sudman (eds.) *Measurement Errors in Surveys.* New York: John Wiley.

SARIS, W. E., de PIJPER, W. M., and NEIJENS, P. (1982) "Some notes on the computer steered interview," in C. Middendorp (eds.) *Proceedings of the Sociometry Meeting* (pp. 306-310). Amsterdam, The Netherlands: Sociometric Research Foundation.

SARIS, W. E., and de ROOY, K. (1988) "What kinds of terms should be used for reference points?" in W. E. Saris (ed.) *Variation in Response Functions: A Source of Measurement Error in Attitude Research* (pp. 199-219). Amsterdam, The Netherlands: Sociometric Research Foundation.

SARIS, W. E., van de PUTTE, B., MAAS, K., and SEIP, H. (1988) "Variation in response function: Observed and created," in W. E. Saris (ed.) *Variation in Response Function: A Source of Measurement Error* (pp. 165-178). Amsterdam, The Netherlands: Sociometric Research Foundation.

SCHUMAN, H., and PRESSER, S. (1981) *Questions and Answers in Attitude Surveys: Experiments on Question Form Wording and Context.* London: Academic Press.

SHANKS, J. M. (1989) "Information technology and survey research: Where do we go from here?" *Journal of Official Statistics* 5: 3-21.

SIKKEL, D. (1985) "Models for memory effects." *Journal of the American Statistical Association* 80: 835-841.

SILBERSTEIN, A. R. (1989) "Recall effects in the U.S. consumer expenditure interview survey." *Journal of Official Statistics* 5: 125-142.

SOCIOMETRIC RESEARCH FOUNDATION. (1988, Spring) "New facilities of INTERV for panel research." *SRF Newsletter.*

SPAETH, M. A. (1990) "CATI facilities at academic research organizations." *Survey Research* 2(2): 11-14.

STEVENS, S. S. (1975) *Psychophysics: Introduction to Its Perceptual Neural and Social Prospects.* New York: John Wiley.

SUDMAN, S., and BRADBURN, N. M. (1973) "Effects of time and memory factors on responses in surveys." *Journal of the American Statistical Association* 68: 805-815.

SUDMAN, S., and BRADBURN, N. M. (1974) *Response Effects in Surveys.* Hawthorne, NY: Aldine.

THORNBERRY, O., ROWE, B., and BIGGER, R. (1990, June) *Use of CAPI with the U.S. National Health Interview Survey.* Paper presented at the meeting of the International Sociological Association, Madrid, Spain.

THORNTON, A., FREEDMAN, D. S., and CAMBURN, D. (1982) "Obtaining respondent cooperation in family panel studies." *Sociological Methods and Research* 11: 33-51.

TORTORA, R. (1985) "CATI in agricultural statistical agency." *Journal of Official Statistics* 1: 301-314.

van BASTELAER, A., KERSSEMAKERS, F., and SIKKEL, D. (1988) "A test of the Netherlands continuous labour force survey with hand held computers: Interviewer behaviour and data quality," in D. Sikkel (ed.) *Quality Aspects of Statistical Data Collection* (pp. 67-92). Amsterdam, The Netherlands: Sociometric Research Foundation.

van DOORN, L. (1987-1988) "Het gebruik van microcomputers in panelonderzoek" ["The use of microcomputers in panel research"], in *Jaarboek van de Nederlandse Vereniging Voor Marktonderzoekers* (pp. 7-23).

van DOORN, L., SARIS, W. E., and LODGE, M. (1983) "Discrete or continuous measurement: What difference does it make?" *Kwantitatieve Methoden* 10: 104-120.

VERWEIJ, M. J., KALFS, N. J., and SARIS, W. E. (1986) *Tijdsbestedings-Onderzoek Middels: Tele-Interviewing en de Mogelijkheden Voor Segmentatie [Time-Budget Research Using Tele-Interviewing and the Possibilities for Segmentation]* (Research Memo No. 87031). Amsterdam, The Netherlands: Sociometric Research Foundation.

WEBB, E., CAMPBELL, D. T., SCHWARTZ, R. D., and SECHREST, L. (1981) *Unobtrusive Measures: Nonreactive Research in the Social Sciences.* Boston: Houghton Mifflin.

250

WEEKS, M. F. (1988) "Call scheduling with CATI: Current capabilities and methods," in R. M. Groves, P. P. Biemer, L. E. Lyberg, J. T. Massey, W. L. Nicholls II, and J. Waksberg (eds.) *Telephone Survey Methodology* (pp. 403-421). New York: John Wiley.

WEGENER, B. (1982) *Social Attitudes and Psychophysical Measurement*. Hillsdale, NJ: Lawrence Earlbaum.

WILLENBORG, L. C. R. J. (1989) *Computational Aspects of Survey Data Processing*. Amsterdam, The Netherlands: CWI.

WINTER, D. L. S., and CLAYTON, R. L. (1990) *Speech Data Entry: Results of the First Test of Voice Recognition for Data Collection*. Washington, DC: Bureau of Labor Statistics.

ACKNOWLEDGMENTS

I would like to thank my Ph.D. students for their important contributions to this book in the form of our continuous discussions. I also thank my colleagues Mike Lewis-Beck, Robert Groves, Dirk Sikkel, Mick Couper, Carol House, and Harm Hartman, and two anonymous reviewers for their critical comments on the text.

BASIC CONTENT ANALYSIS

PART IV

ROBERT PHILIP WEBER

1. INTRODUCTION

Content analysis is a research method that uses a set of procedures to make valid inferences from text.[1] These inferences are about the sender(s) of the message, the message itself, or the audience of the message. The rules of this inferential process vary with the theoretical and substantive interests of the investigator, and are discussed in later chapters.

Content analysis can be used for many purposes. The following list points out a few notable examples (adapted from Berelson, 1952):

- disclose international differences in communication content;
- compare media or "levels" of communication;
- audit communication content against objectives;
- code open-ended questions in surveys;
- identify the intentions and other characteristics of the communicator;
- determine the psychological state of persons or groups;
- detect the existence of propaganda;
- describe attitudinal and behavioral responses to communications;
- reflect cultural patterns of groups, institutions, or societies;
- reveal the focus of individual, group, institutional, or societal attention; and
- describe trends in communication content.

The numerous examples presented throughout this monograph mainly show the last three uses of content analysis.

This monograph is an introduction to content analysis methods from a social science perspective.[2] The material covered here will be useful to students and researchers who wish to analyze text. The following chapters assume that the reader has had at least introductory courses in research methods and in data analysis or social statistics.

Compared with other data-generating and analysis techniques, content analysis has several advantages:

- Communication is a central aspect of social interaction. Content-analytic procedures operate directly on text or transcripts of human communications.
- The best content-analytic studies use both qualitative and quantitative operations on texts. Thus content analysis methods combine what are usually thought to be antithetical modes of analysis.
- Documents of various kinds exist over long periods of time. Culture indicators generated from such series of documents constitute reliable data that may span even centuries (e.g., Namenwirth and Weber, 1987)
- In more recent times, when reliable data of other kinds exist, culture indicators can be used to assess quantitatively the relationships among economic, social, political, and cultural change.
- Compared with techniques such as interviews, content analysis usually yields unobtrusive measures in which neither the sender nor the receiver of the message is aware that it is being analyzed. Hence, there is little danger that the act of measurement itself will act as a force for change that confounds the data (Webb, Campbell, Schwartz, and Sechrist, 1981).

Two very different studies summarized below show some ways content analysis has been used. Following chapters explain other studies in greater detail.

Some Content-Analytic Studies

Content analysis has been used to study popular art forms. Walker (1975) analyzed differences and similarities in American black and white popular song lyrics, 1962-1973. Using computer-aided content analysis, Walker investigated differences in narrative form. He found that compared with popular white song lyrics, "rhythm and blues" and "soul" song lyrics showed greater emphasis on action in the objective world, less concern with time, and greater emphasis on what Walker calls "toughmindedness" or "existential concreteness."

The study also investigated changes in narrative focus. Walker found that identification with others increased significantly over time in "soul" and "rhythm and blues" lyrics, but not in popular white song lyrics. This change may reflect increasing self-awareness and positive images within the black community.

Walker's study illustrates that computer-based content analysis may be used to study popular and elite culture. In fact, one important substantive question content analysis might address is the relationship between popular and elite culture. Specifically, do changes in elite culture lead or lag behind changes in mass culture? Unfortunately, one serious difficulty exists in any study addressing this question. Textual materials that survive over long periods often reflect an elite bias.

In another study, Aries (1973; summarized in Aries, 1977), also using computer-aided content analysis, studied differences in female, male, and mixed-sex small groups. She found that differential sex-role socialization and sex-role stereotyping affect thematic content and social interaction. In female groups, women show much concern with interpersonal issues. Women discuss "themselves, their homes and families, and their relationships, defining themselves by the way they relate to the significant others who surround them" (Aries, 1973: 254).

In male groups, members do not address interpersonal matters directly. Instead, men indirectly relate personal experiences and feelings through stories and metaphors. Men "achieve a closeness through the sharing of laughter and stories of activities, rather than the sharing of the understanding of those experiences" (Aries, 1973: 254). Also, all-male groups manifest more themes involving aggression than do all-female groups.

In mixed groups, Aries found that women talked less of their homes and families. Women also spoke less of achievement and institutions. In short, women in these groups "orient themselves around being women with men by assuming the traditional female role" (Aries, 1973: 256). Men in mixed groups expressed their competitiveness less through storytelling than through assuming leadership roles in the group. Moreover, in the presence of women, men shift more toward reflection of themselves and their feelings.

Aries's study illustrates that content analysis may be:

- applied to substantive problems at the intersection of culture, social structure, and social interaction;
- used to generate dependent variables in experimental designs; and
- used to study small groups as microcosms of society.

Changes in sex-role socialization could be assessed by repeating the study. Furthermore, Aries's research could be extended with appropriate modifications to cross-national and cross-language research designs.

Issues in Content Analysis

A central idea in content analysis is that the many words of the text are classified into much fewer content categories. Each category may consist of one, several, or many words. Words, phrases, or other units of text classified in the same category are presumed to have similar meanings.[3] Depending on the purposes of the investigator, this similarity may be based on the precise meaning of the words (such as grouping synonyms together), or may be based on words sharing similar connotations (such as grouping together several words implying a concern with a concept such as WEALTH[4] or POWER). To make valid inferences from the text, it is important that the classification procedure be reliable in the sense of being consistent: Different people should code the same text in the same way. Also, the classification procedure must generate variables that are valid. A variable is valid to the extent that it measures or represents what the investigator intends it to measure. Because of their central importance, the second chapter discusses reliability, validity, and content classification in detail.

In the past, investigators have used a variety of methods to make inferences from text. The third chapter presents a wide range of techniques that have proved useful.[5] Some of the methods are quite simple and, in a sense, linguistically naive.[6] One should not make the mistake, however, of believing that naive procedures must be put to naive uses. Many of these simple techniques produce highly reliable and valid indicators of symbolic content. Other content-analytic techniques are more complex or are used with statistical methods. Chapter 3 explains the use of these techniques, but highly technical matters are handled by notes or references to the literature.

Because of the general proliferation of computers and the growing capacities for microcomputers, Chapter 3 focuses on computer-aided content analysis. Computers can be used to manipulate the text easily, displaying it in various ways that often reveal aspects of symbol usage not otherwise apparent. For example, one can display all sentences or other units of texts containing a particular word or phrase. Another use of computers is to count symbols, such as all occurrences of the phrase *United States*.

Although this monograph presents numerous examples of what was put into and produced by computers, it does not specify the instructions given (i.e., the computer programs). The Appendix, however, discusses several programs for text analysis and includes information on hardware compatibility and software sources. The Appendix also provides some information on publicly available text data bases that are in machine-readable form.

The first three chapters document a solid core of useful knowledge and tools for the analysis of text. There exist, however, several methodological problems that detract from the reliability of the text classification process or from the validity of the consequent interpretations and explanations. These problems — the subject of Chapter 4 — fall into four major categories: measurement, indication, representation, and interpretation.

Concluding Remarks

The spirit of the following material is illustrative and didactic rather than dogmatic. There is no simple *right way* to do content analysis. Instead, investigators must judge what methods are most appropriate for their substantive problems. Moreover, some technical problems in content analysis have yet to be resolved or are the subject of ongoing research and debate; a few of these problems are discussed in Chapter 4. Where possible, this monograph tries to state the problem clearly, to suggest alternative resolutions (if they are known), and to suggest what kinds of information or capacities might help resolve the matter.

Rather than presenting a summary of the existing literature, this monograph deliberately emphasizes material not covered or stressed elsewhere. The goal is to produce a more interesting and useful guide for those planning or actually doing research using content analysis. During the past 20 years, the introduction of inexpensive microcomputers, the introduction of cost-effective devices for making text machine-readable, and the general reduction of computer costs have renewed interest in content analysis. In the 1990s these tools will be applied increasingly to a wide range of social science questions.

As a brief introduction to content analysis, much has been omitted here. Consequently, there are suggestions for further reading at the end of each chapter. These sources address content analysis methods, substantive research, general issues in research methodology, or statistics at a much greater level of detail than is possible or even desirable here.

Suggestions for Further Reading

There are several books on content analysis that should be read by anyone seriously interested in the subject. Krippendorff (1980) surveys the field and its problems. It is especially useful for those doing human-coded content analysis. His discussion of reliability is "must" reading; the book is not up-to-date, however, regarding the use of computers.

Other books contain numerous methodological insights and practical information. One is the original book on the General Inquirer system (Stone, Dunphy, Smith, and Ogilvie, 1966), the first widely used computer system for content analysis. Although the version discussed there is not the current one (see Kelly and Stone, 1975; Zuell, Weber, and Mohler, 1989), the book presents a wide-ranging discussion of content analysis, its problems, and practical solutions. Stone and his associates also present several chapters illustrating the application of computer-aided content analysis to a variety of substantive problems. Namenwirth and Weber (1987) combine an in-depth consideration of content analysis methods with empirical analyses of political documents and speeches. The results are then interpreted and explained using several major social science theories. Another useful resource is a set of conference papers edited by Gerbner, Holsti, Krippendorff, Paisley, and Stone (1969). This interdisciplinary collection addresses many issues still current in content analysis. Also, Holsti's (1969) brief discussion remains worthwhile reading. North, Holsti, Zaninovich, and Zinnes (1963) apply a variety of content-analytic techniques to the study of communications in international relations. There exists an earlier, precomputer body of work on using content analysis, notably Berelson (1952); Lasswell, Leites, et al. (1965); Lasswell, Lerner, and Pool (1952); and Pool (1952a, 1952b, 1959). Smith (1978) employs coding rules and categories related to the Semantic Differential (Osgood, May, and Miron, 1975; Osgood, Suci, and Tannenbaum, 1957).

More popular accounts that use content analysis to assess cultural and social trends include Merriam and Makower (1988) and Naisbitt (1982). Gottschalk (1979) and Gottschalk, Lolas, and Vinex (1986) show the use of content analysis in behavioral and psychological research. Herzog (1973) shows that, over the past few decades, American political discourse has communicated less and less information (see Orwell, 1949). Williams (1985) gives an historical, social, and political account of certain *keywords* that figure prominently in contemporary social and political speech. His account might be useful in the construction of category schemes.

2. CONTENT CLASSIFICATION AND INTERPRETATION

The central problems of content analysis originate mainly in the data-reduction process by which the many words of texts are classified into much fewer content categories. One set of problems concerns the consistency or reliability of text classification. In content analysis, reliability problems usually grow out of the ambiguity of word meanings, category definitions, or other coding rules. Classification by multiple human coders permits the quantitative assessment of achieved reliability. Classification by computer, however, leads to perfect coder reliability (if one assumes valid computer programs and well-functioning computer hardware). Once correctly defined for the computer, the coding rules are always applied in the same way.

A much more difficult set of problems concerns the validity of variables based on content classification. A content analysis variable is valid to the extent that it measures the construct the investigator intends it to measure. As happens with reliability, validity problems also grow out of the ambiguity of word meanings and category or variable definitions.

As an introduction to these problems, consider two sample texts and some simple coding rules. Using commonsense definitions, imagine that the coding instructions define five categories: CITIZENS' RIGHTS, ECONOMIC, GOVERNMENT, POLITICAL DOCTRINE, and WELFARE. Imagine also that coders are instructed to classify each entire paragraph in one category only. Consider first a portion of the Carter 1980 Democratic Platform:

Our current economic situation is unique. In 1977, we inherited a severe recession from the Republicans. The Democratic Administration and the Democratic Congress acted quickly to reduce the unacceptably high levels of unemployment and to stimulate the economy. And we succeeded. We recovered from that deep recession and our economy was strengthened and revitalized. As that fight was won, the enormous increases in foreign oil prices — 120 percent last year — and declining productivity fueled an inflationary spiral that also had to be fought. The Democrats did that, and inflation has begun to recede. In working to combat these dual problems, significant economic actions have been taken. (Johnson, 1982: 38)

Now consider another paragraph from the Reagan 1980 Republican platform:

Through long association with government programs, the word "welfare" has come to be perceived almost exclusively as tax-supported aid to the needy. But in its most inclusive sense — and as Americans understood it from the beginning of the Republic — such aid also encompasses those charitable works performed by private citizens, families, and social, ethnic, and religious organizations. Policies of the federal government leading to high taxes, rising inflation, and bureaucratic empire-building have made it difficult and often impossible for such individuals and groups to exercise their charitable instincts. We believe that government policies that fight inflation, reduce tax rates, and end bureaucratic excesses can help make private effort by the American people once again a major force in those works of charity which are the true signs of a progressive and humane society. (Johnson, 1982: 179)

Most people would code the first excerpt in the ECONOMIC category, but the proper coding of the second is less obvious. This paragraph could be taken to be mainly about the rights of citizens, the desirability of restricting the government's role, the welfare state, or to be the espousal of a political doctrine. In fact, it occurs at the end of a section titled *Improving the Welfare System*.

The difficulty of classifying the second excerpt is contrived partly by the present author, because it results from the lack of clear and detailed coding rules for each category and from the variety of the subject matter. Large portions of text, such as paragraphs and complete texts, usually are more difficult to code as a unit than smaller portions, such as words and phrases, because large units typically contain more information and a greater diversity of topics. Hence they are more likely to present coders with conflicting cues.

These examples show the kind of difficulties investigators face with coding text. The next two sections look more systematically at coding problems, first from the perspective of reliability assessment and then from the perspective of validity assessment.

Reliability

Three types of reliability are pertinent to content analysis: stability, reproducibility, and accuracy (Krippendorff, 1980: 130-154). *Stability* refers to the extent to which the results of content classification are invariant over time. Stability can be determined when the same content is coded more than once by the *same* coder. Inconsistencies in coding constitute unreliability. These inconsistencies may stem from a variety of factors, including ambiguities in the coding rules, ambiguities in the text, cognitive changes within the coder, or simple errors, such as recording the wrong numeric code for a category. Because only one person is coding, stability is the weakest form of reliability.

Reproducibility, sometimes called *intercoder reliability,* refers to the extent to which content classification produces the same results when the same text is coded by *more than one* coder. Conflicting codings usually result from cognitive differences among the coders, ambiguous coding instructions, or from random recording errors. High reproducibility is a minimum standard for content analysis. This is because stability measures the consistency of the individual coder's private understandings, whereas reproducibility measures the consistency of shared understandings (or meaning) held by two or more coders.

Accuracy refers to the extent to which the classification of text corresponds to a standard or norm. It is the strongest form of reliability. As Krippendorff notes (1980: 131), it has sometimes been used to test the performance of human coders where a standard coding for some text has already been established. Except for training purposes, standard codings are established infrequently for texts. Consequently, researchers seldom use accuracy in reliability assessment.

Krippendorff (1980: 132) also points out that many investigators fail totally to assess the reliability of their coding. Even when reliability is assessed, some investigators engage in practices that often make data seem more reliable than they actually are. In particular, where coders have disagreed, investigators have resolved these disagreements by negotiations or by invoking the authority of the principal investigator or senior graduate assistant. Resolving these disagreements may produce judgments biased toward the opinions of the most verbal or more senior of the coders. Consequently, the reliability of the coding should be calculated *before* these disagreements are resolved. Krippendorff goes on to show several ways of calculating reliability for human coders. Readers who plan to do human-coded content analysis should pay close attention to Krippendorff's discussion. Later sections of this chapter return to reliability issues in conjunction with category construction and word classification.

Validity

The term *validity* is potentially confusing because it has been used in a variety of ways in the methods literature (see Brinberg and Kidder, 1982; Brinberg and McGrath, 1985; Campbell and Stanley, 1963; Cook and Campbell, 1979). Two distinctions, however, may help clarify the concept. The first is between validity as correspondence between two sets of things — such as concepts, variables, methods, and data — and validity as generalizability of results, references, and theory (Brinberg and McGrath, 1982). Correspondence and generalizability are themes that run throughout the following discussion of validity.

A second distinction, more specific to content analysis, is between the validity of the classification scheme, or variables derived from it, and the validity of the interpretation relating content variables to their causes or consequences. To assert that a category or variable (ECONOMIC, for example) is valid is to assert that there is a correspondence between the category and the abstract concept that it represents (concern with economic matters). To assert that a research result based on content analysis is valid is to assert that the finding does not depend upon or is generalizable beyond the specific data, methods, or measurements of a particular study. For instance, if a computer-assisted content analysis of party platforms shows a strong relationship between long-term economic fluctuations and concern with the well-being of economy and society, then the validity of the results would be greater to the extent that other data (e.g., newspaper editorials), other coding procedures (e.g., human rather than computer-coded), or other classification schemes (dictionaries) produced substantive conclusions.

Perhaps the weakest form of validity is *face* validity, which consists of the correspondence between investigators' definitions of concepts and their definitions of the categories that measured them. A category has face validity to the extent that it appears to measure the construct it is intended to measure. Even if several expert judges agree, face validity is still a weak claim because it rests on a single variable. Stronger forms of validity involve more than one variable. Unfortunately, content analysts often have relied heavily on face validity; consequently, some other social scientists have viewed their results skeptically.

Much stronger validity is obtained by comparing content-analytic data with some external criterion. Four types of external validity are pertinent.

A measure has *construct validity*[7] to the extent that it is correlated with some other measure of the same construct. Thus construct validity entails the generalizability of the construct across measures or methods. Campbell and Fiske (1959) and others (e.g., Althauser, 1974; Alwin, 1974; Campbell and O'Connell, 1982; Fiske, 1982) further differentiate *convergent* from *discriminant* validity. A measure has high construct validity when it correlates with other measures of the same construct (convergent) and is uncorrelated with measures of dissimilar constructs (discriminant).

The research reported in Saris-Gallhofer, Saris, and Morton (1978) is a fine example of applying these ideas to content-analytic data. The object of this study was to validate a content-analysis dictionary developed by Holsti (1969) using the main categories of the Semantic Differential (Anderson, 1970; Osgood, May, and Miron, 1975; Osgood, Suci, and Tannenbaum, 1957; Snider and Osgood, 1969). The semantic differential is a technique for assessing the primary categories people use in affective evaluation or classification. The details of the technique are not pertinent here. Investigations in this tradition, however, show that in a variety of cultures people use three basic dimensions of classification. Each of these dimensions is anchored by polar opposites:

- *evaluation* (positive versus negative affect)
- *potency* (strength versus weakness)
- *activity* (active versus passive)

Each word in Holsti's dictionary was assigned three numbers, each indicating its classification on one of the three dimensions of the semantic differential. Saris-Gallhofer and her colleagues compared Holsti's assignment of scores with Osgood's and with scores assigned by a group of students. Thus each word (or other unit of text) was classified by three different methods, with each method claiming to classify text on the same constructs. Using statistical techniques designed to assess convergent and discriminant validity, Saris-Gallhofer found that Holsti's scoring for the evaluation and potency dimensions was much more valid than his scoring for the activity dimension. It remains unclear why Holsti's scoring of the activity dimension is less valid than the scores for the other two. Additional research is required to determine the specific factors that affect the validity of content classification. Nonetheless, this study shows that sophisticated statistical techniques useful in accessing validity can be applied to content analysis data.

Hypothesis validity, the second type, relies on the correspondence among variables and the correspondence between these relationships and theory. A measure has hypothesis validity if in relationship to other variables it "behaves" as it is expected to.[8] For example, several studies based on political documents — such as party platform in presidential campaigns — have shown that the preoccupation of society with economic issues increases during bad economic times and decreases when the economy is good (e.g., Namenwirth, 1969b; Namenwirth and Weber, 1987). These results are consistent with theoretical arguments relating the cultural and social processes that generate political documents (such as party platforms) with changes in the economy. Thus the observed inverse relationship between economic fluctuations and concern with economic matters suggests the hypothesis validity of measured variables and of the constructs that they represent.

A measure has *predictive validity,* the third type, to the extent that forecasts about events or conditions external to the study are shown to correspond to actual events or conditions. These predictions may concern future, past (postdiction), or concurrent events. Predictive validity is powerful because the inferences from data are generalized successfully beyond the study to situations not under the direct control of the investigator.

Content-analytic data are seldom shown to have predictive validity,[9] but three examples illustrate the point:

1. Ogilvie, Stone, and Shneidman (1966) analyzed real suicide notes from 33 males who had been matched for age, gender, occupation, religion, and ethnicity with 33 nonsuicidal controls who were asked to produce simulated suicide notes. Using General Inquirer-type computer-aided content analysis, Stone was able to correctly distinguish real from simulated suicide notes in 30 of the 33 pairs (90.9%) of notes.

2. George (1959a) studied inferences made by The Foreign Broadcast Intelligence Service of the FCC from German Propaganda during the Second World War. He found that Allied intelligence analysts often could

anticipate changes in German war tactics and strategy from changes in the content of radio broadcasts and other media.

3. Namenwirth's (1973) analysis of party platforms in presidential campaigns, written in the late 1960s, suggested that America would experience severe economic difficulties that would peak about 1980. Events since seem to confirm this prediction.

Words or other coding units classified together need to possess similar connotations in order for the classification to have *semantic validity*, the fourth and final type. According to Krippendorff (1980: 159ff), semantic validity exists when persons familiar with the language and texts examine lists of words (or other units) placed in the same category and agree that these words have similar meanings or connotations.

Although this seems an obvious requirement for valid content analysis, many difficulties arise because words and category definitions are sometimes ambiguous. For example, some systems for computer-aided content analysis cannot distinguish among the various senses of words with more than one meaning, such as *mine*. Does this refer to a hole in the ground, the process of extraction, or a possessive pronoun? Because of this failure, word counts including the frequency of *mine* lack semantic validity. Various aspects of semantic validity are discussed later in this and in subsequent chapters.

Creating and Testing
a Coding Scheme

Many studies require investigators to design and implement coding schemes. Whether the coding is to be done by humans or by computer, the process of creating and applying a coding scheme consists of several basic steps. If investigators have identified the substantive questions to be investigated, relevant theories, previous research, and the texts to be classified, they next proceed with the following necessary steps:

1. *Define the recording units.* One of the most fundamental and important decisions concerns the definition of the basic unit of text to be classified. There are six commonly used options:

- *Word* — One choice is to code each word. As noted, some computer software for text analysis cannot distinguish among the various senses of words with more than one meaning, and hence may produce erroneous conclusions.

- *Word sense* — Other computer programs are able to code the different senses of words with multiple meanings and to code phrases that constitute a semantic unit, such as idioms (e.g., *taken for granted*) or proper nouns (e.g., *the Empire State Building*). These issues are discussed in detail later.

- *Sentence* — An entire sentence is often the recording unit when the investigator is interested in words or phrases that occur closely together. For example, coders may be instructed to count sentences in which either positive, negative, or affectively neutral references are made to the Soviet Union. A sentence with the phrase *evil empire* would be counted as NEGATIVE EVALUATION, whereas *Talks with the Soviet Union continue* would be coded NEUTRAL EVALUATION, and *The President supports recent efforts to extend economic and political rights in the Soviet Union* would be coded POSITIVE EVALUATION.

- *Theme* — Holsti (1963: 136, emphasis in the original) defines a theme as a unit of text "having *no more than one each of the following elements:* (1) the *perceiver,* (2) the *perceived* or agent of action, (3) the *action,* (4) the *target* of the action." For example, the sentence *The President / hates / Communists* would be divided as shown. Numeric or other codes often are inserted in the text to represent subject / verb / object. This form of coding preserves important information and provides a means of distinguishing between the sentence above and the assertion that *Communists hate the President.*

Sometimes long, complex sentences must be broken down into shorter thematic units or segments. Here, parts of speech shared between themes must be repeated. Also, ambiguous phrases and pronouns must be identified manually. These steps are taken before coding for the content. Holsti (1963: 136-137) gives the following example of editing more complex sentences before coding for themes and content:[10]

> The sentence, "The American imperialists have perverted the peace and are preparing to attack the Socialist Camp," must be edited to read: The American imperialists have perverted the peace + (the Americans) are preparing to attack the Socialist Camp."

This form of coding is labor-intensive, but leads to much more detailed and sophisticated comparisons. See Holsti (1963, 1966, 1969) for further details.

- *Paragraph* — When computer assistance is not feasible and when resources for human coding are limited, investigators sometimes code entire paragraphs to reduce the effort required. Evidence discussed later in this chapter shows that it is more difficult to achieve high reliability when coding large units, such as paragraphs, than when coding smaller units, such as words.

- *Whole text* — Unless the entire text is short — like newspaper headlines, editorials, or stories — it is difficult to achieve high reliability when coding complete texts.

2. *Define the categories.* In creating category definitions, investigators must make two basic decisions. (Other related issues are taken up later.) The first is whether the categories are to be mutually exclusive. Most statistical procedures require variables that are not confounded. If a recording unit can be classified simultaneously in two or more categories and if both categories (variables) are included in the same statistical analysis, then it is possible that, because the basic statistical assumptions of the analysis are violated, the results are dubious. This is likely to be the case when using common multivariate procedures such as factor analysis, analysis of variance, and multiple regression.

The second choice concerns how narrow or broad the categories are to be. Some categories are limited because of language. For example, a category indicating self-references defined as first person singular pronouns will have only a few words or entries. A category defined as concern with ECONOMIC matters may have many entries. For some purposes, however, it may make sense to use much more narrow or specific categories, such as INFLATION, TAXES, BUDGET, TRADE, AGRI-CULTURE, and so on.

3. *Test coding on sample of text.* The best test of the clarity of category definitions is to code a small sample of the text. Testing not only reveals ambiguities in the rules, but also often leads to insights suggesting revisions of the classification scheme.

4. *Assess accuracy or reliability. Accuracy* in this sense means the text is coded correctly by the computer, not in the sense of the type of reliability that was discussed earlier. If human coders are used, the reliability of the coding process should be estimated *before* resolving disputes among the coders.

5. *Revise the coding rules.* If the reliability is low, or if errors in computer procedures are discovered, the coding rules must be revised or the software corrected.

6. *Return to Step 3.* This cycle will continue until the coders achieve sufficient reliability or until the computer procedures work correctly.

7. *Code all the text.* When high coder reliability has been achieved or when the computer programs are functioning correctly, the coding rules can then be applied to all the text.

8. *Assess achieved reliability or accuracy.* The reliability of human coders should be assessed after the text is classified. Never assume that if samples of text were coded reliably then the entire corpus of text will also be coded reliably. Human coders are subject to fatigue and are likely to make more mistakes as the coding proceeds. Also, as the text is coded, their understanding of the coding rules may change in subtle ways that lead to greater unreliability.

If the coding was done by computer, the output should be checked carefully to insure that the coding rules were applied correctly. Text not in the sample(s) used for testing may present novel combinations of words that were not anticipated or encountered earlier, and these may be misclassified.

Dictionaries and Computerized Text Classification

Content analysts have used several strategies to create categories and variables. Some investigators have counted by hand a few key words or phrases. Tufte (1978: 75), for example, counted certain words in the 1976 Democratic and Republican party platforms, including indicators of distributional issues (such as *inequity, regressive, equal,* and *redistribution*) and indicators of concern with inflation (such as *inflation, inflationary, price stability,* and *rising prices*).

Others have constructed a set of content categories on the basis of a single concept. For example, the early version of Stone's General Inquirer computer system was used to analyze achievement imagery (McClelland's N-Achievement; Stone, Dunphy, Smith, and Ogilvie, 1966: 191ff). This approach offers several advantages. It permits the intensive and detailed analysis of a single theoretical construct. It also provides an explicit rationale not only for what is retained, but also for what is excluded from the analysis. Furthermore, single-concept coding schemes often have high validity and reliability.

Another approach to content analysis involves the creation and application of general dictionaries.[11] Content-analysis dictionaries consist of category names, the definitions or rules for assigning words to categories, and the actual assignment of specific words. This strategy provides the researcher with numerous categories (60 to 150+) into which most words in most texts can be classified.[12] Once created, general dictionaries are advantageous because they:

- provide a wide range of categories to choose from (see Stone et al., 1966: 42-44)
- minimize the time needed for dictionary construction, validation, and revision
- standardize classification
- encourage the accumulation of comparable results when used in many studies[13]

It is worth noting that dictionary construction commonly is misperceived to be merely a preface or preparatory step for quantification. While researchers frequently use dictionaries to define variables for quantification, they also use categories to locate and retrieve text by finding occurrences of semantically equivalent symbols. Chapter 3 presents examples of retrievals based on categories.

Certain problems arise in the creation of *any* content category or set of categories. These problems stem from the ambiguity of both the category definitions and the words that are to be assigned to categories. To aid discussion of these difficulties, two general dictionaries are used as examples: the Harvard IV Psychosocial Dictionaries, developed by Dexter Dunphy and his associates (Dunphy, Bullard, and Crossing, 1989; Kelly and Stone, 1975; Zuell, Weber, and Mohler, 1989), and the Lasswell Value Dictionary (LVD), developed and extended by J. Zvi Namenwirth and his associates (Namenwirth and Weber, 1987; Zuell et al., 1989). Both dictionaries are used with Stone's General Inquirer system for the analysis of English language text.[14]

Tables 2.1 and 2.2 present definitions of selected content categories from the LVD and Harvard IV-4 dictionaries, respectively.[15] Categories often are represented by abbreviations or tags, which appear in these tables. The process of classifying words in texts is often called *tagging*. The categories that appear in these tables show similarities and differences between the dictionaries and introduce the analysis of sample text presented below and in Chapter 3.

For instance, one set of LVD categories contains those words, word senses,[16] and idioms that denote wealth-related matters. Another category contains wealth words indicating a transaction or exchange of

TABLE 2.1

Selected Lasswell Value Dictionary Categories

Tag	Full Name and Definition
ENLSCOP	ENLIGHTENMENT-SCOPE-INDICATOR: Words indicating concern with wisdom, knowledge, etc. as a fundamental goal rather than a means to other ends.
ENLTOT	ENLIGHTENMENT-TOTAL: Indicates concern with knowledge, insight and information concerning cultural and personal relations. Includes all entries denoting and describing academic matters and the processes that generate and communicate information, thought, and understanding.
NTYPE	N-TYPE WORDS: Relatively high frequency words that often lack semantic meaning, e.g., *a, the, to,* forms of the verb *to be.*
SCOPIND	SCOPE-INDICATOR: Indicates concern with ultimate ends rather than with means.
SELVES	SELVES: First person plural pronouns.
SKLTOT	SKILL-TOTAL: SKILL is defined as proficiency in any practice whatever, whether in arts or crafts, trade or profession. Indicates a concern with the mastery of the physical environment and the skills and tools used to that purpose.
SURE	SURE: Sentiment category containing words that indicate certainty, sureness, and firmness.
TIMESP	TIME-SPACE: General time and space category. Contains directions, e.g., *up, down,* etc., and time indicators, e.g., *hour, early, late.*
UNDEF	UNDEFINED: Includes words with value implications that vary from context to context, and which, notwithstanding disambiguation routes, cannot be assessed reliably by present procedures.
UNDEF*	UNDEFINABLE: Includes entries which have no value implications or which have value meaning which cannot be defined in terms of the present category scheme.
WLTOTH	WEALTH-OTHER: Entries denoting the wealth process not classified as PARTICIPANT or TRANSACTION are classified here.
WLTPT	WEALTH-PARTICIPANT: Contains the generic names of the trades and professions in the wealth process. Also includes social roles related to wealth processes, e.g., *banker.*
WLTTOT	WEALTH-TOTAL: Wealth is defined as income or services of goods and persons accruing to the person in any way whatsoever. All references to production resources and the accumulation or exchange of goods and services have been included in this category.
WLTXACT	WEALTH-TRANSACTION: Contains references to the creation or exchange of wealth, mainly verbs.
XACT	TRANSACTION: Residual category indicating value transactions not classified elsewhere because it could not be determined reliably whether the transaction resulted in a gain or loss or what was the object of the transaction.

TABLE 2.2

Selected Harvard IV Dictionary Categories

Tag	Full Name and Definition
AFFIL	AFFILIATION: All words with the connotation of affiliation or supportiveness.
BEGIN	BEGIN: Words indicating beginning.
CAUSAL	CAUSAL: Words denoting presumption that occurrence of one phenomenon necessarily is preceded, accompanied, or followed by the occurrence of another.
COLL	COLLECTIVITY: All-collectivities excluding animal collectivities (ANIMAL).
COMFORM	COMMUNICATION FORM: All processes and forms of communication, excluding finite, concrete, visible, and tangible objects for communication, e.g., *book*, but does include words such as *essay, fare*, and *chapter*, where the emphasis is more on the communication transaction than on the object itself.
COMN	COMMUNICATION: All forms and processes of communication.
DOCTR	DOCTRINE: Organized systems of belief or knowledge. Includes all formal bodies of knowledge (*astronomy, agriculture*), belief systems (*Christianity, stoicism*), the arts.
ECON*	ECONOMIC: All words which relate to economic, commercial, and industrial matters. Includes all economic roles, collectivities, acts, abstract ideas, and symbols. Also includes references to technical industrial processes and to economic commodities such as coal and aluminum.
EXCH	EXCHANGE: Words indicating economic processes and transactions such as buying and selling.
GOAL	GOAL: Names of end-states toward which striving, muscular or mental, is directed.
IMPERS	IMPERSONAL: All impersonal nouns.
INCR	INCREASE: Words indicating increase.
INTREL	INTERRELATE: Interpersonal action words involving changing relationships between people, things, or ideas. Abstract nouns derived from these verbs are to be found generally in VIRTUE or VICE.
OUR	OUR: All pronouns which are inclusive self-references.
OVRST	OVERSTATE: Words providing emphasis in the following areas: speed, frequency, inevitability, causality, inclusiveness of persons, objects, or places, quantity in numerical and quasi-numerical terms, accuracy and validity, importance, intensity, likelihood, certainty, and extremity.
POLIT*	POLITICAL: All words with a clearly political character. Includes political roles, collectivities, acts, ideas, ideologies, and symbols.
POWER	POWER: All words with the connotation of power, control, or authority.

value (WEALTH-TRANSACTIONS), such as forms of the verbs *buy, sell,* and *mortgage.* A third category contains words that name a role or person involved in wealth matters (WEALTH-PARTICIPANTS), such as *banker, buyer,* and *seller.*

Reliability and Classification Schemes

As noted, the construction of valid and useful content categories depends on the interaction between language and the classification scheme (Namenwirth and Weber, 1987). For example, one often can think of categories for which only a few words exist, such as a category for first person singular pronouns (e.g., SELF in the LVD). To avoid difficulties in statistical estimation[17] resulting from categories with limited numbers of words, the LVD aggregates the remaining wealth-related words, word senses, and idioms indicating a concern with wealth into a WEALTH-OTHER category. Finally, all the WEALTH subcategories are combined into a category indicating the overall concern with economic matters, WEALTH-TOTAL. In comparison (Table 2.3), the Harvard IV-4 dictionary scheme provides only two similar categories, ECONOMIC and EXCHANGE. Another perspective on classification schemes is gained by examining the assignment of words to categories. Table 2.3 presents a portion of the alphabetic list of nouns assigned to WEALTH-OTHER. The LVD originally was constructed primarily for the analysis of political documents, such as newspaper editorials and party platforms. Thus the WEALTH-OTHER category includes many nouns that refer to commodities, such as *corn, tin,* and so forth because in political documents references to these commodities occur in an economic context (e.g., *The price of corn declined for the seventh consecutive month*).

The numbers at the end of some words indicate the particular sense number of a word with more than one meaning (i.e., a homograph). They are not immediately useful without a corresponding list of the various senses of each homograph, but space limitations preclude an extensive discussion here (the interested reader is referred to Kelly and Stone, 1975; Zuell et al., 1989).

Although categories about economic matters generally have high internal consistency in the sense that all the words have similar connotations, this is not necessarily the case with other categories. For example, the LVD lumps together words related to temporal and spatial relations. The justification for this has always been vague, and perhaps there should be a separate category for each. Similarly, the Harvard

TABLE 2.3

Alphabetical Listing of WEALTH-OTHER Nouns,

(Lasswell Value Dictionary)

NOUNS	DEPRESSION#2	IRRIGATION	RESOURCE
ABUNDANCE	DOLLAR	LEDGER	RETAIL#1
ACCOUNT#2	EARN#2	LIABILITY#1	RETIREMENT
ACRE	ECONOMICS	LIVESTOCK	RETURN#3
AFFLUENCE	ECONOMIST	LOAN#1	RICH#6
AGRICULTURE	ECONOMY	LOT#3	ROAD#1
ALLOWANCE	ELECTRICITY	LOW-COST	ROYALTY#2
ANNUITY	EMPLOYMENT	LUXURY	RUBBER
APPROPRIATION	END#6	MANUFACTURE#1	SALARY
ARTICLE#2	ENDOWMENT	MANUFACTURER	SALESMANSHIP
AUTO	ENERGY	MARKET#1	SAVE#3
AUTOMOBILE	ENGINE	MARKET#2	SCARCITY
BACKWARDNESS	ENTERPRISE	MERCHANDISE	SECURITY#2
BALE	EQUITY	MINE#2	SECURITY#3
BANKRUPTCY	ESTATE	MINERAL	SELL#2
BARGAIN#1	EXPENDITURE	MINT	SHIFT#2
BELONG#2	EXPENSE#1	MONEY	SHOP#1
BENEFIT#1	EXPORT#1	MORTGAGE#1	SHOP#3
BILL#2	FACTORY	OIL	SILK
BONUS	FARM#1	ORE	STEEL
BOOKKEEPING	FARM#3	OUTPUT#1	STERLING
BOUNTY	FERTILIZER	OWNERSHIP	STOCK
BRANCH#2	FINANCE#1	PARITY	STORE#1
BRASS	FOREST	PAY#2	STORE#3
BREAD	FORESTRY	PAYROLL	SUPPLIER
BUDGET	FORTUNE#2	PENNY	SUPPLY#1
BUSINESS#1	FREIGHT	PENSION	SURPLUS
BUY#2	FRUGALITY	PIECE#2	TARIFF
CAPITAL	FUND#1	PLANT#2	TAX#1
CAR	FUND#2	PLANTATION	TAX#3
CARTEL	FUR	POOR#5	TAX#4
CASH#1	GARDEN#1	POPULATION	TAXATION
CATTLE	GARDEN#2	PORT	TEXTILE
CENT	GIFT	POULTRY	TIMBER
CHARGE#4	GOLD	POUND#1	TIN
CHECK#1	GOODS	POVERTY	TRAIN#1
CHEQUE	GRAIN	PRESENT#5	TRANSPORT#1
CLEAR#10	GRANT#1	PRICE	TRANSPORTATION
COAL	HERD#1	PROCEED#3	TREASURE#1
COFFEE	HIDE#3	PRODUCE#2	TREASURER
COIN	HIGHWAY	PRODUCER	TREASURY
COLLATERAL	HOLD#N	PRODUCTIVITY	TRUST#5
COMMERCE	HORTICULTURE	PROPERTY	UNEMPLOYMENT
COMMODITY	HOUSEHOLD	PROSPERITY	WAGE#1
COPPER	INCENTIVE	RANCH	WEALTH#1
COPYRIGHT	INCOME#1	RANCHER	WHEAT
CORN	INDEMNITY	RATE#1	WHOLESALE
COTTON	INDUSTRIALISM	REAL#3	WIN#3
CROP#1	INDUSTRY	RECEIPT	WOOD#1
CURRENCY	INFLATION	RECLAMATION	WOOD#2
CUSTOM#2	INPUT	REDEVELOPMENT	WOOL
DEBT	INTEREST#2	REFUND#1	WORTH#3
DEFICIT	INVENTORY	REMUNERATION	
DEPARTMENT#2	INVESTMENT	RENT#1	
DEPRECIATION	IRON#1	RENTAL	

dictionary classifies words that refer to political ideologies and to political actors in the same category. Again, the justification for this strategy is unclear.

Whether to extend the effort required to resolve these kinds of difficulties will depend on the goals of specific investigations. For example, if *time* is an important concept, then separate categories for *space* and *time* will be desirable.

Even if the ambiguity of category definitions and word classifications can be overcome, other potential sources of error remain. As noted, one of the most serious problems in some computer programs for content analysis is that they cannot deal with words that have more than one meaning (i.e., homographs). For example, does *kind* refer to class of objects or a benevolent disposition? For English-language text, these problems are resolved by the latest version of the General Inquirer system (Kelly and Stone, 1975; Zuell et al., 1989). These computer programs and their associated dictionaries — the Harvard IV and the LVD — incorporate rules that distinguish among the various senses of homographs according to the context of usage. Technically known as *disambiguation rules,* these procedures lead to an important increase in the precision of text classification. In this context, higher precision refers to higher accuracy resulting from more or finer distinctions.[18]

Another problem in text analysis arises from phrases or idioms that constitute a single unit of meaning. Some of these are proper noun phrases — for example, *Sage Publications, United Nations,* or *United States of America.* Others are idioms or phrases such as *bleeding-heart liberals, point of no return,* or *a turn for the worst.* Whereas the earliest forms of the General Inquirer included the capability to handle idioms, the latest version uses the same flexible features for handling homographs to handle idioms. Thus the investigator can choose from among the individual word, word sense (of homographs), or phrase as the appropriate semantic unit.[19]

Although some computer systems handle the ambiguity of homographs, there exist other unresolved difficulties with this type of text classification. Because this software operates on only one sentence at a time, it cannot determine the referents of pronouns and ambiguous phrases (such as *we* or *dual problems* in the last sentence of the first example at the beginning of this chapter). Two resolutions of this problem have been commonly employed. The first is to ignore it, with the consequence that some category counts are slight underestimations. The second strategy is to edit the text so that the referent is placed immediately after the pronoun or phrases. This method is labor-intensive, but leads to more accurate counts.[20] Here is an excerpt from the 1886 address of the British monarch before Parliament (similar to our State of the Union address) discussing Home Rule for Ireland with the referent of *it* identified by the investigator (adapted from Namenwirth and Weber, 1987: 108):

> I have seen with deep sorrow the renewal, since I last addressed you, of the attempt to excite the people of Ireland to hostility against the legislative union between that country and Great Britain. I am resolutely opposed to any disturbance of the fundamental law, and in resisting it [any disturbance of the fundamental law] I am convinced that I shall be heartily supported by my Parliament and my people.

TABLE 2.4

Sample Text with LVD Tags

Word	Categories
SENTENCE 7 ** DOCUMENT 1 ** IDENTIFICATION AD1980	
THE	N-TYPE
EFFECT#1	SCOPE-INDICATOR
ON	N-TYPE
OUR	SELVES
ECONOMY	WEALTH-OTHER WEALTH-TOTAL
MUST#1	UNDEFINED
BE#1	N-TYPE
ONE#2	UNDEFINABLE
WHICH	N-TYPE
ENCOURAGE#1S	POWER-INDULGENCE POWER-TOTAL
JOB	SKILL-OTHER SKILL-TOTAL
FORMATION	UNDEFINED
AND	N-TYPE
BUSINESS#1	WEALTH-OTHER WEALTH-TOTAL
GROWTH.	SCOPE-INDICATOR
*** START NEW DOCUMENT..	
SENTENCE 8 ** DOCUMENT 2 ** IDENTIFICATION AR1980	
TAX#1ES.	WEALTH-OTHER WEALTH-TOTAL
SENTENCE 9 ** DOCUMENT 2 ** IDENTIFICATION AR1980	
ELSEWHERE	TIME-SPACE
IN	N-TYPE
THIS#1	N-TYPE
PLATFORM#1	POWER-OTHER POWER-TOTAL
WE	SELVES
DISCUSS	ENLIGHTENMENT-SCOPE-INDICATOR ENLIGHTENMENT-TOTAL
THE	N-TYPE
BENEFIT#3S	BASE-INDICATOR
FOR	N-TYPE
SOCIETY	COLLECTIVE-PARTICIPANT
AS#1	N-TYPE
A	N-TYPE
WHOLE#2,	UNDEFINED
OF	N-TYPE
REDUCED	TRANSACTION
TAXATION,	WEALTH-OTHER WEALTH-TOTAL
PARTICULAR#4LY	SURE
IN	N-TYPE
TERM#1S	ENLIGHTENMENT-OTHER ENLIGHTENMENT-TOTAL
OF	N-TYPE
ECONOMIC	WEALTH-OTHER WEALTH-TOTAL
GROWTH.	SCOPE-INDICATOR

Table 2.4 presents a few sentences from the 1980 party platforms. Each word is followed by a list of assigned LVD categories.[21] As in the previous table, the numbers next to some words indicate the particular sense of homographs. A significant portion of the text consists of words that are important for the construction of sentences, but are not assigned to substantive LVD categories. These N-TYPE words include articles (e.g. *a, the*) and some prepositions (e.g., *in, of*). Indices usually are constructed after subtracting the number of N-TYPE words from the total number of words. For example, dividing the number of words in a document classified in a particular category by the total minus N-TYPE number of words in the document yields a measure interpreted as the proportion of words with relevant semantic information classified in that category.

Additional problems arise because some words may be classified in two categories, where one is a total and the other is a subcategory. *Economy,* for example, is classified as WEALTH-OTHER and WEALTH-TOTAL. As noted, to maintain the mathematical independence of the content variables, investigators should analyze either the total category or one or more subcategories, but not both the total and one or more subcategories in the same statistical procedure.

A major advantage of computer-aided content analysis is that the same text can be analyzed easily using more than one category scheme. Also, because of errors or because changes seem justified in light of the particular text being analyzed, the text can be reclassified after making modifications to an existing dictionary. Table 2.5 presents the text from Table 2.4 classified according to the categories of the Harvard IV-4 dictionary. Again, the output consists of words with the sense numbers of homographs and a list of assigned Harvard IV categories.[22]

Several ways of manipulating, classifying, and analyzing text are presented in Chapter 3. The remainder of this chapter discusses several important problems in the construction of category schemes and text classification.

Single Versus Multiple Classification

In classifying a word or other recording unit into a particular dictionary category, one really answers the question: Does the entry generally have a certain attribute (or set of interrelated attributes)? Two answers to this question exist: yes, the entry does, and therefore it is classified thus; or no, and therefore the entry is not classified under this heading.

TABLE 2.5

Sample Text with Harvard IV Tags

Word	Categories
SENTENCE 7 ** DOCUMENT 1 ** IDENTIFICATION AD1980	
THE	ARTICLE
EFFECT#1	ABSTRACT CAUSAL PSV
ON	SPACE
OUR	AFFILIATION OUR
ECONOMY	DOCTRINE ECONOMIC
MUST#1	OUGHT
BE#1	BE
ONE#2	INDEF OTHER
WHICH	INDEF INT RLTVI
ENCOURAGE#1S	INTERRELATEL AFFILIATION PSTV ACTV
JOB	MEANS ECONOMIC
FORMATION	MEANS STRNG
AND	CONJ1
BUSINESS#1	DOCTRINE ECONOMIC
GROWTH.	STRNG INCR PSV
*** START NEW DOCUMENT..	
SENTENCE 8 ** DOCUMENT 2 ** IDENTIFICATION AR1980	
TAX#1ES.	MEANS POLIT ECONOMIC
SENTENCE 9 ** DOCUMENT 2 ** IDENTIFICATION AR1980	
ELSEWHERE	SPACE
IN	SPACE
THIS#1	DEM DEM1
PLATFORM#1	DOCTRINE POLITICAL
WE	PLRLP OUR
DISCUSS	PSTV COMFORM
THE	ARTICLE
BENEFIT#3S,	GOAL PSTV STRNG
FOR	CONJ CONJ2
SOCIETY	COLL POLITICAL
AS#1	CONJ2 CAUSAL
A	ARTICLE
WHOLE#2,	QUAN STRNG OVRST
OF	PREP
REDUCED	DECR STRNG
TAXATION,	MEANS POLIT ECONOMIC
PARTICULAR#4LY	OVRST
IN	SPACE
TERM#1S	COM COMFORM
OF	PREP
ECONOMIC	POLIT DOCTRINE ECONOMIC
GROWTH.	STRNG INCR PSV

This formulation points at two complications. First, having one attribute logically does not exclude the possession of another. Second, not all entries need have the same attribute to the same extent; the qualities by which words are classified may be continuous rather than dichotomous, thus leading to variation in intensity.[23] Double or multiple classification of entries resolves the first problem, but creates others.

Different strategies have been followed to resolve these issues. For example, the design of the Lasswell dictionary assumes that the gain in semantic precision does not outweigh the loss of logical distinctiveness and exclusiveness (Namenwirth and Weber, 1987; Zuell et al., 1989). Logical exclusiveness is a precarious precondition of all classification for subsequent statistical analysis. Therefore, in the Lasswell dictionary, if an entry can be classified under more than one category it is classified in the category that seems most appropriate — most of the time — for most texts. As for intensity, although it is true that not all entries will reflect the category to the same extent, Namenwirth and Weber (1987) chose a dichotomous rather than a weighted classification scheme because no reliable method for assigning weights or intensity scores could be perfected.

The category scheme of the current Harvard dictionaries was constructed using a very different strategy (Dunphy et al., 1989). They have a set of *first-order* categories to which entries can be assigned on a hierarchical basis if warranted. These first-order categories represent the basic analytic categories. Figure 2.1 illustrates the hierarchical nature of the Harvard IV-4 first-order categories that deal with psychological states. Two categories, NEED and PERCEIVE, have no subcategories, but FEEL, THINK, and EVALUATE do.

The Harvard dictionary contains another set of categories, called *second-order* categories that are independent of the first, and provide alternative modes of classification. For example, there is a set of second-order categories derived from the Osgood semantic differential discussed earlier. How, then, are words classified using this architecture? The word *abstract* is classified in both THINK and its subcategory KNOW. *Absence* is categorized in the same two categories with the addition of WEAK, one of the Osgood categories. *Acceptable* is classified in the first-order THINK and EVALUATE, the EVALUATE subcategory VIRTUE, and the Osgood POSITIVE category.

Although this type of scheme provides a multitude of possibilities for the investigator, great care must be taken if multivariate statistical

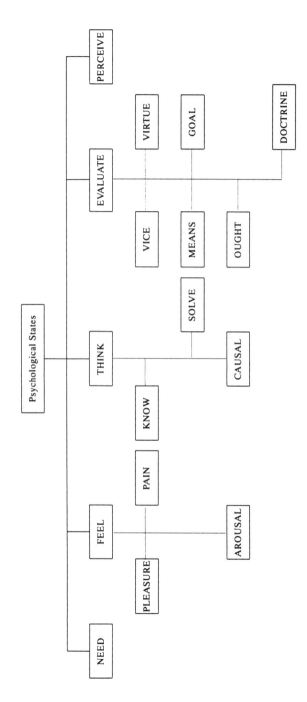

Figure 2.1. Harvard IV Dictionary First-Order Categories: Psychological States.

procedures will be used to analyze category counts, because the categories and the variables based on them may not be mutually exclusive.

Even if the category definition is precise, the decision to classify a particular word in a category often is difficult because of ambiguities in word meaning. Word ambiguity poses two problems. As noted above, a word may have multiple meanings. Also, a word may not seem as strong an indicator of a category as other similar words. Consider the LVD category SURE (similar to the Harvard category OVERSTATE), which contains words indicating certainty, sureness, and firmness. Words such as *certainly, sure,* and *emphatically* fit the definition quite well. But what about *authoritative* and *doctrinaire,* which in one thesaurus are also listed under "certainty"? In the LVD, *authoritative* is categorized with words indicating a concern with authoritative power (POWER-AUTHORITATIVE), whereas *doctrinaire* is categorized with words indicating a concern with doctrines and ideologies (POWER-DOCTRINE).

In some instances the investigator may decide that certain words clearly represent a particular category, that other words indicate or represent a category less strongly than words in the first group, while still other words seem to belong in more than one category. Many proposals exist to resolve these problems (Namenwirth and Weber, 1987: chapter 8), but none are entirely satisfactory. One solution is to weight each word depending on how well it connotes the category. Advocates of this strategy, however, never have provided a convincing argument demonstrating how valid weights can be determined reliably. An alternate solution is to categorize some words in more than one category. This strategy may lead to conceptually fuzzy categories, which, as noted, lack statistical independence.

Perhaps the best practical strategy is to classify each word, word sense, or phrase in the category where it most clearly belongs. If there is sufficient ambiguity, the word should be dropped from the category and — if necessary — from analysis. This tactic restricts categories to those words that unmistakably indicate concern with the category, thereby maximizing validity. Some words of substantive interest, however, may not be analyzed because they are not clear indicators of a particular category. Each investigator will have to find the resolution that makes the most sense in light of the goals of the analysis.

Assumed Versus Inferred Categories

Compared with hand coding, computer-based content analysis has the advantage that one set of texts can be classified easily by more than one dictionary. This, however, generates multiple descriptions of the same textual reality. Consequently, an important debate exists over whose classification scheme should be used. Some (Dunphy et al., 1989; Stone et al., 1966) hold that the category scheme should be justified theoretically; therefore, the investigator's categories should be used. For example, the earliest Harvard Psychosocial dictionaries were based in part on Parsonian and Freudian concepts (Stone et al., 1966) whereas the Lasswell Value Dictionary (Namenwirth and Weber, 1987; Zuell et al., 1989) is predicated on Lasswell and Kaplan's (1950) conceptual scheme for political analysis.[24]

Others (e.g., Cleveland, McTavish, and Pirro, 1974; Iker and Harway, 1969; Krippendorff, 1980: 126) argue that assumed category schemes impose the reality of the investigator on the text and that the better course of action uses the categories of those who produced the text.[25] These categories frequently are inferred from covariation among high-frequency words using factor analysis or similar techniques.[26]

This dispute stems both from difficult methodological problems and from conceptual confusion. Specifically, let the term *category* be reserved for groups of words with *similar* meanings and/or connotations (Dunphy et al., 1989; Stone et al., 1966). The words *banker, money,* and *mortgage* might be classified in a WEALTH or ECONOMIC category. Now let the term *theme* refer to clusters of words with *different* meanings or connotations that taken together refer to some theme or issue. For instance, the sentence *New York bankers invest money in many industries both at home and abroad* in part reflects concern with an economic theme. This disagreement over categories is largely a dispute between those who define categories as words with different meanings or connotations that covary empirically (inferred categories) and those who define categories as words with similar meanings or connotations that do not covary (assumed categories). Words classified as ECONOMIC, for example, will tend to covary with words in other categories, say POWER, UNCERTAINTY, or WELL-BEING, rather than with other ECONOMIC words.

Terminology aside, in studies using inferred categories, different category schemes arise from different sets of texts. Advocates of inferred categories have failed to recognize that this multitude of categories requires a theory of categories. Such a theory would explain the range of possible categories and the empirically observed variation in category schemes (Namenwirth and Weber, 1987). Without such a theory, research using inferred categories is unlikely to lead to the cumulation of comparable results.

Alternate Classification Schemes and Substantive Results

The choice of classification schemes is in part predicated on theoretical considerations. For example, if one wishes to study exclusively a particular construct, such as McClelland's Need Achievement (Nach), then one might construct a dictionary that scores only that variable (e.g., Stone et al., 1966: 191ff). General dictionaries follow a different strategy based on many commonsense categories of meaning. These categories are chosen to reflect the wide range of human experience and understanding encoded in language.

Having decided to use the strategy of general dictionaries, the choice of one rather than another content classification scheme has little or no effect on the substantive results. That is, if the same text is classified using different general dictionaries (and analogous measurement models; see Namenwirth and Weber, 1987: chapter 8), then one will arrive at the same substantive conclusions.

Empirical evidence supports this point (Namenwirth and Bibbee, 1975: 61). In their analysis of newspaper editorials, Namenwirth and Bibbee classified the text using two different dictionaries and then factor analyzed the two sets of scores separately. Comparing the results across dictionaries, they found that the factors had similar interpretations. Furthermore, irrespective of which dictionary was used, Namenwirth and Bibbee arrived at similar substantive conclusions.[27]

This evidence is suggestive rather than conclusive. Consequently, future research should investigate the relationship between the dictionary used to classify text and the substantive conclusions. Texts can be classified with more than one dictionary and the results compared. If the results only partially replicate across dictionaries, additional research should determine the circumstances under which the results are similar and variant. Also, if the substantive conclusions do not depend on the particular category scheme, researchers reluctant to use one or another existing dictionary that does not operationalize their particular conceptual scheme might now be persuaded to do so. In addition, those who might create dictionaries in languages other than English might be persuaded to use existing category schemes to maintain cross-language comparability of results.

Units of Aggregation Problems

After assigning the words in the text to various categories, the investigator usually counts the words in each category in each document. In turn, these summary measures represent the intensity of concern with each category in a given document.[28] The choice of document as the logical aggregate unit of analysis, however, is only one of several possibilities. There is some evidence (Grey, Kaplan, and Lasswell, 1965; Saris-Gallhofer et al., 1978) indicating that the reliability of content categories varies by the level of aggregation: In a comparison of hand- and computer-coded content analysis of the same texts, sentences and documents had the highest reliabilities, whereas the reliability for paragraphs was slightly lower. In addition, the reliability at all levels of aggregation was substantially less than the reliabilities for specific words or phrases.

Using people to code *New York Times* editorials that appeared during the Second World War, Grey et al. (1965) found that the substantive conclusions were affected by the type of recording unit. They coded a sample of editorials using four different units of text:

- symbols, which correspond to words or short phrases
- paragraphs
- units of three sentences
- whole editorials

They also coded each unit of text as being favorable, neutral, or unfavorable toward the symbol. Controlling for the total number of each type, they found that longer coding units (paragraphs, entire editorials) produced a greater proportion of units scored favorable or unfavorable and fewer units scored neutral than did the shorter units.

These findings question long-standing practices regarding aggregation of words into larger units in both hand-coded and computer-aided content analysis. Future research should investigate the relationships among substantive conclusions, reliability, validity, and different levels of aggregation.

Concluding Remarks

Some problems of content analysis are well-known; others require further investigation (see Chapter 4). The paper by Saris-Gallhofer and her associates (1978) mentioned above remains a model of the kind of research that is required if content analysis is to be put on a more solid footing. Even though much basic research remains to be done, the accumulated results of the last 20 years suggest that, for many kinds of problems, existing techniques of content analysis lead to valid and theoretically interesting results. Many of these techniques are discussed in the next chapter.

Suggestions for Further Reading

The symposium papers edited by Gerbner, Holsti, Krippendorff, Paisley, and Stone (1969) address many methodological issues and are still valuable reading. Kelly and Stone (1975) discuss problems in distinguishing among the various senses of words with multiple meanings. They developed one solution to this problem using procedures that are sensitive to the semantic context in which each word appears. Dunphy et al. (1989) discuss the validation of the Harvard IV-4 General Inquirer dictionary.

Validity and reliability in their most general sense are discussed in Brinberg and Kidder (1982), Campbell and Stanley (1963), Carmines and Zeller (1982), Cook and Campbell (1979), Lord and Novick (1968), Zeller and Carmines (1980), and some of the papers in Blalock (1974), to cite several possibilities. The *Sociological Methodology* series, originally published by Jossey-Bass and now published by Basil Blackwell, includes many articles on validity and reliability assessment.

3. TECHNIQUES OF CONTENT ANALYSIS

Compared with human-coded or interpretive modes of text analysis, one of the most important advantages of computer-aided content analysis is that the rules for coding text are made explicit. This public nature of the coding rules yields tools for inquiry that, when applied to a variety of texts, generate formally comparable results. Over time, this comparability should lead to the cumulation of research findings.

A second major advantage of computer-aided content analysis is that, once formalized either by computer programs and/or content-coding schemes, the computer provides perfect coder reliability in the application of coding rules to text. High coder reliability then frees the investigator to concentrate on other aspects of inquiry, such as validity, interpretation, and explanation.

Even with the assistance of computers, however, a remaining difficulty is that there is too much information in texts. Their richness and detail preclude analysis without some form of data reduction. The key to content analysis — in fact, to all modes of inquiry — is choosing a strategy for information loss that yields substantially interesting and theoretically useful generalizations while reducing the amount of information analyzed and reported by the investigator.

Researchers must, of course, tailor their methods to the requirements of their research by selecting specific techniques and integrating them with other methods, substantive considerations, and theories. To aid in that selection process, this chapter presents a wide variety of techniques for analyzing text that researchers may find useful. The central focus here is on computer-based content analysis as a means of text manipulation, data reduction, and data analysis in which the word or phrase is the basic unit.[29] Several ways of manipulating text are illustrated, including word-frequency counts, key-word-in-context (KWIC) listings, concordances, classification of words into content categories, content category counts, and retrievals based on content categories and co-occurrences. Some of these procedures are also useful in analyzing human-coded text.

The most important uses of content analysis are in research designs that relate content to noncontent variables. Other more advanced approaches to content analysis use exploratory and confirmatory factor analysis to identify themes in texts. Analysis of variance and structural equation models are often used to relate these themes to other variables. For instance, this chapter discusses research indicating that the content of newspaper editorials varies according to the type of newspaper (mass or elite). Another example shows how the content of the speeches of the German Kaiser responded to changing economic conditions. These advanced examples are discussed in some detail to clarify the logic of inquiry they entail and to clarify the substantive issues addressed.

Although this chapter presents examples drawn mainly from political sociology and political science, the techniques shown here can be applied to documents from myriad sources.

Document Selection and Sampling

Although some studies use an entire population of documents, most do not. Sampling is used primarily for the sake of economy. For content analysis, three sampling populations exist:

- communication sources
- documents
- text within documents

The sampling scheme employed will depend in large part on the population to be sampled and the kind of inferences to be made from the text. Among the communication sources that might be sampled are newspapers, magazines, and authors. To draw a sample, the universe must first be identified. For example, the universe of newspapers published in America is listed in the *Ayer Directory of Publications* (1983) and more recently (from 1987 onward) in the *Gale Directory of Publications and Broadcast Media* (1989).

Investigators interested in editorial opinions in American newspapers could take a simple random sample[30] that represented the population of newspapers. Suppose empirical evidence or theory suggested, however, that editorial opinions varied by region of the country and by frequency of publication (weekly versus daily). To insure that the sample included an adequate number of weekly and daily papers in each region, the sampling design might call for stratified sampling.[31] Here, the population of newspapers would first be divided by region and frequency of publication. Each of the resulting subpopulations would then be sampled randomly. This type of sampling design ensures that the final sample contains adequate numbers of newspapers from each subpopulation, and, more importantly, that the final sample represents the universe of daily and weekly newspapers in each region.

After identifying the communication sources to be studied, the investigator may reduce the amount of text to be analyzed by sampling documents. To avoid reaching biased or erroneous conclusions, however, researchers must take into account the conditions under which the documents were produced. For instance, consider a sample of editorials from two newspapers published both on weekdays and on Sunday. Suppose that the sample is to represent editorials in both papers over a two-year period. Also suppose that the purpose of the study is to compare and contrast editorial concerns. The investigator should consider several factors: First, newspapers usually publish several editorials per day and generally order them by importance on the editorial page. Second, editorials may vary by day of the week, with the less serious ones coming on weekends rather than on weekdays. Also, editorial writers often take note of major holidays and the arrival of and departure of the seasons. The sampling design must control for these systematic sources of variation in editorial content. For example, one might want to analyze only the first editorial that appears in each newspaper each nonholiday of a randomly selected week within each of the 24 months covered by the study.

Editorials are short documents. For longer texts, such as speeches or books, economy may suggest that sampling be employed. Here again the investigator must consider the nature of the texts. For example, speeches such as presidential acceptance speeches, State of the Union addresses, and the British Monarch's Speech from the Throne tend to have forms or organizations that reflect the partly ritualized nature of these texts. Often there exist routine introductions and closings. Domestic and financial affairs may be addressed before foreign affairs.

Where possible, the entire text should be analyzed. This preserves the semantic coherence of texts as units. If sampling is required, however, then the investigator must consider the structure of the text. For instance, the introductory and closing sections might be excluded. Portions dealing with domestic and foreign matters might be sampled separately. If the researcher must sample text within documents, each sample should consist of one or more entire paragraphs. This preserves some degree of semantic coherence. Sentences should *not* be sampled, because analyzing sentences in isolation — even ones drawn from the same text — destroys semantic coherence, making later validation and interpretation extremely difficult, if not impossible.

Text Encoding

After selecting the documents to be analyzed, the investigator must convert the text to a format and on a medium readable by the computer (i.e., machine-readable). In the early days of computers this process was notoriously costly and error-prone. The text was encoded by punching different patterns of holes in cards to represent different letters, numbers, and special characters (e.g., dollar signs and ampersands). Often the same text was punched twice to locate errors, a process called *verification*. It was not unusual for text entry to take up a large part of a modest research budget. For example, one project took about 9 person-months to keypunch, proofread, and correct almost a half million words and punctuation marks. Today, researchers can use optical scanners that read almost any typed or printed page and then transfer the text to an electronic storage medium such as tape or disk.

Key-Word-In-Context
Lists and Concordances

One of the first things the investigator wants to know is which words appear in the text and how they actually are used. Key-word-in-context (KWIC) lists (Table 3.1) show the context in which each word appears. This information can be used in a variety of ways. First, KWIC lists draw attention to the variation or consistency in word meaning and usage.[32] Second, KWIC lists provide structured information that is helpful in determining whether the meaning of particular words is dependent on their use in certain phrases or idioms. If so, the investigator will have to analyze the phrase or idiom as a single semantic unit.

Table 3.1 presents excerpts from the KWIC listing for the word *rights* in the 1980 party platforms. The two rightmost columns in the table, the document identification field (e.g., *American Democrats 1980*) and the sentence number within each document, exist for cross-reference. The computer program used to generate the KWIC list does not deal with word endings (suffixes); consequently, suffixes remain intact. Thus retrieval of sentences with *rights* excludes sentences that contain only *right*. Note that the KWIC list shows the larger context of word usage,[33] and makes syntactical and semantic differences in usage more apparent. For instance, *rights* occurs most frequently as a noun, but there are a few occasions when it functions as an adjective, as in *equal rights amendment*.

Table 3.2 presents a KWIC list for the word *state* after a computer has distinguished among its various senses and idioms. The instructions contained in this particular dictionary permit the identification of four different senses[34] of *state*:

(text continues on page 291)

TABLE 3.1

Selected Key-Word-In-Context Records for Word *Rights*, 1980 Republican and Democratic Party Platforms

1980 Reagan Republican Platform

Left context	KEY	Right context	Source	No.
YOUNG PEOPLE WANT THE OPPORTUNITY TO EXERCISE THE	RIGHTS	AND RESPONSIBILITIES OF ADULTS. THE REPUBLICAN PA	AR1980	372
ACTERIZED BY THE HIGHEST REGARD FOR PROTECTING THE	RIGHTS	OF LAW-ABIDING CITIZENS, AND IS CONSISTENT WITH T	AR1980	1004
OF THEIR SCHOOL SYSTEMS. WE WILL RESPECT THE	RIGHTS	OF STATE AND LOCAL AUTHORITIES IN THE MANAGEMENT	AR1980	333
RIGHTS AND THE HELSINKI AGREEMENTS WHICH GUARANTE	RIGHTS	SUCH AS THE FREE INTERCHANGE OF INFORMATION AND T	AR1980	1391
UALLY AND STEADFASTLY COMMITTED TO THE EQUALITY OF	RIGHTS	FOR ALL CITIZENS, REGARDLESS OF RACE. AS THE PART	AR1980	206
S ISSUES, IS ULTIMATELY CONCERNED WITH EQUALITY OF	RIGHTS	UNDER THE LAW. THERE CAN BE NO DOUBT THAT THE QUE	AR1980	284
SE WHO SUPPORT OR OPPOSE RATIFICATION OF THE EQUAL	RIGHTS	AMENDMENT. WE ACKNOWLEDGE THE LEGITIMATE EFFORTS	AR1980	227
SSION ARE IN THE COURTS. RATIFICATION OF THE EQUAL	RIGHTS	AMENDMENT IS NOW IN THE HANDS OF STATE LEGISLATUR	AR1980	232
REAFFIRM OUR PARTY'S HISTORIC COMMITMENT TO EQUAL	RIGHTS	AND EQUALITY FOR WOMEN.	AR1980	228
XEMPTION FROM THE MILITARY DRAFT. WE SUPPORT EQUAL	RIGHTS	AND EQUAL OPPORTUNITIES FOR WOMEN, WITHOUT TAKING	AR1980	229
ON POLICY MUST BE BASED ON THE PRIMACY OF PARENTAL	RIGHTS	AND RESPONSIBILITY. FEDERAL EDUCATI	AR1980	322
N'S COMMITMENT TO DEFEND THEM. INDIVIDUAL	RIGHTS	AND SOCIETAL VALUES ARE ONLY AS STRONG AS A NATIO	AR1980	152
MULTIRACIAL SOCIETY WITH GUARANTEES OF INDIVIDUAL	RIGHTS	IS POSSIBLE AND CAN WORK. REPUBLICANS BELIEVE THA	AR1980	1557
VE ECONOMIC SECURITY. HISPANICS SEEK ONLY THE FULL	RIGHTS	OF CITIZENSHIP -- IN EDUCATION, IN LAW ENFORCEMEN	AR1980	213
UNITIES FOR WOMEN, WITHOUT TAKING AWAY TRADITIONAL	RIGHTS	OF WOMEN SUCH AS EXEMPTION FROM THE MILITARY DRAF	AR1980	229
ING STRONG, EFFECTIVE ENFORCEMENT OF FEDERAL CIVIL	RIGHTS	STATUTES, ESPECIALLY THOSE DE DURING THE NEXT FOU	AR1980	209
CARE IS DEREGULATION AND AN EMPHASIS UPON CONSUMER	RIGHTS	AND PATIENT CHOICE. THE PRESCRIPTION FOR GOOD HEA	AR1980	350
IMPLEMENT THE UNITED NATIONS DECLARATION ON HUMAN	RIGHTS	AND THE HELSINKI AGREEMENTS WHICH GUARANTEE RIGHT	AR1980	1391
THEIR EMIGRATION IS A FUNDAMENTAL AFFRONT TO HUMAN	RIGHTS	AND THE U.N THE DECLINE IN EXIT VISAS TO SOVIET J	AR1980	1394
BEEN DURING THE CARTER ADMINISTRATION. HUMAN	RIGHTS	IN THE SOVIET UNION WILL NOT BE IGNORED AS IT HAS	AR1980	1398
N'S RHETORIC, THE MOST FLAGRANT OFFENDERS OF HUMAN	RIGHTS	INCLUDING THE SOVIET UNION, VIETNAM, AND CUBA HAV	AR1980	1072
NS LINKED TO ITS UNDIFFERENTIATED CHARGES OF HUMAN	RIGHTS	VIOLATIONS. YET, THE CARTER ADMINISTRATION'S POLI	AR1980	1473

(continued)

TABLE 3.1 Continued

1980 Carter Democratic Platform

FAIR SHARE OF OUR ECONOMY. WE PLEDGE TO SECURE THE	RIGHTS	OF WORKING WOMEN, HOMEMAKERS, MINORITY WOMEN AND	AD1980 255
CH ARE IN OUR CURRENT LAWS IN ORDER TO VIOLATE THE	RIGHTS	OF THOSE ATTEMPTING TO ORGANIZE. WE CAN NO LONGER	AD1980 194
.AS THAT EFFORT PROCEEDS, WE MUST ENSURE THAT THE	RIGHTS	OF WORKERS TO ENGAGE IN PEACEFUL PICKETING DURING	AD1980 1042
.EPENDENT CONSUMER PROTECTION AGENCY.'TO PROTECT THE	RIGHTS	AND INTERESTS OF CONSUMERS. WE PLEDGE CONTINUED S	AD1980 301
EMPHASIZED THE INTENT OF CONGRESS.''TO PROTECT THE	RIGHTS	OF STATE AND LOCAL GOVERMENTS AND PUBLIC AND PRI	AD1980 579
MENT OF THE CYPRUS PROBLEM BASED ON THE LEGITIMATE	RIGHTS	OF THE TWO COMMUNITIES. WE AGREE WITH SECRETARY G	AD1980 1627
H MANY AMERICANS HAVE ABOUT ABORTION. REPRODUCTIVE	RIGHTS	-- WE FULLY RECOGNIZE THE RELIGIOUS AND ETHICAL C	AD1980 374
UILDING TRADES WORKERS THE SAME PEACEFUL PICKETING	RIGHTS	CURRENTLY AFFORDED INDUSTRIAL WORKERS. LEGISLATIO	AD1980 203
ORTS. BOTH THE ERA AND DISTRICT OF COLUMBIA VOTING	RIGHTS	AMENDMENTS TO THE CONSTITUTION MUST BE RATIFIED A	AD1980 858
ST ENFORCE VIGOROUSLY THE AMENDMENTS TO THE VOTING	RIGHTS	ACT OF 1975 TO ASSIST HISPANIC CITIZENS. TO END D	AD1980 861
TO BARGAIN COLLECTIVELY, WHILE ENSURING THE LEGAL	RIGHTS	OF FARMERS. FARM LABOR--WE MUST VIGOROUSLY ENFORC	AD1980 1286
TION TO RESPECT FULLY THE HUMAN AND CONSTITUTIONAL	RIGHTS	OF ALL WITHIN OUR BORDERS. THE DEMOCRATIC PARTY A	AD1980 846
E TO THAT NEW HORIZON IS RATIFICATION OF THE EQUAL	RIGHTS	AMENDMENT.	AD1980 819
EQUAL	RIGHTS	AMENDMENT. THE PRIMARY ROUT	AD1980 809
ING, EDUCATION, WELFARE AND SOCIAL SERVICES, CIVIL	RIGHTS	, AND CARE FOR THE DISABLED, ELDERLY AND VETERANS,	AD1980 335
S OF GOVERNMENT WITH FULL PROTECTION FOR THE CIVIL	RIGHTS	AND LIBERTIES OF AMERICAN CITIZENS LIVING AT HOME	AD1980 873
THE FAIR HOUSING ACT AND TITLE VI OF THE CIVIL	RIGHTS	ACT MUST BE AMENDED TO INCLUDE THE HANDICAPPED.	AD1980 901
NITY PROGRAMS, TITLE VI AND TITLE VII OF THE CIVIL	RIGHTS	ACT, THE FAIR HOUSING LAWS, AND AFFIRMATIVE ACTIO	AD1980 834
T INVESTIGATION AND PROSECUTION OF SUSPECTED CIVIL	RIGHTS	VIOLATIONS. ATTORNEYS' OFFICES, AND SWIF	AD1980 1060
ONVENTION AND THE INTERNATIONAL COVENANTS ON HUMAN	RIGHTS	AS SOON AS POSSIBLE. WE SUPPORT SENATE RATIFICATI	AD1980 1529
D GUARANTEE FULL PROTECTION OF THE CIVIL AND HUMAN	RIGHTS	OF ALL WORKERS. WE MUST RECOGNIZE THE VALUE OF CU	AD1980 862
TIONS, WE WILL ACTIVELY PROMOTE THE CAUSE OF HUMAN	RIGHTS	AND EXPRESS AMERICA'S ABHORRENCE OF THE DENIAL OF	AD1980 1732
DING SOUTH AFRICA. WE MUST BE VIGILANT ABOUT HUMAN	RIGHTS	VIOLATIONS IN ANY COUNTRY IN WHICH THEY OCCUR INC	AD1980 1527
GROUPS, ASSERT OUR SUPPORT OF THE COURAGEOUS HUMAN	RIGHTS	ADVOCATE, NOBEL PEACE PRIZE WINNER, DR. WE SALUTE	AD1980 1478
ETWEEN OUR TWO COUNTRIES. WE WILL PURSUE OUR HUMAN	RIGHTS	CONCERNS AS A NECESSARY PART OF OVERALL PROGRESS	AD1980 1474
980 IS NOT ONLY IDENTIFIED WITH THE CAUSE OF HUMAN	RIGHTS	AND DEMOCRACY, BUT ALSO WE HAVE OPENED A NEW CHAP	AD1980 1748
LEGISLATION DESIGNED TO GIVE PROTECTION AND HUMAN	RIGHTS	TO THOSE WORKÉRS AFFECTED BY PLANT CLOSINGS. WE S	AD1980 208
ON OF UNIVERSALLY RECOGNIZED AND FUNDAMENTAL HUMAN	RIGHTS	THROUGHOUT THE AMERICAS BY URGING THAT THE SENATE	AD1980 1758
EXCEPT FOR CLEARLY HUMANITARIAN PURPOSES TO HUMAN	RIGHTS	VIOLATORS. WE WILL UPHOLD OUR OWN LAW AND TERMINA	AD1980 1760

TABLE 3.2

Selected Key-Word-In-Context Records for Word *State*, 1980 Republican and Democratic Party Platforms, Disambiguated Text

1980 Reagan Republican Platform

Left context	Keyword	Right context	Source	No.
ERNMENT OF NICARAGUA . WE DO2 NOT SUPPORT1 UNITE2D	STATES	ASSISTANCE TO2 ANY1 MARXIST GOVERNMENT IN THIS1 H	AR1980	1423
NOW , WE HAVE2 TO1 PUT1 THE UNITE2D	STATES	BACK1 ON THE WORLD EXPORT1 MAP .	AR1980	1535
NUCLEAR POWER1 WOULD OVERTAKE THAT2 OF THE UNITE2D	STATES	BY THE EARLY1 1980 S , THREATENING THE SURVIVAL O	AR1980	1099
STRENGTH . REPUBLICANS BELIEVE1 THAT1 THE UNITE2D	STATES	CAN ONLY2 NEGOTIATE WITH THE SOVIET UNION3 FROM A	AR1980	1329
ND EVENTUALLY A MILITARY CATASTROPHY . THE UNITE2D	STATES	CANNOT ABDICATE THAT1 ROLE WITHOUT INDUCING A DI	AR1980	1113
UTION TO2 THE PROBLEM OF INEQUALITY OF THE UNITE2D	STATES	CITIZENS OF PUERTO RICO WITHIN THE FRAMEWORK OF T	AR1980	295
AT1 THE MOST1 EFFECTIVE WEAPONS AGAINST CRIME ARE1	STATE1	AND LOCAL AGENCYIES . ALTHOUGH WE RECOGNIZE THE V	AR1980	533
FAMILYIES INTOLERABLE PRESSURE1S WILL1 BUILD1 ON	STATE1	, LOCAL , AND FEDERAL BUDGETS AS1 TAX1 REVENUE1S D	AR1980	504
OF TURN3ING THE POOR5 INTO PERMANEN1 WARDS OF THE	STATE1	, TRADE2ING THEIR POLITICAL SUPPORT2 FOR CONTINUE	AR1980	213
CIAL1 WELFARE2 AGENCIES AND STRENGTHEN1 LOCAL AND	STATE1	ADMINISTRATIVE FUNCTION2S , AND - BETTER3 COORD1N	AR1980	148
ADMIT1TED INTO THE UNION1 AS1 A FULL4LY SOVERE1GN1	STATE1	AFTER1 THEY FREE3LY SO1 DETERMINE1 . THE REPUBLIC	AR1980	294
EQUAL1 RIGHT1S AMENDMENT 1S1 NOW IN THE HANDS OF	STATE1	LEGISLATURES , AND THE ISSUE3S OF THE TIME1 EXTEN	AR1980	246
WLEDGE THE FUNDAMENTAL RIGHT2 TO2 EXISTENCE OF THE	STATE1	OF ISRAEL 1S1 WRONG1 . THE IMPUTATION OF LEGITIMA	AR1980	1397
E1 · WE BELIEVE1 THE ESTABLISHMENT OF A PALESTINIAN	STATE1	ON THE WEST BANK2 WOULD BE2 DESTABILIZING AND HAR	AR1980	1399
1 · GOVERNMENT1S WHICH WILL1 NOT DESTROY TRADITIONAL	STATE1	SUPREMACY IN WATER1 LAW . WE MUST1 DEVELOP A PART	AR1980	774
1 A STATE1 . THIS1 ENACTMENT WILL1 ENABLE THE NEW1	STATE1	OF PUERTO RICO TO1 STAND1 ECONOMICALLY ON AN EQUA	AR1980	299
AND EFFORTS TO1 RETURN1 DECISION-MAKING POWER1 TO1	STATE1	AND LOCAL ELECTED OFFICIAL1S . WE PLEDGE TO1 REV	AR1980	1021
LP2 RETURN1 CONTROL1 OF WELFARE2 PROGRAM1S TO2 THE	STATE1S	. WE SUPPORT1 A BLOCK1 GRANT2 PROGRAM1 THAT2 WIL	AR1980	151
SUE CLOSE1 TIE3S AND FRIENDSHIP WITH MODERATE ARAB	STATE1S	. WHILE2 REEMPHASIZING OUR COMMITMENT TO2 ISRAEL	AR1980	1411
L4LING INFLUENCE1 OVER2 THE REGIONS' RESOURCE-RICH	STATE1S	. AND THEREBY TO1 GAIN1 DECISIVE POLITICAL AND E	AR1980	1391
AS3 LEFT3 , THE U.S. ARMED1 FORCE2S AT THEIR LOW2EST	STATE2	OF PREPARE[D]NESS SINCE1 1950 . SERIOUSLY COMPROMIS	AR1980	1249
OPMENT . , IN OUR PLATFORM1 FOUR YEAR1S AGO , WE	STATE3D	THAT2 , THE GROWTH OF CIVILIAN NUCLEAR TECHN	AR1980	1319
US TO1 CATCH4 UP . THE SECRETARY2 OF DEFENSE HAS3	STATE3D	THAT3 . EVEN5 IF WE WERE1 TO1 MAINTAIN1 A CONSTANT	AR1980	1151
THE MINIMUM QUANTITYIES THE ARMED1 SERVICE1S HAVE3	STATE3D	THEY NEED1 . YET3 FUNDING REQUEST1S FOR SUFFICI	AR1980	1248

(continued)

TABLE 3.2 Continued

1980 Carter Democratic Platform

Context (left)	Keyword / context (right)	Ref	Line
NCENTIVES TO1 MAKE1 ALL1 RESIDENCES IN THE UNITE2D	STATES ENERGY EFFICIENT , THROUGH2 UPGRADED INSULATION ,	AD1980	1195
ATION OF THE LEADERSHIP ROLE TAKEN1 BY THE UNITE2D	STATES IN THE AREA OF HUMAN RIGHTS AND URGE1 THAT1 THE	AD1980	1576
RE . WITH THOSE1 TREATYIES RATIFYIED , THE UNITE2D	STATES IN 1980 IS1 NOT ONLY2 IDENTIFYIED WITH THE CAUSE3	AD1980	1762
AL REGIME IN THE WEST BANK2 AND GAZA . THE UNITE2D	STATES IS1 A FULL1 PARTNER IN NEGOTIATIONS BETWEEN ISRAE	AD1980	1620
COLLECTIVE DEFENSE EFFORTS . IN 1977 , THE UNITE2D	STATES JOIN2ED WITH NATO TO1 DEVELOP , FOR THE FIRST1 TI	AD1980	1455
2 TERM1S IN THE LAST1 THREE YEAR1S . THE UNITE2D	STATES NON-FARM EXPORT1S HAVE3 RISEN1 50 PERCENT IN REAL	AD1980	157
AN ASSAULT1 ON THE VITAL INTEREST1S OF THE UNITE2D	STATES OF AMERICA AND SUCH1 AN ASSAULT1 WILL1 BE3 REPELL	AD1980	1495
ASSISTANCE . IT IS1 UNACCEPTABLE THAT1 THE UNITE2D	STATES RANKS 13TH AMONG 17 MAJOR1 INDUSTRIAL POWER1S IN	AD1980	1733
DING TO1 FERMENT IN THE THIRD1 WORLD . THE UNITE2D	STATES SHOULD BE1 A POSITIVE FORCE1 FOR PEACEFUL CHANGE2	AD1980	1437
PORT1S AND REDRESS TRADE1 IMBALANCES , THE UNITE2D	STATES SHOULD CONFORM WITH THE PRACTICE2S OF OTHER1 MAJO	AD1980	1029
18-YEAR-OLD S IS3 INTEND1ED TO1 ENABLE THE UNITE2D	STATES TO1 MOBILIZE MORE RAPID2LY IN THE EVENT3 OF AN EM	AD1980	1483
N3 STRENGTHEN1ED . AT THE SAME TIME1 , THE UNITE2D	STATES' COMMITMENT TO2 THE INDEPENDENCE , SECURITY1 , AN	AD1980	1622
OME COUNTRY1IES . WE WILL1 CONTRIBUTE1 THE UNITE2D	STATES' FAIR5 SHARE1 TO2 THE CAPITAL OF THE MULTILATERAL	AD1980	1736
WE OPPOSE1 CREATION OF AN INDEPENDENT1 PALESTINIAN	STATE1 - MORE THAN $10 BILLION - HAS3 BEEN3 REQUEST2ED D	AD1980	1630
D1 TO2 ISRAEL SINCE1 ITS CREATION AS1 A SOVEREIGN1	STATE1 AND LOCAL GOVERNMENT , REPRESENTATIVE1S OF LABOR2	AD1980	1623
ICH ACTIVE2LY INVOLVE3D THE ELECT2ED OFFICIAL1S OF	STATE1 AND COMMUNITY GROUP1S , AND - AMENDMENTS TO2 THE	AD1980	783
TION AND TREATMENT ACT1 WHICH PROVIDE1S FUND1S TO1	STATE1 AND LOCAL GOVERNMENTS ; THE FEDERAL GOVERNMENT WI	AD1980	982
F PROVIDE1ING IMMEDIATE1 FEDERAL FISCAL RELIEF TO1	STATE1 AND LOCAL GOVERNMENTS FOR THEIR WELFARE2 COST1S A	AD1980	550
HE OPPOSITE - TO1 PROVIDE1 GREATER ASSISTANCE TO1	STATE1 AND LOCAL GOVERNMENT IN SETTING POLICY AND IN RE	AD1980	569
FICANT ADMINISTRATIVE AND ORGANIZATIONAL ROLES FOR	STATE1S IN PURSUEING HUMAN RIGHT1S , DEMOCRACY , AND ECO	AD1980	371
HE REGION . WE WILL1 JOIN2 WITH OTHER1 LIKE-MINDED	STATE1S IN THE PACIFIC1 BASIN PLAY2 , IN THE SOLIDIFICATIO	AD1980	1775
HE U. S. TERRITORY1IES AND OTHER1 EMERGEIING ISLAND	STATE1S IN THE REGION TO1 SUPPORT1 THE HISTORIC EFFORTS	AD1980	1801
BUILD1 A COMPREHENSIVE PEACE1 . WE CALL1 UPON ALL1	STATE1S NOT PROVIDEIING ASSISTANCE TO2 UNIFYIED FAMILYIE	AD1980	1639
M OUR SUPPORT2 FOR THE 1962 ACTION AND URGE1 THAT1	STATE3D : EVEN2 DURING PERIODS OF NORMAL ECONOMIC1 GROWT	AD1980	562
NATIONAL ECONOMIC1 PROSPERITY . OUR 1976 PLATFORM1	STATE3D IN THE 1976 PLATFORM2 , THE DEMOCRATIC PARTY2 RE	AD1980	129
ITS HOLY PLACE1S PROVIDE1D TO2 ALL1 FAITH1S . AS1	STATE3D THAT1 THE COMPOSITION OF AMERICAN1 SOCIETY IS1 A	AD1980	1635
OUS TO2 A BEAUTIFUL MOSAIC . PRESIDENT CARTER HAS3	STATE3D	AD1980	1008

- state (noun; body politic or area of government)
- situation (e.g., *state of science*)
- to state (verb; to declare)
- "united states" (idiom; handled by the second sense of *United*)

A KWIC list can be thought of as a concordance, a listing by word of each word in the text together with its context (Burton, 1981, 1982; Hockey and Marriott, 1982; Hockey and Martin, 1987; Preston and Coleman, 1978). Often used in literary or biblical studies, concordances provide a rich data base for detailed studies of word usage in all kinds of texts. For example, the KWIC lists shown in Tables 3.1 and 3.2 illustrate excerpts from a much larger KWIC list for party platforms from 1968 to 1980. This larger data base can be used to study detailed differences and similarities in symbol usage in party platforms from this period.

Concordances do not automatically show the referents of pronouns and ambiguous phrases. Furthermore, unlike retrievals from text based on category assignments (which are discussed later in this chapter) concordances do not organize the text according to synonyms or words with similar connotations. A concordance or KWIC list with sentence identification numbers, however, makes it easy for the investigator to examine a sentence in its larger textual context. This examination often will reveal synonyms or pronouns that need to be taken into account.

Although concordances and KWIC lists provide essential information concerning symbol usage, they are, at least initially, data-expanding rather than data-reducing techniques. If the concordance presents each word with three words to the left or the right, for example, the original text is expanded by a factor of six. How, then, can investigators narrow their focus? Concordances lend themselves to the intensive study of a few specific symbols, such as *equal rights amendment* or *women*. Consequently, investigators will have to translate substantive hypotheses into concern with specific symbols.

Word-Frequency Lists

Researchers can view texts from another perspective by examining the highest-frequency words. Because each accounts for a relatively large proportion of the text, many content analysts focus their efforts primarily on the most frequently occurring words. Table 3.3 presents ordered word-frequency lists for the 1976 and 1980 Democratic and

TABLE 3.3

Ordered Word-Frequency Lists,
1976-1980 Democratic and Republican Party Platforms

Jimmy Carter, 1976			Gerald Ford, 1976			Jimmy Carter, 1980			Ronald Reagan, 1980		
Rank	Word	Frequency	Rank	Word	Frequency	Rank	Word	Frequency	Rank	Word	Frequency
1	OUR	222	1	OUR	318	1	OUR	430	1	OUR	347
2	MUST	140	2	MUST	148	2	MUST	321	2	THEIR	161
3	SHOULD	130	3	SHOULD	109	3	DEMOCRATIC	226	3	ADMINISTRATION	131
4	DEMOCRATIC	90	4	GOVERNMENT	100	4	FEDERAL	177	4	GOVERNMENT	128
5	GOVERNMENT	87	5	STATES	86	5	SUPPORT	144	5	REPUBLICAN	126
6	ECONOMIC	78	6	FEDERAL	75	6	PARTY	139	5	FEDERAL	126
6	SUPPORT	78	7	UNITED	74	7	GOVERNMENT	133	6	AMERICAN	119
7	FEDERAL	74	8	SUPPORT	73	8	PROGRAMS	129	7	REPUBLICANS	116
8	ALL	72	9	ALL	70	9	ADMINISTRATION	127	8	CARTER	112
9	STATES	69	10	THEIR	66	10	ALL	122	9	MUST	104
9	UNITED	69	11	NATIONAL	61	10	ECONOMIC	122	10	ECONOMIC	101
10	POLICY	67	12	POLICY	60	11	THEIR	112	11	POLICY	100
10	PROGRAMS	67	13	AMERICAN	56	12	CONTINUE	109	12	SOVIET	98
11	PARTY	66	14	PROGRAMS	52	13	ENERGY	107	13	STATES	93
12	ENERGY	62	15	REPUBLICAN	51	14	SHOULD	99	14	MILITARY	89
13	NATIONAL	59	16	PEOPLE	49	15	OTHER	96	15	TAX	85
14	PUBLIC	51	17	CONGRESS	48	16	POLICY	89	16	SUPPORT	83
15	AMERICAN	48	18	WORLD	46	17	EFFORTS	87	17	ENERGY	81
16	PEOPLE	47	19	MORE	45	17	DEVELOPMENT	87	17	MORE	81
17	THEIR	46	20	SYSTEM	44	18	RIGHTS	86	18	PARTY	79
18	HEALTH	45	21	DEMOCRATIC	43	19	HEALTH	85	19	PEOPLE	74
19	OTHER	44	22	DEVELOPMENT	42	20	AMERICAN	84	20	UNITED	73
20	INTERNATIONAL	43	23	ECONOMIC	41	21	PROGRAM	81	21	PROGRAMS	72
21	DEVELOPMENT	42	23	ENERGY	41	21	MORE	81	21	THEY	72
22	NEEDS	40	23	OTHER	41	22	NATIONAL	80	22	ALL	70
23	POLICIES	39	24	THEY	40	23	NEW	79	22	POLICIES	70
23	TAX	39	25	NEW	39	24	STATES	73	23	AMERICANS	68
24	MORE	38	26	CONTINUE	37	25	SECURITY	72	24	SHOULD	64
24	SYSTEM	38	27	THROUGH	36	26	WOMEN	70	25	NEW	63
25	NEW	37	28	LOCAL	35	27	WORK	69	26	BELIEVE	62
26	ADMINISTRATION	36	29	AMERICANS	33	28	EDUCATION	65	26	DEFENSE	62
26	EFFORTS	36	29	NATIONS	33	29	YEARS	64	26	NATIONAL	62
26	WORLD	36	30	TAX	33	30	NEEDS	62	26	WHO	62
27	HOUSING	34	30	WORK	32	30	PEOPLE	32	27	PLEDGE	61
28	FULL	33	31	CARE	30	31	ALSO	30	28	FOREIGN	60
29	CITIZENS	32	31	FOREIGN	30	32	THEY	30	29	GROWTH	58
30	BOTH	31	31	MOST	30	32	WORLD	30	30	OTHER	55
30	FORCES	31	31	NOW	30	33	SOVIET	30	31	MOST	53
30	RIGHTS	31	32	RESOURCES	29	34	HUMAN	30	31	SECURITY	53
31	AREAS	30	32	THERE	29	35	PROVIDE	29	32	YEARS	51
31	PROVIDE	30	32	USE	29	35	UNITED	29	33	THROUGH	50
31	SOCIAL	30	33	RIGHTS	28	36	INTERNATIONAL	29	34	INFLATION	49
31	WORK	30	33	SHALL	28	36	AREAS	28	34	PRIVATE	49
31	YEARS	30				36	CARE	28	35	JOBS	48

Republican party platforms.[35] Three aspects of this table deserve mention. First, the computer program that generated these lists was instructed to omit certain frequently occurring words that are usually substantively uninteresting; for example, articles such as *a* and *the,* and forms of the verb *to be* such as *is* and *was.*[36] These words, however, could easily have been included. The program also omitted one- and two-letter words, such as *I* and *we.* Second, as with the KWIC lists, the computer program used to generate word frequencies does not deal with word endings (suffixes). Consequently, *Republican* and *Republicans* appear as separate entries. Third, there are many more low-frequency than high-frequency words. In the 1980 Republican Platform, for example, there are 4619 different word forms, of which 2307 — or slightly less than half — occur only once (data not shown). This large proportion of infrequently occurring word forms is found in all naturally occurring texts, that is, those not conducted for special purposes such as linguistic analysis (Zipf, 1932, 1965). Analyzing the many low-frequency words is not very efficient, and, as noted, researchers often focus their attention on the fewer high-frequency words.

Examining the list for the 1976 platforms suggests that the Carter and Ford documents used similar words with about the same relative frequencies. For example, the two most frequent words in each platform are identical, and there are obvious similarities in the top 10 words. Nevertheless, noticeable differences exist. *Economic* and *health* are ranked 6th and 18th in the Carter platform, whereas in the Ford platform *economic* ranks only 23rd and *health* is not among the most frequent words.

Comparison of the 1976 with the 1980 platforms reveals striking differences. *Soviet, military,* and *defense* rank high in Reagan's platform but are not among the most frequent words in either of the 1976 platforms. *Soviet* ranks 33rd in the 1980 Carter platform, but the other two words fail to make this short list. *Health, women,* and *education* rank high in the 1980 Carter document but are not among the high-frequency words in the Reagan document.

This table confirms that the Reagan platform articulated a very different set of priorities and concerns than either the Carter campaign, or the previous Ford Republican platform. The relationship between articulations and actions remains to be investigated thoroughly. In a great many instances, however, the Reagan platforms advocated policies that were a radical departure from the policies articulated by the Ford and Carter campaigns. Similar data can be generated over long periods of time to study the relationships among articulations, policy changes, and voter responses.

Ordered word-frequency lists provide a convenient way of getting at gross differences in word usage. Table 3.3 illustrates that these differences may be between

- the same message source at different points in time;
- different message sources at the same time; or
- both.

Several assumptions underlie this mode of analysis. An obvious one is that the most frequently appearing words reflect the greatest concerns. This is likely to be generally true, but two cautions must be noted. First, one word may be used in a variety of contexts or may have more than one meaning, so that word frequencies may suggest far greater uniformity in usage than actually exists, thus questioning the validity of inferences from word-frequency data. For instance, *states* appears frequently in all four platforms. One cannot tell from just the word-frequency list whether the platform addresses states' rights, the United-States, sovereign states, or the state of affairs. To augment a word-frequency list, however, a concordance can often help the researcher to assess the uniformity of word usage and to generate counts of specific phrases.

Second, the use of synonyms and/or pronouns for stylistic reasons may lead to the underestimation of actual concern with particular words or phrases. For example, in Democratic platforms the pronoun *we* may refer to the party or to an incumbent administration. If one were interested in counting self-references, perhaps the best index would be the sum of references to *we* in the former sense (the phrase *Democratic Party*) and perhaps references to *our party*. Thus counts of any one, rather than all, of these words or phrases will yield less valid indicators of self-reference. No simple, widely available resolution of this problem currently exists, especially one for large amounts of text. Key-word-in-context lists discussed in the previous section do provide the basis for valid indicators of concepts such as party self-reference. For studies using numerous indicators, however, this may be an impractical, time-consuming answer.[37]

The previous chapter noted the ability of some computer software to distinguish among words with more than one meaning or to treat phrases as a single semantic unit. Table 3.4 presents ordered word-frequency lists for the 1976 and 1980 party platforms based on disambiguated text. *Support,* for example, moves from 5th to 23rd and 25th in the 1980 Carter platform. The first sense of *support* is the verb form; the second sense is the noun form, meaning sustain, provide for, or encouragement, as in *The bill has our support.* The ranking of most words, however, does not change greatly. Consequently, the overall conclusions would not be very different because of disambiguation. Nevertheless, because this text classification procedure is more precise, the data in Table 3.4 have greater semantic validity than the data in the previous table.

Although word-frequency lists reveal changes or differences in emphasis between documents, they must be used with caution. Word frequencies do not reveal very much about the associations among words. For example, although it may be interesting to know that *support* ranks higher in the 1980 Carter than in the 1980 Reagan platform, one cannot tell whether the platforms differ in their support of democratic

TABLE 3.4

Ordered Word-Frequency Lists,
1976-1980 Democratic and Republican Party Platforms,
Disambiguated Text

Jimmy Carter, 1976			Gerald Ford, 1976			Jimmy Carter, 1980			Ronald Reagan, 1980		
Rank	Word	Frequency	Rank	Word	Frequency	Rank	Word	Frequency	Rank	Word	Frequency
1	OUR	222	1	OUR	318	1	OUR	430	1	OUR	347
2	MUST1	140	2	MUST1	148	2	MUST1	321	2	THEIR	161
3	SHOULD	130	3	SHOULD	109	3	DEMOCRATIC	226	3	GOVERNMENT	128
4	DEMOCRATIC	90	4	GOVERNMENT	100	4	FEDERAL	177	4	FEDERAL	126
5	GOVERNMENT	87	5	FEDERAL	75	5	GOVERNMENT	133	4	REPUBLICAN	126
6	ECONOMIC1	78	6	THEIR	67	6	PROGRAM1S	129	5	ADMINISTRATION1	125
7	FEDERAL	74	7	STATES	65	7	ADMINISTRATION1	124	6	AMERICAN1	117
8	POLICY	67	7	UNITE2D	65	8	ECONOMIC1	122	7	REPUBLICANS	116
8	PROGRAM1S	67	8	NATIONAL	61	9	PARTY2	116	8	CARTER	112
9	PARTY1	66	9	POLICY	60	10	THEIR	112	9	MUST1	104
10	ENERGY	62	10	AMERICAN1	56	11	CONTINUE1	109	10	ECONOMIC1	101
11	ALL1	59	11	ALL1	53	12	ENERGY	107	11	POLICY	100
11	NATIONAL	59	12	PROGRAM1S	52	13	ALL1	106	12	SOVIET	98
12	UNITE2D	55	13	REPUBLICAN	51	14	SHOULD	99	13	MILITARY	89
13	STATES	54	14	PEOPLE1	49	15	OTHER1	96	14	ENERGY	81
14	PEOPLE1	47	15	WORLD	46	16	POLICY	89	14	MORE	81
15	AMERICAN1	46	16	SUPPORT1	45	17	DEVELOPMENT	87	15	TAX1	80
15	THEIR	46	17	SYSTEM	44	17	EFFORTS	87	16	PEOPLE1	74
16	HEALTH	45	18	DEMOCRATIC	43	18	HEALTH	85	17	PROGRAM1S	73
17	PUBLIC1	44	19	DEVELOPMENT	42	19	AMERICAN1	84	18	THEY	72
18	INTERNATIONAL1	43	20	ECONOMIC1	41	19	MORE	81	19	POLICYIES	70
19	DEVELOPMENT	42	21	THEY	40	20	PROGRAM1	81	20	UNITE2D	69
19	OTHER	42	22	CONGRESS1	38	21	NATIONAL	80	21	AMERICAN1S	68
20	SUPPORT1	41	22	NEW1	38	22	NEW1	79	22	STATES	67
21	POLICYIES	39	23	CONTINUE1	37	23	SUPPORT1	75	23	SHOULD	64
22	MORE	38	23	OTHER1	37	24	WOMEN	72	24	DEFENSE	62
22	THESE1	38	24	LOCAL	35	25	SUPPORT2	71	24	NATIONAL	62
22	SYSTEM	38	25	AMERICAN1S	33	26	EDUCATION	65	24	NEW1	62
22	TAX1	38	25	NATIONS	33	26	RIGHT1S	65	24	WHO	62
23	SUPPORT2	37	26	TAX1	31	27	YEAR1S	64	25	BELIEVE1	61
23	NEW1	37	27	FOREIGN1	30	28	PEOPLE1	62	25	PLEDGE	61
24	EFFORTS	36	27	NOW	30	29	ALSO	61	26	FOREIGN1	60
24	WORLD	36	28	RESOURCES	29	30	WORLD	60	27	ALL1	59
25	HOUSE4ING	34	28	THROUGH2	29	30	THEY	60	28	GROWTH	58
26	FULL1	33	29	RIGHT1S	28	31	SOVIET	58	29	PARTY3	56
26	ADMINISTRATION1	33	29	SUPPORT2	28	32	HUMAN	57	30	MOST1	51
27	CITIZENS	32	30	INTERNATIONAL1	27	33	PROVIDE1	56	31	YEAR1S	51
28	AREAS	30	31	COMMUNITY	26	34	AREAS	55	31	OTHER1	50
28	NEED2S	30	31	HEALTH	26	34	CARE1	55	32	SUPPORT1	50
28	YEAR1S	30	31	PARTY1	26	34	INTERNATIONAL1	55	32	INFLATION	49
28	PROVIDE1	30	31	PROVIDE1	26	34	PERCENT	55	32	PRIVATE1	49
28	EMPLOYMENT	30	32	NATION	25	35	NEED2S	54	33	JOBS	48
29	REPUBLICAN	29				36	ASSISTANCE	51	33	PERCENT	48
29	MILITARY	29				36	RESOURCES	51	33	SYSTEM	48

principles, of the equal rights amendment, or of foreign countries that have pro-Western authoritarian regimes. Having used ordered word-frequency lists to identify words of potential interest, the investigator should use KWIC lists for retrievals from text to test hypotheses concerning the larger context of symbol usage.

Retrievals from Coded Text

With computer-aided content analysis, the investigator easily may search through the text to retrieve portions meeting specific criteria (see Ogilvie, 1966; Stone, Dunphy, Smith, and Ogilvie, 1966: 121ff). One way of searching text is to retrieve sentences by the occurrence of at least one word in a particular category, for example, all sentences with one WEALTH word. Some investigators (DeWeese, personal communication) strongly feel that counts and retrievals based on the co-occurrence[38] or combination of categories or words in a single sentence are the most useful indicators. Of course, one difficulty is knowing in advance which combinations will be particularly useful. Presumably, substantive hypotheses suggest appropriate combinations, but induction usually prevails in these instances. Another difficulty in analyzing co-occurrences is that infrequently occurring combinations might be of substantive interest, for example, references to *individual rights,* which occurred only twice in the 1980 Reagan platform and not at all in the 1980 Carter platform (Table 3.1). In the social science literature there is little, if any, systematic research on retrievals; hence, only a brief example will be given.

Using party platforms 1844-1864, the computer was instructed to retrieve all sentences with at least one WEALTH word that was a noun and that also had any word in the category WELL-BEING-DEPRIVATION. The latter category indicates a concern with the loss of well-being, either of a person or a collectivity. Table 3.5 presents a sample of nine sentences meeting this criterion.[39] The criterion words are underscored. The program retrieved sentences addressing two different subjects. Some sentences mention economic difficulties; others mention pensions for the survivors of the war dead and for the disabled. The third sentence in the table contains both themes.

Obviously, the diversity of sentences retrieved can be narrowed or expanded by varying the criteria of selection: more criteria will result in fewer retrievals, and fewer criteria will result in more. But the primary difficulty is that the results depend on an interaction among the text, the category scheme, and the assignment of words to categories. Thus each investigator will have to experiment with retrievals to find the most helpful approach. No general guidelines now exist.

Finally, why use retrievals based on categories? Why not use retrievals based on words? Certainly the computer is capable of doing either. For example, one could retrieve all sentences containing the words *pension* or *pensions.* This might retrieve some sentences, however, dealing with the pensions of postal workers. Instead, sentences with *pension* and *disability* could be retrieved, but this would miss the second sentence in Table 3.5, which is similar in content to the others dealing with pensions for veterans and their survivors. Synonyms frequently are used that would be missed by a purely word-oriented approach to retrievals, but they are captured more easily in a category-based system.

TABLE 3.5

Selected Retrievals, Democratic and Republican Platforms: Sentences with WEALTH Nouns and WELL-BEING-DEPRIVATION, 1844-1964

DOC# 15   SENT# 12   ID=D1868
AND A TARIFF FOR REVENUE UPON FOREIGN1 IMPORTS, SUCH2 AS WILL2 AFFORD1 INCIDENTAL PROTECTION TO2 DOMESTIC MANUFACTURE1S; AND AS1 WILL1, WITHOUT IMPAIRING THE REVENUE, IMPOSE THE LEAST2 BURDEN1 UPON, AND BEST PROMOTE AND ENCOURAGE1 THE GREAT1 INDUSTRIAL INTERESTS OF THE COUNTRY1.
*** END DOCUMENT, NUMBER RETRIEVALS=   1

DOC# 18   SENT# 23   ID=R1872
THEIR PENSIONS ARE1 A SACRED DEBT OF THE NATION, AND THE WIDOW1S AND ORPHANS OF THOSE2 WHO DIED FOR THEIR COUNTRY1 ARE3 ENTITLED TO2 THE CARE1 OF A GENEROUS AND GRATEFUL PEOPLE1.
*** END DOCUMENT, NUMBER RETRIEVALS=   1

DOC# 22   SENT# 16   ID=R1880
AND THAT1 THE LIBERTY SECURE1D TO2 THIS1 GENERATION SHOULD BE3 TRANSMITTED UNDIMINISHED TO2 OTHER1 GENERATIONS, THAT1 THE ORDER2 ESTABLISHE1D AND THE CREDIT1 ACQUIRE2D SHOULD NEVER BE3 IMPAIRED, THAT1 THE PENSIONS PROMISE2D SHOULD BE3 PAID1, THAT1 THE DEBT SO1 MUCH REDUCED SHOULD BE3 EXTINGUISHED BY THE FULL1 PAYMENT OF EVERY DOLLAR.
*** END DOCUMENT, NUMBER RETRIEVALS=   1

DOC# 24   SENT# 31   ID=R1884
THE GRATEFUL THANK2S OF THE AMERICAN PEOPLE1 ARE1 DUE1 TO2 THE UNION1 SOLDIERS AND SAILORS OF THE LATE2 WAR1 AND THE REPUBLICAN PARTY1 STAND1S PLEDGED TO2 SUITABLE PENSIONS FOR ALL2 WHO WERE1 DISABLED, AND FOR THE WIDOW1S AND ORPHANS OF THOSE2 WHO DIED IN THE WAR1.
*** END DOCUMENT, NUMBER RETRIEVALS=   1

DOC# 24   SENT# 33   ID=R1884
SO2 THAT1 ALL1 INVALID SOLDIERS SHALL SHARE1 ALIKE, AND THEIR PENSIONS BEGIN1 WITH THE DATE1 OF DISABILITY OR DISCHARGE1, AND NOT WITH THE DATE1 OF APPLICATION.
*** END DOCUMENT, NUMBER RETRIEVALS=   2

DOC# 29   SENT# 50   ID=D1896
RECOGNIZE1ING THE JUST3 CLAIM1S OF DESERVE1ING UNION1 SOLDIERS, WE HEARTILY INDORSE THE RULE1 OF THE PRESENT1 COMMISSIONER OF PENSIONS THAT1 NO1 NAME1S SHALL BE3 ARBITRARY1LY DROP3PED FROM1 THE PENSION ROLL1, AND THE FACT1 OF ENLISTMENT AND SERVICE1 SHOULD BE3 DEEMED CONCLUSIVE EVIDENCE1 AGAINST DISEASE AND DISABILITY BEFORE ENLISTMENT.
*** END DOCUMENT, NUMBER RETRIEVALS=   1

DOC# 30   SENT# 21   ID=R1896
WE BELIEVE1 THE REPEAL OF THE RECIPROCITY ARRANGEMENTS NEGOTIATED BY THE LAST1 REPUBLICAN ADMINISTRATION1 WAS1 A NATIONAL CALAMITY, AND DEMAND2 THEIR RENEWAL AND EXTENSION ON SUCH1 TERM3S AS1 WILL1 EQUALIZE OUR TRADE1 WITH OTHER1 NATIONS, REMOVE THE RESTRICTIONS WHICH NOW OBSTRUCT THE SALE OF AMERICAN PRODUCT1S IN THE PORTS OF OTHER1 COUNTRY1IES+
*** END DOCUMENT, NUMBER RETRIEVALS=   1

DOC# 30   SENT# 35   ID=R1896
WE ARE3 UNALTERABLELY OPPOSE2D TO2 EVERY MEASURE1 CALCULATE2D TO1 DEBASE OUR CURRENCY OR IMPAIR THE CREDIT1 OF OUR COUNTRY1
*** END DOCUMENT, NUMBER RETRIEVALS=   3

DOC# 31   SENT# 67   ID=D1900
WE ARE1 PROUD OF THE COURAGE AND FIDELITY OF THE AMERICAN SOLDIERS AND SAILORS IN ALL1 OUR WAR1S, WE FAVOR2 LIBERAL2 PENSIONS TO2 THEM AND THEIR DEPENDENTS, AND WE REITERATE THE POSITION1 TAKEN1 IN THE CHICAGO PLATFORM2 OF 1896 THAT1 THE FACT1 OF ENLISTMENT AND SERVICE1 SHALL BE3 DEEMED CONCLUSIVE EVIDENCE1 AGAINST DISEASE AND DISABILITY BEFORE ENLISTMENT
*** END DOCUMENT, NUMBER RETRIEVALS=   1

298

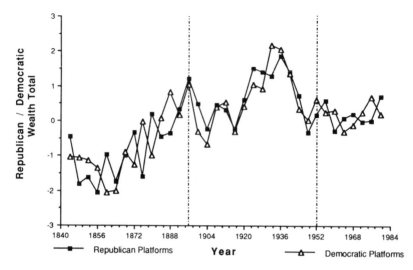

Figure 3.1. Republican and Democratic Concern with WEALTH-TOTAL, 1844-1980

Category Counts

Another approach to analyzing text counts words that have been classified into categories. As noted above, counting assumes that higher relative counts (proportions, percentages, or ranks) reflect higher concern with the category.

Counting is often useful because it may reveal aspects of the text that would not be apparent otherwise. For instance, one substantive question that arises in the analysis of party platforms is: Over time, how do the Democrats and Republicans vary with respect to each other in their concerns? Figure 3.1 shows each party's concern with WEALTH-TOTAL 1844-1980.[40] For each party, the data consist of the percentage of words in each platform categorized in WEALTH-TOTAL.[41]

Between 1844 and about 1952 there is a general rise in the percentage of each platform devoted to economic matters (Figure 3.1). This increase probably reflects greater importance of the state in the management of economic affairs. Second, from 1952 or so to the present there is a relatively constant level of concern with economic matters. Third, and more important, since 1844 the character of competition between the parties has changed qualitatively in dramatic ways.[42] From 1844 through the election of 1892 (the left vertical reference line) the parties

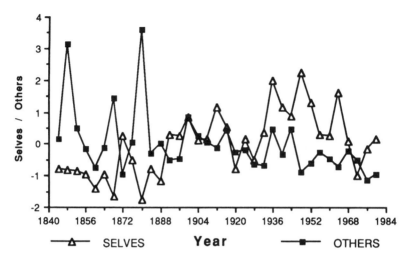

Figure 3.2. Democratic Concern with SELVES and OTHERS, 1844-1980

have varied opposite to each other in their concern with economic matters. Between 1896 and 1952 (the right vertical reference line) the parties manifest similar levels of economic concerns. Between 1952 and 1980, however, they move opposite each other again, although the overall variation in this time period is relatively small. The break points of 1894 and 1952 are congruent with Burnham's (1970) and others' interpretations of periodic realignments of the American party system (see Namenwirth and Weber, 1987: chapter 4).

Not only may simple counts reveal differences between message sources but they also may show how the communication content from one message source varies over time. From the Democratic party, Figure 3.2 illustrates how party platforms vary with respect to first-person plural pronouns (SELVES) and third person plural pronouns (OTHERS). As might be expected, these categories vary inversely with each other: When the Democrats emphasize their own accomplishments and programs, they de-emphasize those of the opposition. For Republican platforms, similar results were found (figure not shown here). Even though these examples are drawn from political sociology, comparing simple percentages has been used in other realms to great advantage. For example, Aries (1973, 1977) analyzed conversations in small groups to make inferences about sex-role differences in group interactions (see Chapter 1 for a summary).

Measurement Models

Although the preceding methods often work quite well, investigators have used a variety of multivariate data analysis techniques to analyze data based on text. One often-used technique is known as *factor analysis*,[43] a general name for several related mathematical procedures that summarize the variation of many observed or measured variables in terms of fewer underlying or latent variables that are called *factors*. The variation in these underlying factors usually is assumed to cause the variation in the observed variables. In content-analytic research, the observed variables are often categories and the factors often are assumed to be underlying themes in the text. The extent to which an observed variable is correlated to a latent variable or factor is called a *factor loading*, which is similar to a correlation coefficient. These ideas are illustrated in the following example.

This section reports some of the factor-analysis results in a study of American and British newspaper editorials (Namenwirth and Bibbee, 1975) and then considers interpretive problems. The next section outlines and critiques the substantive results based on the themes described here.

Using the General Inquiry computer system (Stone et al., 1966) and the Namenwirth Political Dictionary[44] (Namenwirth, no date), 288 randomly selected editorials concerning the Korean War from mass (*New York Daily News, Boston Daily Record,* and *Washington Daily News*) and elite (*New York Times, Christian Science Monitor,* and *Washington Post*) newspapers were classified into categories. For each editorial the computer reported the percentage of words in each of 40 categories retained for analysis.[45] Principal components analysis[46] produced four interpretable factors (accounting for 33% of the total variance). Table 3.6 presents factor loadings on the first two factors for each category. These numbers may be interpreted as the correlation between the category and the factor (loadings < .30 are omitted).

Categories that correlate (load on) with the same factor tend to vary together and investigators usually interpret them as representing a theme in the text. For example, editorials that have frequent references to American leaders and topics (AMERICAN) will also contain frequent references to words with higher status connotations (HIGHER STATUS)

TABLE 3.6
Selected Themes in Korean War Editorials in
Mass and Prestige (Elite) Newspapers

Theme 1: Control of the Social Environment — Parochialism Versus Cosmopolitan

Parochialism Categories	Loadings	*Cosmopolitan* Categories	Loadings*
American	.85	International Institution	−.53
Higher Status	.80	Approach	−.44
Job Role	.79	Sign Accept	−.42
Male Role	.68	Danger Theme	−.34
Selves	.43	Static	−.32
Sign Authority	.55		

Theme 2: Control of the Physical Environment — Economic Versus Military

Economic Categories	Loadings	*Military* Categories	Loadings
Sign Authority	.68	Death Theme	−.44
Collective Static	.64	Social Place	−.33
Action Norm	.55	Natural World	−.31
Guide	.47		
Ought	.46		
Control	.45		
Ideal Value	.41		
Work	.40		
Individual Static	.39		
Collective Dynamic	.35		
Sign Accept	.35		
Economic	.31		
Technological	.30		

SOURCE: Adapted from Namenwirth and Bibbee (1975)
* Loadings < |.30| are omitted.

and occupational references (JOB ROLE). Other editorials manifest concern with INTERNATIONAL INSTITUTIONS, conciliatory feelings and moods (APPROACH), words implying interpersonal acceptance (SIGN ACCEPT), words connoting alarm or concern with danger (DANGER THEME), and words concerned with maintaining the status quo (STATIC).

What do these themes mean or signify, and how can the investigator validate their interpretation? A discussion of factor interpretation is beyond the scope of this section. Some practical guidelines, however, may be helpful. For each editorial, the factor analysis procedure computes a score for each factor or theme that indicates the extent to which the editorial reflects the factor. To determine if these themes are real rather than statistical artifacts, these steps should be taken. First, the analyst should examine those editorials that have the highest positive and the highest negative factor scores. Typically, texts with similar scores manifest similar concerns. Second, the analyst should determine how the words in these exemplary texts are classified. There should be many words classified in the categories that have high loadings on the factor. Third, the analyst should compare the texts with extreme positive and negative factor scores with each other and with texts that have scores of nearly zero for that theme (factor). These contrasts should show that texts with high positive scores are quite different in content from those with zero scores, and that they are in some sense opposite to those with high negative scores.

Furthermore, each factor can be thought of as representing a controversy of some sort. The themes at the positive and negative poles typically are opposing resolutions of the underlying controversy. Examination of editorials with extreme positive and negative scores on Factor 1 suggested to Namenwirth and Bibbee that this controversy addresses control of the social environment. Editorials propose two alternative solutions, which they label *parochial* versus *cosmopolitan.* The parochial theme "stresses a fortress America stance: nationalism and isolationism best serve American interests and world peace" (Namenwirth and Bibbee, 1975: 53), as illustrated by this excerpt from the *Boston Daily Record,* May 4, 1951, titled "Now Let Us Have Facts:"

> More than 10,500 Americans are dead in Korea because these three men [Truman, Acheson, and Marshall][47] had a vested interest in their own mistakes. . . . Our concern is our sons in Korea. We frankly do not want any more Americans to die on that Asian peninsula seven thousand miles away from our shores, to protect the synthetic reputations of Acheson and Truman. Our sole concern is America and Americans. And that, we truly believe, is the concern of 99 percent of the American people. (Namenwirth and Bibbee, 1975: 53)

The cosmopolitan theme emphasizes "the need for an active role in world affairs, urging constant diplomatic initiative, coordination, and conciliation" (Namenwirth and Bibbee, 1975: 53), as illustrated by this excerpt from the December 3, 1952, *Christian Science Monitor* editorial titled "Unity in the UN:"

To the [anti-communists] the [communist rejection of the Indian Truce Plan] should suggest the possibility of a considerable strain between Moscow and Peking on this matter, a strain which free world diplomacy may exploit to advantage in the future. . . . It would be a great mistake for the anti-communist world to ignore the possibility [of future Chinese independence from Moscow], as it would be unrealistic for the neutral world to expect too much from it too soon. . . . Meanwhile, the precarious unity of the non-communist countries, as shown in the UN vote, can best be maintained as the United States demonstrates how far it is from seeking to dominate its friends and allies in the iron-fisted Moscow manner. (Namenwirth and Bibbee, 1975: 54)

The second issue or theme (Table 3.6) concerns contrasting approaches to control of the physical environment: Some editorials stress economic problems whereas other editorials stress military problems. Economic concerns mainly address inflation and the government's instituting and administering of a wartime system of price controls. Several categories correlate positively with this factor: normative patterns of social behavior (ACTION NORM); social/emotional actions consisting of assistance and positive direction (GUIDE); words indicating a moral imperative (OUGHT); words about limiting action (CONTROL); task activity (WORK); culturally defined virtues, goals, valued conditions, and activities (IDEAL VALUE); the ECONOMIC and TECHNOLOGICAL rules, actions, and contexts,[48] concern with the maintenance of the status quo, with the collectivity as agent or object of preferred action (COLLECTIVE STATIC); and the same as the former, but indicating a concern with the change of the status quo (COLLECTIVE DYNAMIC).

The ECONOMIC theme is illustrated by this portion of the August 16, 1950, *Washington Post* editorial titled "Defense Organization:"

The limited authority [Truman] has requested to allocate scarce materials, give priority to defense orders, tighten credit controls, and increase taxes certainly does not require any additional control machinery. . . . For the present, the existing organizational setup seems adequate to establish effective controls over allocations of the limited number of raw materials in short supply. . . . However much we may dislike the prospect, any effective general control over prices and living costs would necessitate the creation of a huge bureaucratic agency comparable to the Office of Price Administration. The government would also need new agencies to settle labor disputes, control and adjust wages. (Namenwirth and Bibbee, 1975: 55)

Editorials manifesting the opposing theme are mainly concerned with the cost of military intervention in terms of wounded and mutilated soldiers (DEATH THEME) and military solutions for these emergencies. These problem solutions are also seen as part of nature rather than society (SOCIAL PLACE, NATURAL WORLD). The following passage, from an editorial titled "Saving the Wounded" that appears in the April 5, 1952, *New York Times,* illustrates this military theme:

> Good news from the Korean battle front was reported in a recent address in Los Angeles by Major General George E. Armstrong, Army Surgeon General. He said that United States soldiers, wounded in Korea, who reach hospitals near the front had more than twice as good a chance of recovery as did soldiers wounded in the Second Word War. The medical corps, which has always been long on good hard work and short on publicity, warrants special commendation for this record. General Armstrong indicated that although body armor experiments had been favorable, teamwork between the medical corps, rescue troops, and helicopters had been an important factor in the diminishing death rate. (Namenwirth and Bibbee, 1975)

The essential point is that interpretations of statistical manipulations based on quantified text *must* be validated by reference to the text itself. Examination of exemplary texts, here identified by extreme factor scores, will provide direct evidence for or against particular interpretations. Similar themes in those editorials with similar extreme factor scores provide direct textual evidence that the same "story" is found repeatedly in a subset of texts, and consequently that the substantive conclusions are not artifacts of the content classification or statistical techniques employed. Also, examination of the texts may suggest the need to revise or discard the initial interpretation of the factor.

Note that interpretation is in part an art. Those who naively believe that data or texts speak for themselves (the doctrine of radical empiricism) are mistaken. The content analyst contributes factual and theoretical knowledge to the interpretation (see Namenwirth and Weber, 1987).

Interpretation cannot be the only goal of content analysis. As Krippendorff (1980) rightly stresses, the content of texts, however interpreted, must be related either to the context that produced them or to some consequent state of affairs. The following section shows that variation in the two sets of themes identified by Namenwirth and Bibbee (1975) is related to the type of newspaper in which they appeared.

TABLE 3.7

Prestige (Elite) Versus Mass Newspapers as a
Determinant of Selected Themes in Editorials

	Factor 1: Control of the Social Environment	
	Mass Newspapers	*Prestige Newspapers*
Mean Factor Score:	1.56	−1.56
	$F = 112.70$, df = 1,270, $p < .05$, ω^2 (%) = 77	
	Factor 2: Control of the Physical Environment	
	Mass Newspapers	*Prestige Newspapers*
Mean Factor Score:	−.75	.75
	$F = 20.24$, df = 1,270, $p < .05$, ω^2 (%) = 38	

SOURCE: Adapted from Namenwirth and Bibbee (1975)

Accounting for Content 1:
Characteristics of the Message Producers

As evidence of validity, many content analysis studies rely on internal consistency (i.e., showing that the textual evidence is more consistent with the interpretation). Even when explanations are offered, researchers seldom determine how strongly content-analytic variables are related to external factors. This section presents further results showing that variation in the themes documented above depends in part on characteristics of the message source (newspapers).

Namenwirth and Bibbee (1975) used an analysis of variance design[49] to assess the effect of newspaper type (elite or mass) on variation in themes, while simultaneously controlling for city (Boston, New York, or Washington) and time period during the Korean War.[50]

As Table 3.7 indicates, type of newspaper accounts for substantial variation in concern with control of the social environment and control of the physical environment: 77% and 38%, respectively. Mass newspapers stress parochial themes; prestige newspapers stress cosmopolitan ones. In addition, the mass press stresses military themes; the prestige press stresses economic problems. This result may not be surprising, because few sons of the elite classes were dying in Korea and because economic problems and controls directly affected the economic basis of the elite classes and their institutions.

The amount of variance in the dependent variables explained by type of newspaper is much larger than in most studies not using time-series analysis (econometricians routinely account for 90% or more of the variance in the dependent variable). Two other themes reported by Namenwirth and Bibbee, however, did less well: Type of newspaper accounted for only 15% and 6% of the variance, respectively. Also, not all of the variance of the first two themes was accounted for by type of newspaper. This means, first, that other causes of newspaper content were not included in the design and hence were not controlled. Second, some variance was accounted for by the two control variables, city and time. Third, error variance was not excluded from the factor scores,[51] and some unreliability remains.[52] This unreliability probably attenuates the relationship between themes and other variables.

Accounting for Content 2:
Changes in the Socioeconomic System

One of the most interesting and important applications of content analysis may be in cross-language designs. This section briefly describes findings from a small study undertaken to assess the cross-language validity of one content analysis dictionary.[53]

The development of valid and reliable content-analytic instruments for the analysis of German-language text is a prerequisite for comparing quantitatively the relationships between changes in symbol usage, economy, society, and polity in German and English-speaking countries. Consequently, the investigators carried out a small study to evaluate the cross-language validity and reliability of some content categories from the Lasswell Value Dictionary (Namenwirth and Weber, 1987: chapter 2; Zuell, Weber, and Mohler, 1989). Their immediate empirical question concerned the relationship between concern with wealth in the speeches of the German Kaiser 1871-1912 and economic fluctuations.

Specifically they hypothesized two theoretical concepts: *wealth concerns* and *economic performance*. Each of these unobserved or latent variables is measured by two or more observed variables. Three WEALTH categories of the Lasswell Value Dictionary measure wealth concerns: WEALTH-PARTICIPANTS, WEALTH-TRANSACTIONS, and WEALTH-OTHER. As noted in Chapter 2, the first category contains the names of those persons or positions involved in the creation, maintenance, and transfer of wealth, such as *banker*. The TRANSACTIONS category contains references to exchanges of wealth, such as *buying, selling,* and *borrowing*. The WEALTH-OTHER category contains wealth-related words not classified in the other two categories.

The measurement of economic performance in the period 1871-1912 is difficult because reasonably valid and reliable economic data from this period are usually lacking. The investigators were fortunate, however, to locate the prices of wheat and rye on the Berlin wholesale grain market between 1871 and 1912. Grain prices have two qualities important for the study: First, they are public information well-known to most people, either directly or indirectly through the price of bread and other grain products. Second, grain prices are less likely to be subject to measurement errors than are composite price indices or national accounts data based on aggregation across many units, such as estimates of gross national product. Although there may have been some regional variation in grain prices, the investigators believe that the data accurately represent the prices of these two widely used commodities.

What is the relationship between grain prices and economic performance? Prices are related positively to economic performance; that is, the price of grain and the economy tend to rise and fall together because price levels are in part an indicator of the inflation that often occurs in expanding economies. It is certainly true that other factors — such as weather, foreign trade, and the availability of substitutes — influence prices. Only that part of variation in wheat and rye prices that the two variables have in common, however, is used in the composite measure of economic performance. The remaining variance in wheat and rye prices is considered to be error variance consisting of measurement errors and variance because of factors other than economic performance.

If grain prices are an indicator of economic performance, then what is the relationship between economic performance and wealth concerns? Previous analyses of American and British political documents and economic change (Namenwirth, 1969b; Namenwirth and Weber, 1987) show that economic performance and wealth concerns are related inversely: As the economy improves there is less concern with wealth, whereas a declining economy is associated with increasing wealth concerns. In short, higher levels of concern with economic matters are associated with economic adversity. Thus the investigators were pleased to find that the data showed a negative relationship between economic performance and wealth concerns in the Kaiser's speeches from 1871 to 1912—that is, changes in the rate of change of the economy (acceleration) were negatively related to wealth concerns.[54]

Figure 3.3 shows the structure of the causal model and the parameters to be estimated from the data. These unknown parameters (coefficients) are estimated using the LISREL approach to the analysis of covariance structures (Jöreskog and Sörbom, 1979, 1984). The general LISREL model consists of two parts: the measurement model and the structural equation model. The measurement model defines how the latent or unobserved variables are related to observed variables. The structural equation model specifies the structure of causal relationships among latent variables and among the error variances. In the model proposed above, the observed variables are content categories, and the latent variables are economic performance and wealth concerns.

Besides estimating the measurement and structural equation models simultaneously, the LISREL model also estimates how well the predicted covariance matrix reproduces or fits the observed covariance (or correlation) matrix. This indicator is an approximation to chi square with appropriate degrees of freedom for the number of free and constrained parameters. The lower the chi square, the better the fit of the model to the data.

Table 3.8 and Figure 3.3 present the results.[55] Some caution is necessary in the interpretation of these results, because the LISREL goodness-of-fit statistics assume large sample sizes. The chi square for the overall fit of the model is not significant (.905 with 4 df, $p < .9238$), which suggests that there is a very small probability of finding a better fitting model. Almost all the estimated parameters are twice their standard errors. The t statistic for the causal coefficient between economic performance and wealth concerns is just under 2, at 1.98. Also, the t statistic for the error variance of the dependent variable (wealth concerns) is .667, which in this case suggests that there is very little error variance left (i.e., the residual or error variance is not different from zero). This is not surprising because economic performance accounts for 73% of the variance in wealth concerns. The coefficient indicating the loading of WEALTH-PARTICIPANTS on wealth concerns (LY3) is not significant, but given the overall results of the model and the low number of cases, the researchers decided to leave this variable in the model.

Finally, the magnitude and direction of the relationship between wealth concerns and economic performance show that the WEALTH categories the investigators constructed for German text are quite reli-

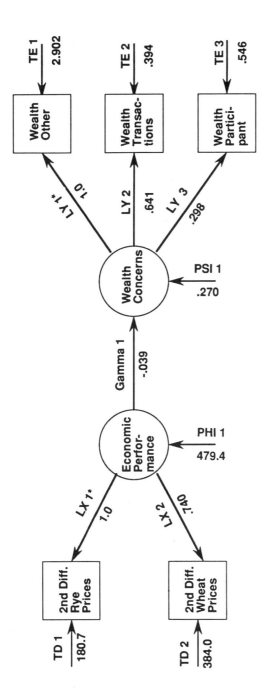

Note: R^2 = .730; * = Fixed Parameter

Figure 3.3. Structural Model Relating Economic Performance and Wealth Concerns in Kaiser Speeches, 1871-1912
SOURCE: Adapted from Weber (1984a)

309

TABLE 3.8

LISREL Parameter Estimates: Economic Performance and
Wealth Concerns in Kaiser Speeches, 1871-1912*

Parameter	Unstd. Coef.	Std. Err.	t
LX1**	1.000		
LX2	.740	.275	2.690
TDI	180.700	155.100	1.165
TD2	384.000	128.000	3.000
PHI1	479.400	220.800	2.171
GAMMA1	−.039	.020	1.980
PSI1	.270	.404	.667
LY1**	1.000		
LY2	.641	.296	2.166
LY3	.298	.195	1.528
TE1	2.902	.859	3.378
TE2	.394	.184	2.143
TE3	.546	.150	3.646

LISREL Estimates, $N = 31$

*See Figure 3.3 for structure of model.
** Parameter fixed to 1 for purposes of identification.
SOURCE: Adapted from Weber (1984a)

able and valid. As predicted, this relationship is negative. The size of
the coefficient (−.039) suggests that a 10-mark change in the rate of
change of prices caused an increase (or decrease) of 4 wealth words per
1000. Because of the content-analytic procedures employed, it is likely
that the size of the unstandardized coefficient understates the relationship between wealth-related issues and economic performance. The
investigators counted only those words that by themselves indicate
wealth concerns rather than total words in sentences dealing with
economic problems. Had the latter been done, the size of the coefficient
might be substantially higher because the variance of the dependent
variable would be higher. It is also worth noting that if all the observed
and latent variables had zero means and standard deviations of 1.0, then
the coefficient between economic performance and wealth concerns
would be −.855, which is certainly a substantial relationship.[56]

Concluding Remarks

The techniques presented in this chapter illustrate several possibilities for content analysis ranging from detailed analysis of word or

phrase usage (KWIC lists and concordances) to multivariate analysis based on quantification. Other quantitative means of analysis were omitted because of space limitations. These include regression analysis, time-series regression models, discriminant analysis, and cluster analysis.

The spirit of the preceding presentation is illustrative and didactic. It is worth repeating that there is no single right way to do content analysis. Instead, investigators must judge what methods are appropriate for their substantive problems. Given the ubiquity of computers, there is a real danger that as software for content analysis becomes distributed more widely, as the costs of encoding texts in machine-readable form continue to decline, and as the opportunity for capturing texts directly from other electronic media increases (e.g., newspaper editing and composing systems, word processors and typesetters, and newswires), the danger of mindless content analysis will also increase. One reason content analysis is not used more widely is that it is difficult and time-consuming to do well. Computers eliminate some of the drudgery, but time, effort, skill, and art are required to produce results, interpretations, and explanations that are valid and theoretically interesting.

Suggestions for Further Reading

Anyone thinking of doing content analysis would be well advised to look carefully at Stone et al. (1966). Namenwirth and Weber (1987) apply updated versions of these techniques to political documents, newspaper editorials, and speeches. Related methodological concerns are addressed in Kelly and Stone (1975) and Zuell et al. (1989). Rosengren (1981) presents several studies of the Swedish symbol system using human-coded content analysis. The early classics of Berelson (1952), Lasswell (e.g., Lasswell, Leites, et al., 1965; Lasswell, Lerner, and Pool, 1952), and Pool (1951, 1952a, 1952b, 1959) are still worthwhile reading to see what kind of problems they addressed and how they resolved them.

There is also a large "computers and the humanities" literature, including a journal by that title currently published by the Paradigm Press. Papers from several conferences on computers and the humanities also have been published, including Ager, Knowles, and Smith (1979); Aitken, Bailey, and Hamilton-Smith (1973); Jones and Churchhouse (1976); and Wisbey (1971). A related text is Oakman (1980).

Salton (1989) discusses text processing from a computer-science perspective focusing on information retrieval. There is a huge and still-growing literature on natural language processing and computational linguistics. Allen (1987) provides an excellent introduction to modern methods for computer processing of language. Winograd and Flores (1986) provide an important philosophical and social critique of such endeavors.

4. ISSUES IN CONTENT ANALYSIS

Content analysis procedures create quantitative indicators that assess the degree of attention or concern devoted to cultural units such as themes, categories, or issues. The investigator then interprets and explains the results using relevant theories. This chapter considers four key aspects of the content analysis process:

- *measurement* — the assignment of numbers that stand for some aspect of the text
- *indication* — the inference by the investigator of some unmeasured quality or characteristic of the text from those numbers
- *representation* — techniques for describing syntactic, semantic, or pragmatic aspects of texts
- *interpretation* — the translation of the meaning in text into some other abstract analytical or theoretical language

For each of these processes, difficulties exist that may detract from the reliability of the procedures or from the validity of substantive conclusions based on them. This chapter discusses some of these problems in order to help researchers make more informed choices about their procedures, to help in understanding the limitations of currently available content analysis procedures, and to suggest new lines of research that may (at least in part) resolve these problems.

Measurement

In content analysis, measurement consists of counting the occurrences of meaning units such as specific words, phrases, content categories, and themes. Regardless of whether the text is coded by humans or by computers, two standard measurement practices are using the percentage (or proportion) transformation to control for document length[57] and counting each occurrence of a word or other meaning unit equally. Each of these practices leads to serious difficulties that require attention.

The Percentage Transformation. This section addresses four specific problems that arise from using the percentage transformation to control for document length. First, the percentage or proportion has limited range and is asymptotic; consequently, the resulting measurement is not linear (for example, an increase from 5% to 10% is not the same as an increase from 60% to 65%).

Second, statisticians have shown that the mean and variance of percentages are not independent. Therefore, when used as the dependent variable in analysis of variance designs, proportions are subjected to an arcsin square root transformation, a procedure recommended by statisticians to make the mean and variance independent (see, e.g., Freeman and Tukey, 1950; Schuessler, 1971: 411-416). Additional research is required to determine if percentages based on textual data — with or without transformation — create problems in statistical estimation and inference when used with multivariate procedures other than ANOVA, such as factor analysis or the LISREL approach to structural equation models.

Third, different measurement strategies may imply different theoretical assumptions. For example, the percentage distribution may be inconsistent with the hypothesis that concern with secular rather than sacred themes increases linearly over time. Extended far enough into the future, such a trend must eventually exceed 100%. Investigators therefore should consider whether their measurement procedures unwittingly conflict with their epistemological and methodological assumptions and substantive theories.

Fourth, many of the statistical procedures used by content analysts make distributional assumptions that probably are violated by the percentage distribution. For example, content analysis data are unlikely to be either univariate or multivariate normal.

Rather than using percentages or proportions, some colleagues (in personal communications) have suggested instead modeling frequency counts generated by content analysis as a Poisson process and then using statistical estimation procedures based on this distribution. Most content-analytic studies thus far have relied on the robustness of factor analysis, curve-fitting, ANOVA, and other statistical procedures combined with validation techniques based on examination of the original text. Still, additional research is needed to assess whether the robustness of these statistical methods really compensates for the deviations of most content analysis data from the Gaussian normal distribution.

Counting Occurrences Equally. The standard practice of counting equally each occurrence of a given semantic unit engenders two different problems. The first is that each of the words classified in a given category may not reflect that category to the same extent. The second is that subsequent mentions of a category or topic may require greater effort than the first few mentions.

To explain: The measurement procedures of content analysis are based on frequency counts of semantically equivalent textual units such as words, word senses, phrases, issues, or themes. The semantic equivalence that underlies the procedures described earlier in this volume is *connotative categorical equivalence.*[58] Textual units are connotative categorically equivalent if they signify or suggest certain meanings, ideas, and so forth in addition to their explicit or primary meanings. For example, in one category scheme, both *bonus* and *allowance* are classified in the category WEALTH because they share a common connotation — namely, economic matters.

Each word classified in a particular category need not equally represent the category content. Nevertheless, counting each entry equally is desirable because we currently lack procedures that reliably and validly assign weights indicating the unequal representation of category content by different entries in a single category (see Namenwirth and Weber, 1987: chapter 8). Neither can we now handle situations where the degree of representation may vary across sets of documents or over time.[59]

A different problem arises when investigators count equally each occurrence of each entry in the same category in a given document. For example, the 25th occurrence of an entry in the category AFFECTION is given the same weight or importance as the 5th occurrence or as the 125th. Equal counting is a practical simplification that content analysts believe works well in most circumstances, but reality is probably much more complicated.

Specifically, content analysts long have assumed that the more a text contains mentions of a particular category, the more it is concerned with it. Philip J. Stone (personal communication) has conjectured that the initial mention of a word (or category, theme, or topic) required more effort or energy than successive mentions. Put another way, raising a new topic requires more energy or effort than continuing the previous one (topic avoidance is addressed later). If raising the topic at all requires an effort, what about continuing the topic through succeeding mentions? There exists a point after which each succeeding mention requires more rather than less effort. This is so because:

- Stylistic considerations may cause authors to substitute pronouns where possible.[60]
- Continuing concern with a particular category (e.g., WEALTH) may lead to redundancy or repetition so that the amount of information being communicated declines as the text continues.
- If there are contextual constraints on text length — for example, the amount of time available for a State of the Union address — continued attention to one issue, theme, or category, precludes attention to other topics.
- Even if there are not contextual constraints, the resources available for text production are surely finite. Text producers therefore typically will allocate their efforts to a range of issues and themes.

Not all topics are equally difficult to raise. In contemporary America, for example, it may well be easier for political parties to address economic issues such as trade and deficits than the history and current plight of Native Americans living precariously on reservations. Thus some topics may require much more effort to raise than others. For reasons noted above, however, continued attention to a topic requires still greater effort. Therefore, equal counting of each instance does not reflect changes in the level of effort required to maintain the topic.

Also, the assertion that zero mention requires no effort is plainly wrong at times. Keeping issues from being mentioned may also require much effort. The Freudian notions that unconscious ego urges drive us and that we must repress ourselves and others to maintain civilization are relevant here. Under circumstances that have yet to be explored systematically, the lack of mention therefore can be of great significance.

These ideas suggest that further research should examine the consequences of equal counting on validity and reliability in general, and on measurement in particular.

Indication

As noted earlier, the term *indication* refers to inferences made by the investigator of some unmeasured or latent characteristics of text using numbers that represent some manifest aspect of the text. For example, as shown in the previous chapter, factor analysis often is used to infer themes in text. More subtle examples are presented shortly. Some critics believe that indication is problematic because they question the reliability and validity of all inferences concerning latent characteristics of text, or of such inferences in the absence of accompanying detailed syntactic and semantic information.

This section addresses two important aspects of indication. The first concerns the rationale for analyzing latent characteristics of the text at all. The second concerns latent characteristics of texts that may not be discernible through detailed semantic analysis without quantification.

In social science research we often use statistical procedures (such as factor analysis, structural equation models, and simple correlations) that suggest or assume the existence of unmeasured or latent variables. As most often applied in content analysis, the unit of analysis in these statistical procedures is the entire document.[61] Therefore, latent variables indicate features of each entire text (or other coding or analytic unit, such as paragraphs, chapters, or document sections). These latent-variable models raise interesting problems and possibilities not often met in social research (Mohler, personal communication). In latent-indicator models of mental ideas such as attitudes, for example, the investigator can never observe directly mental states that validate the interpretation of the results (and given the problematic relationships between attitudes and behavior, it is not possible to infer the former from the latter, either). A different situation, however, exists in content analysis. Here the investigator *can* examine the relationship between latent variables and the original text being analyzed.

If one has observables such as text, why bother with quantification and latent-indicator models at all? There are several reasons. First, counting generates results that allow for more precise comparisons among texts. Second, we want to know how much more (or less) attention is devoted to some issues than to others. Third, quantitative analytical procedures often reveal similarities and differences among texts that would be difficult, if not impossible, to detect otherwise.

Investigators often find that covariation among observed variables suggests substantively interesting features of texts that otherwise would not be apparent. The fact that latent variables so inferred actually are derived from observable texts makes them no less useful. Rather, examining the observable text is an important opportunity to improve the interpretation and validation of the substantive findings.

As noted in the introductory chapter, the coding and quantitative techniques discussed in this volume often are criticized because they do not make much use of the syntactical and semantic information in each sentence. Nevertheless, these quantitative methods often permit inferences that probably could not be made by other means.

For example, several studies (Namenwirth and Weber, 1987: chapter 9) have found similar positive correlations between four pairs of categories: (1) IF and SURE (or UNDERSTATE[62] and OVERSTATE), (2) POSITIVE AFFECT and NEGATIVE AFFECT, (3) POWER CONFLICT and POWER COOPERATION, and (4) POWER AUTHORITATIVE and POWER AUTHORITATIVE PARTICIPANTS. What do these correlations tell us?

- If a document uses many UNDERSTATE words, such as *ambiguous, apparent,* and *little,* it is also likely to use many OVERSTATE words, such as *absolute, natural,* and *necessary.* But this finding leaves open whether these classes of words do or do not occur in the same sentence or paragraph context. Furthermore, Namenwirth and Weber (1987: chapter 9) interpret this correlational finding itself as *indicating* that those documents high in OVERSTATE and UNDERSTATE words discuss matters very defensively compared with those documents with few words in these categories. But this is not to say that such documents explicitly state that they are defensive about whatever they discuss. In fact, they rarely do.

- Similarly, the positive correlation between POSITIVE AFFECT (*attachment, beneficial,* and *inspire*) and NEGATIVE AFFECT (*adverse, neglect,* and *obnoxious*) first suggests that documents are most often either affect-laden or affect-neutral, and, second, indirectly tells whether and to what extent particular documents are of one kind or another. Documents rarely will state this fact outright. Instead, these correlations suggest something about the mood, tone, or style of documents.

- Third, several studies have found a positive correlation between POWER CONFLICT (*agitate, encroachments,* and *rebellion*) and POWER COOPERATION (*solidarity, supporter,* and *unanimous*). Thus documents with a high frequency of one will displace a high frequency of the other.

- We also find that POWER COOPERATION and POWER CONFLICT are usually correlated negatively with another pair of categories, namely, POWER AUTHORITATIVE (*administer, reign, statute*) and POWER AUTHORITATIVE PARTICIPANT (*administrator, regiment, tribunal*). The latter positively correlated cluster indicates a concern with consensual power that is a facility of the entire society (Lehman, 1977; Namenwirth and Weber, 1987: 149). These findings show that documents are preoccupied with either consensual or conflictual power concerns, but not both at the same time. More important, whatever their power concerns, documents rarely state them explicitly: they "merely" are indicated.

Thus our commonsense impressions about the utility of semantic information in narrow contexts reflect a limited (but still important) truth, as these examples also show. In fact, content-analytic procedures that restrict themselves to themes that are stated explicitly would certainly miss many of these important indications.

Representation

The kind of text classification and content analysis described in this volume is criticized sometimes for not utilizing essential syntactic or semantic features of language or text in the analysis. These critics often call attention to the fact that both human-based coding procedures and the computer systems described here do not encode or represent the richness of language or of specific texts. One way that the meaning of words, phrases, or other textual units is represented is through classification into a set of categories. In assigning meaning units to categories, not all connotations or nuances of meaning are pertinent. It does not make much sense to insist on linguistic distinctions that are more fine-grained than the distinctions made by the category scheme. Thus content classification procedures safely ignore irrelevant distinctions. But what is a relevant distinction?

In the early and mid-1970s, Stone and his collaborators (Kelly and Stone, 1975; Zuell, Weber, and Mohler, 1989) developed an improved version of the General Inquirer computer system for content analysis that can differentiate among the various senses of homographs. For example, is the word *frame* a noun or a verb? Does *kind* refer to a class of objects or a benevolent disposition? Consider the word *state*. The General Inquirer distinguishes six different senses or uses:

- state (noun; body politic or area of government)
- situation (e.g., *state of science*)
- "to state" (verb; to declare)
- "state of affairs" (idiom; situation)
- "united states" (idiom; handled by *United*)
- "ship of state" (idiom; government, handled by *ship*)

Kelly and Stone's (1975) disambiguation of *state* is itself a simplification.[63] The *Random House Dictionary of the English Language* (college edition) lists 17 different senses for *state*. The *Oxford English Dictionary* lists at least 41 different meanings. Not every shade of meaning or nuance, however, will be relevant to a particular investigation. Thus in the interest of parsimony, perhaps only 5 or 10 usages of *state* may be sufficient.

In short, although more powerful text analysis systems will be useful, some distinctions may not be worth maintaining. Convenience and parsimony are important factors in deciding how much detail to maintain.

Interpretation

Interpretation consists of translating one set of linguistic or linguistically expressed elements into another (Namenwirth and Weber, 1987: chapters 2 and 8). This translation or "mapping" procedure leads to several difficulties that are explored best through an example.

Weber analyzed British Speeches from the Throne 1689-1972 (Namenwirth and Weber, 1987: chapters 4 and 5; Weber, 1981, 1982). For each of the documents, the content analysis procedures created quantitative measures of attention devoted to various content categories. Subsequent analysis of these quantitative data suggested the existence of political issues or themes that recurred periodically in these texts. For example, Weber (Namenwirth and Weber, 1987: chapter 4) identified four issues or themes that recurred approximately every 72 years[64] during the period 1689-1795. Consider the following excerpt from the speech of 1690 (Namenwirth and Weber, 1987):

It is sufficiently known how earnestly I have endeavored to extinguish, or at least compose, all differences amongst my subjects, and to that end, how often have I recommended an Act of Indemnity to the last Parliament; but since that part of it which related to the preventing of private suits, is already enacted, and because debates of that nature must take up more of your time than can now be spared from the dispatch of those other things which are absolutely necessary for our common safety, I intend to send you an Act of Grace, with exceptions of some few persons only, but such as may be sufficient to show my great dislike of their crimes; and, at the same time, my readiness to extend protection to all my other subjects, who will thereby see that they can recommend themselves to me by no other methods, than what the law prescribes, which shall always be the only rules of my government.

Now compare the preceding with excerpt with the following one given in 1757:

I have had such ample experience of the loyalty and good affections of my faithful subjects towards me, my family, and government, in all circumstances, that I am confident they are not to be shaken. But I cannot avoid taking notice of that spirit of disorder, which has shown itself amongst the common people, in some parts of the Kingdom. Let me recommend it to you, to do your part in discouraging and suppressing such abuses and for maintaining the law, and lawful authority. If anything shall be found wanting, to explain or enforce what may have been misunderstood or misrepresented, I am persuaded it will not escape your attention. Nothing can be so conducive to the defense of all that is dear to us, as well as for reducing our enemies to reason, as union and harmony amongst ourselves.

Many readers will agree that these excerpts address the same underlying issue or theme, but might disagree over what to name it. Let us briefly postpone naming the common theme until after we consider interpretation itself.

The process of interpretation constitutes translation from one language to another (Namenwirth and Weber, 1987). Each language consists of a set of rules that define what constitutes a valid sentence in the language. Using these rules, speakers of the language can generate a virtually infinite number of sentences. Considering a text in one language, translation consists in large part of mapping the syntactic and semantic structures that comprise the text in the first language into structures that are valid for the second and that convey the meaning of the first.

As is well-known, translation can be a difficult process (Steiner, 1975). A procedure, however, for checking the validity of a translation exists — namely, back-translation. Here the text in the target language is translated back into the original and then compared with the original. When the back-translation and the original text are the same, then the first translation is valid. Note that this kind of translation is bidirectional or reversible: Once investigators have translated the text into the second language they usually can reconstruct the original text. Note also that there may be only one or very few translations that are valid. Not all translations, however, are reversible.

The primary concern here is with irreversible or unidirectional transformations that map the content of texts into more abstract, usually theoretical structures. For content analysis, this specialized language is usually the social science theory (or theories) used by the investigator to interpret the text and explain the substantive results. Here the mapping is from the many words of the text into fewer and more abstract categories and into relations suggested by the theory.

Note that in the excerpts above, the words — let alone the syntax — used to convey the basic themes are hardly identical. For example, the first excerpt begins by discussing differences among subjects of the King, whereas the second excerpt begins by discussing the loyalty and good affections of the subjects. Some differences reflect differing historical circumstances. Coming two years after the Glorious Revolution of 1688, the first excerpt discusses an Act of Indemnity and Act of Grace. Given during the Seven Years' War, the second excerpt ends with a reference to foreign enemies and internal cohesion.

These differences aside, sociologists and political scientists usually would choose one of two principal theoretical and conceptual frameworks for labeling the common underlying issue. Marxists and other conflict theorists might say that these excerpts deal with conflict between the common people on the one side and the aristocracy, commercial interests, and the incipient capitalist classes on the other.[65] Weber (Namenwirth and Weber, 1987: chapter 4) chose to interpret the common underlying issue as reflecting what Bales and Parsons refer to as *integrative* concerns, whose principle focus is the coordination of the various subgroups in society (or other social system).[66]

As this example illustrates, there is no one-to-one mapping between text and theory. Also, the translation from text to theory is not reversible. One could generate virtually an infinite number of excerpts whose interpretation is as an instance of integrative themes in the Bales/Parsons sense. Thus the strategy of back-translation is not available to us as a means of validating the mapping from text to theory.

Given that differing, perhaps antithetical theoretical frameworks can be used to interpret these texts, what should we conclude? First, a variety of interpretations usually will be available and the investigator must choose. It is inappropriate to pursue a fruitless quest in search of the "true" or the "valid" interpretation. As Slater (1966) points out, it is not the validity of an interpretation per se that is at issue, but rather the salience of an interpretation given one or another theory. Second, just as it is true that quantitative data do not speak for themselves (i.e., that the doctrine of radical empiricism is false), so is it true that texts do not speak for themselves either. The investigator must do the speaking and the language of that speech is the language of theory.

Concluding Remarks

This chapter addressed several problems that arise when text is analyzed for social science purposes. These difficulties are inherent in the fundamental processes of content analysis — namely, measurement, indication, representation, and interpretation. Not only are they fundamental to content analysis, these processes are fundamental to most inquiry in the humanities and sciences. Interpretation and representation, for example, entail difficulties that are neither understood widely nor resolved easily. A much more sustained, interdisciplinary effort is required.

Suggestions for Further Reading

The techniques discussed in this volume were developed before recent advances in other disciplines concerning language and understanding. The literature has grown huge, but some of the literature not mentioned here previously includes Boden (1987, 1988), Brady and Berwick (1983), Dyer (1983), Weizenbaum (1976), and Winograd (1983).

APPENDIX
Computer Software and Text Data Archives

TEXTPACK, a comprehensive software system for text analysis, is now being distributed for a nominal charge by the Computer Department/ ZUMA/ The Center for Surveys, Methods, and Analysis/ B2,1/ D-6800 Mannheim 1/ Federal Republic of Germany. This software will run on microcomputers, workstations, minicomputers, and mainframes provided they have a FORTRAN compiler that supports the 1977 standard. A version for MS-DOS personal computers is now available from ZUMA. TEXTPACK documentation is available in either English or German.

As desired by the investigator, TEXTPACK V will perform or generate frequency counts of words, key-word-in-context (KWIC) lists, key-word-out-of-context (KWOC) lists, comparisons of vocabularies, cross-references, procedures for iterative dictionary construction, retrievals of text units, reduction of text via go-stop lists, and tagging (OR function for all systems: OR, AND, NOT, BEFORE, AFTER, NOT functions for IBM and Siemens versions). In addition, there are interfaces for the major statistical packages. Full disambiguation, however, is not available at this time.

The General Inquirer III system for classifying and analyzing text by computer is now available from ZUMA at the address above. This software classifies the many words of texts into content categories by looking up each word in a content analysis dictionary. The dictionary contains a list of words — a vocabulary — and for each word the category or categories in which it is to be classified.

The General Inquirer is written in the PL/1 language for IBM MVS and VM operating systems. Although the PL/1 source code is distributed, the system should not be considered portable to other (and especially non-IBM) computing environments. The General Inquirer was created many years ago when batch computer systems prevailed. Thus the system is not particularly user-friendly. The full documentation for the system and related material is now available as a ZUMA publication (Zuell, Weber, and Mohler, 1989). Together with the General Inquirer software, ZUMA is distributing three large and well-established dictionaries, namely, the Lasswell Value Dictionary and two versions (IV-3 and IV-4) of the Harvard Psychosociological Dictionary. These are documented in Zuell et al. (1989). The General Inquirer runs on all IBM mainframes using MVS or VM operating systems; a PL/1 compiler must be available because the system is delivered as program source code and must therefore be compiled; the system SORT utility is required by some General Inquirer routines.

The current version of the Oxford Concordance Program for mainframes is version 2. This is distributed by Oxford University Computing Service. Please address inquiries to OCP, Oxford University Computing Service, 13 Banbury Road, Oxford OX2 6NN, England, e-mail OCP@VAX.OX.AC.UK. Micro-OCP is a version of OCP for the IBM PC and compatibles. It requires at least 512K, a hard disk, and DOS 3.0

or higher. It is completely compatible with mainframe OCP V2 (i.e., files can be transferred from the PC to mainframe and run without change). Micro-OCP is published by Oxford Electronic Publishing, Oxford University Press, Walton Street, Oxford OX2 6DP, England. The program is documented in Susan Hockey and Jeremy Martin's *OCP Users' Manual Version 2*, Oxford University Computing Service; *Micro-OCP Manual*, obtainable from Oxford University Press, address above—this is not sold in bookstores, only by mail order from OUP; and Hockey and Martin (1987).

Software for text analysis often is described in the journal *Computers and the Humanities*, currently published by Paradigm Press, P. O. Box 1057, Osprey, FL 33559-1057.

At this writing, few text data sets have been archived and made publicly accessible. The ICPSR at the University of Michigan has at least two text data sets created by Holsti and North. One contains a sample of the replies to the British Speeches from the Throne given at the opening of each session of Parliament. Another file contains the speeches of the German Kaiser. The latter data set was found to be incomplete and contains numerous errors. The former data set is documented poorly.

The entire texts of Democratic and Republican (Whig) Party platforms 1844-1964 have been archived at the Roper Center, University of Connecticut, Storrs, CT 06268. They are available on computer tape through the Roper Center for a small fee. These data are also available in Europe from the Zentralarchiv für Empirische Sozialforschung/Bachmer Strasse 40/D-5000 Köln 31/FRG. In addition, British Speeches from the Throne at the opening of Parliament 1689-1972 have been archived at the same institutions.

NOTES

1. Various authors have proposed format definitions of content analysis. For example, Stone et al. (1966: 5) state: "Content analysis is any research technique for making inferences by systematically and objectively identifying specified characteristics within text." Krippendorff (1980: 21) defines the method as follows: "Content analysis is a research technique for making replicative and valid inferences from data to their context." Krippendorff is right to emphasize the relationship between the content of texts and their institutional, societal, or cultural contexts. See Chapter 3 and Namenwirth and Weber (1987) for extended discussions.

2. Other perspectives on text analysis include linguistics, psychology, and artificial intelligence. As noted in Chapter 3, there is also a large "computers and the humanities" literature that partly overlaps the concerns of this volume.

3. *Meaning* refers to shared as opposed to private understandings.

4. Category names are shown in small capital letters.

5. Another, more qualitative or clinical tradition of content analysis is not emphasized here. See, for example, George (1959a, 1959b), Berelson (1952: chapter 3), and some of the articles in a special issue of Qualitative Sociology, 1984 (volume 7, numbers 1 and 2).

6. Various systems for computer-aided content analysis are more or less successful in distinguishing among various word meanings and connotations. This problem and several resolutions are discussed later.

7. *Construct validity* has been used to refer to two different types of validity; hence there is some confusion over the term. Cook and Campbell (1979: 59) use the term to refer to "the possibility that the operations which are meant to represent a particular cause or effect construct can be construed in terms or more than one construct." Others, following Cronbach and Meehl (1955) use the term *construct validity* to refer to the fit between data and constructs suggested by theory. The present discussion uses the former definition, and following Brinberg and McGrath (1982), refers to the latter definition as *hypothesis validity*, which is discussed below.

8. This is what Janis (1965) refers to as *indirect* validation, which he suggests is the main form of validation for content analysis. Hypothesis validity, however, has an important weakness: If the relationship between a content and a noncontent variable is counter to theory, does this invalidate the variables or the hypothesis?

9. There is nothing inherent in content-analysis techniques to limit predictive validity; rather, investigators seldom include assessments of predictive validity in their research designs.

10. This form of coding is based on Osgood, Suci, and Tannenbaum's (1957) evaluation assertion analysis (also see Holsti, 1966, 1969). A more sophisticated form is used by Axelrod (1976) and his collaborators in the coding of cognitive maps of political elites. Appendix One in that volume gives detailed coding rules.

11. Holsti (1969: 104-116) gives numerous examples of broad and narrow category schemes for content analysis.

12. It is routine to classify 90 to 95% of the words in most nonspecialized texts using general dictionaries. Also, they can be modified easily to handle highly specialized texts, such as the speeches of the presidents of American scientific associations (Namenwirth and Weber, 1987: chapter 7).

13. One reason content analysis did not blossom the way survey research did was that the lack of standardized procedures and measuring instruments worked against the accumulation of comparable results. See Namenwirth and Weber (1987: 195-196) for further discussion.

14. Many of the examples presented here use the General Inquirer system. At present, the TEXTPACK program mentioned in the Appendix will do everything that the General Inquirer can do, except disambiguation.

15. Table 2.1 is adapted from Namenwirth and Weber (1987) and Zuell et al. (1989). Table 2.2 is adapted from Dunphy et al. (1989).

16. Current computer software can distinguish the various senses of words with more than one meaning. This is discussed later.

17. For example, low-variance or oddly shaped distributions often cause problems in statistical estimation.

18. These distinctions are often semantic, but may also be syntactic — for example, identifying syntactic categories such as verbs, nouns, and modifiers. More precise classification results from correctly classifying modifiers, for example, into more specific classes such as adjectives and adverbs.

19. TEXTPACK V also has some capabilities for dealing with idioms.

20. Natural language-processing techniques developed in artificial intelligence and computer science are likely to provide a proper solution to the problem, but the software and hardware required will not be widely available for some time.

21. For simplicity, this and the next table omit the syntactic and marker categories assigned to each word. The latter are used in the disambiguation rules, and are not used normally in substantive interpretations.

22. Except for subcategory/category-total assignments (e.g., WEALTH-OTHER/WEALTH-TOTAL), the LVD is a single-classification dictionary. Words or word senses are assigned only to one substantive category. The Harvard IV-3 and Harvard IV-4 are multiple-classification dictionaries in which word senses may be assigned to more than one substantive category.

23. Intensity might be taken into account by multivariate models such as factor analysis and multidimensional scale. In that case intensity is indicated by magnitude of the factor loadings or MDS weights. See Namenwirth and Weber (1987: chapter 8) for a more technical discussion.

24. Note "Weber's Paradox" (Namenwirth and Weber, 1987: 36, 208n; Weber, 1983): Results using the Lasswell dictionary have not been interpreted or explained using Lasswell's theory, and results using the Harvard dictionary have not been interpreted or explained using Freudian or Parsonian theory. At present, general dictionaries should be considered useful, commonsense category schemes rather than the operationalization of a formal theory.

25. Krippendorff (1980: 157) distinguishes between "emic or indigenous rather than etic or imposed" categories, asserting without evidence that only the former are semantically valid. This raises sticky problems concerning both category schemes and manifest versus latent content. See Namenwirth and Weber (1987) for an extended discussion.

26. Factor analyzing word counts to infer themes has a long history, which is reviewed by Iker (1974). Stefflre (1965) is an early programmatic statement. Moreover, each approach entails a different measurement model. Specifically, first-order exploratory factor analysis is the statistical model that corresponds to inferring themes from word covariation. The measurement model for single-classification-assumed dictionaries corresponds to a restricted second-order confirmatory factor analysis (Namenwirth and Weber, 1987: chapter 8). I am unaware of any attempt to analyze the same texts using both measurement models. Therefore, it is uncertain whether these different approaches yield similar or different substantive findings.

27. Both the Harvard and Lasswell dictionaries emphasize institutional aspects of social life. In addition, Zvi Namenwirth played a large role in the creation of the Lasswell and early Harvard dictionaries. Therefore, it is not surprising that his results did replicate across dictionaries.

28. Usually percentages or proportions are used to standardize for the length of the document or other unit of text. These create other problems for analysis, however, that are addressed in Chapter 4.

29. Several useful indicators of content are not discussed here. For example, one might assume that words, topics, or themes mentioned near the beginning of the text are more important than those mentioned near the end of the text. Also, as Holsti (1969) shows, one can code text for positive or negative (favorable or unfavorable) assertions. These examples were suggested by an anonymous reviewer.

30. In choosing a simple random sample, each member of the universe or population to be sampled has an equal probability of being included in the sample.

31. In choosing a stratified random sample, each member of each subclass of the population has an equal probability of being included in the sample, but a different proportion of each subclass may be chosen. Put another way, the probability of a particular member of the population being chosen depends on which subclass that member belongs to.

32. Where the meaning of a word changes over time, KWIC lists often reflect these changes. Usually this poses no problem, because new meanings frequently entail additional usages such as the change from verb to noun, noun to adjective, and so forth. As shown later, computers can distinguish the various senses of homographs. Consequently, changes in meaning can be taken into account.

33. This version of KWIC prints the keyword with all or most of the sentence in which it appears. In principle, however, there is no limit other than utility of the size of the context provided.

34. Depending on the goals of the content analysis, other senses could be distinguished (see Chapter 4).

35. The utility of ordered word-frequency lists was suggested by Ronald D. Brunner (personal communication). The number of words included in the table was determined by space limitations rather than substantive or methodological considerations.

36. In studies of disputed authorship, however, these types of words have been found to distinguish accurately between authors (e.g., Mosteller and Wallace, 1964).

37. A second assumption is that differences in word frequencies reflect differences in the attention of the message source. This is likely to be true for rank orders but not for absolute frequencies, because absolute frequencies are partly a function of document length.

38. In the computers and humanities literature these are called *collocations* (e.g., Berry-Rogghe, 1973; Firth, 1957; Geffroy, Lafon, Seidel, and Tournier, 1973; Haskel, 1971).

39. Very long sentences were broken up; plus signs represent semicolons.

40. This and the following section draw on a larger text data base consisting of Democratic and Republican party platforms 1844-1980 (Johnson, 1979, 1982) developed in collaboration with J. Zvi Namenwirth. See the Appendix for information regarding archived text data.

41. For each party, the data were standardized to a mean of zero and a standard deviation of 1.0 to eliminate differences of scale in the figure.

42. These results replicate and extend some of Namenwirth's (1969b) findings for the period 1844-1964.

43. Iker (1965, 1974; Iker and Harway, 1969), for example, factor-analyzed word-frequency counts. Another approach (Namenwirth, 1969a, 1970; Namenwirth and Bibbee, 1975; Namenwirth and Weber, 1987) applies factor analysis to category counts to identify themes in texts. The relative merits of these approaches have been discussed extensively elsewhere (Namenwirth and Weber, 1987: chapter 8; Weber, 1983).

44. This is a modification of the Harvard III Psychosocial dictionary documented in Stone et al. (1966: 169ff).

45. Some categories were eliminated because of low variance or because they did not discriminate between mass and elite papers.

46. The principal-components method is often confused with true factor analysis. The former excludes unique variances, but retains common and error variances. True factor analysis excludes both unique and error variances. Most, if not all factor analysis solutions, however, do not produce unique factor scores; the principal components method does (Kim and Mueller, 1978; Rummel, 1970).

47. Pronouns and ambiguous references were identified in the text.

48. These definitions are from Stone et al. (1966: 174-176). The remaining definitions are from Namenwirth (no date).

49. ANOVA is used in the analysis of categorical independent and continuous dependent variables (e.g., see Rosenthal and Rosnow, 1984).

50. There were three time periods corresponding to June 25, 1950, to October 31, 1950 (the beginning of hostilities until the intervention of the Chinese); November 1, 1950, to July 7, 1951 (the Chinese intervention until the beginning of truce talks); and July 8, 1951, to August 11, 1953 (the onset of truce talks until 15 days after signing the truce agreement).

51. The principal components method was used, which, as noted, excludes unique variances but retains common and error variances (Kim and Mueller, 1978; Rummel, 1970).

52. One can calculate the reliability of factor scores obtained through principal components by calculating the Theta reliability coefficient (Armor, 1974).

53. This research was conducted by Hans-Dieter Klingemann at Freie Universitat Berlin, Peter Philip Mohler, and the present writer.

54. The idea of acceleration or changes in the rate of change may not be intuitively obvious, and so a few examples may help to clarify the matter. For each year the acceleration (or deceleration) of the economy is derived from prices for three years. If wheat prices are 50, 65, and 55 marks per ton in 1871, 1872, and 1873 respectively, then for 1872 and 1873 the first differences are 15 and –10 respectively. The second difference for 1873 is –25 (–10 – 15). Hence concern with wealth in 1873 is likely to be somewhat higher than average. This is intuitively plausible because the economy was improving between 1871 and 1872 and declining between 1872 and 1873. Consider another series of prices: 50, 55, and 65. Here the first differences are 5 and 10, and the second difference is 5. This would show that the economy is growing at an increasing rate of change, and hence one would expect that in the third year the level of wealth concerns would be lower than average.

55. Figure 3.3 presents the values of various coefficients and the symbols frequently used to represent them in LISREL models. These are (see Jöreskog and Sörbom, 1979, and Long, 1983a, 1983b, for a technical discussion and more detailed explication):

1. Lambda Y (LY): factor loadings of the observed Y's on the unobserved dependent variables;
2. Lambda X (LX): factor loadings of the observed X's on the unobserved independent variables;
3. Theta Delta (TD): covariance matrix of the residuals or error term for the measurement model of the latent independent variables;

4. Theta Epsilon (TE): covariance matrix of the residuals or error term for the measurement model of the latent dependent variables;
5. Beta (BE): causal coefficients among the dependent variables;
6. Gamma (GA): causal coefficients linking dependent and independent variables;
7. Phi (PH): covariance matrix of the latent independent variables; and,
8. Psi (PS): covariance matrix of the residuals in the structured model.

56. Using the data reported above, however, Jan-Bernd Lohmoller and Herman Wold (1984) estimated our model using two alternative procedures, canonical correlation and partial least-squares "soft modeling" (Wold, 1975, 1981). Using procedures that make weaker statistical assumptions, they found weaker relationships between economic performance and wealth concerns. I believe, however, that the stronger assumptions incorporated in the LISREL model are justifiable. In any event, this research is still in the exploratory phase and — irrespective of estimation technique — the hypothesized negative relationship between economic performance and wealth concerns is confirmed.

57. Chapter 3 shows that these measures are, in turn, sometimes analyzed using statistical techniques such as factor analysis to generate indicators of themes, issues, and dilemmas. Namenwirth and Weber (1987: chapter 8) address problems resulting from different measurement models for indicators of themes.

58. Another form of categorical equivalence is *denotative categorical equivalence*. Textual units are denotative categorically equivalent if they have the same meaning, such as *purchase* and *buy*.

59. When words take on new meanings, the disambiguation procedures noted earlier generally handle large differences of meaning; the discussion here concerns less obvious differences.

60. In some content analysis research (e.g., Namenwirth and Weber, 1987), referents of pronouns and other anaphoras were edited manually into the text.

61. There is nothing inherent in the text classification procedures described above that requires the unit of analysis to be the entire document. Other units can be used, such as paragraphs or sentences. In related research, Saris-Gallhofer and her colleagues (1978) found that shorter coding units, such as words, yielded higher validity than longer coding units such as sentences, paragraphs, or entire texts. An area for future research, however, is the consequences for validity and reliability of aggregating word counts at various levels, such as sentences or paragraphs.

62. UNDERSTATE and OVERSTATE are categories from the Harvard dictionary (Dunphy et al., 1989; Stone et al., 1966; Zuell et al., 1989). OVERSTATE contains words providing emphasis in the following areas: speed, frequency, inevitability, causality, inclusiveness of persons, objects, or places, quantity in numerical and quasi-numerical terms, accuracy and validity, importance, intensity, likelihood, certainty, and extremity. UNDERSTATE contains words providing de-emphasis in the following areas: speed, frequency, inevitability, causality, inclusiveness of persons, objects or places, quantity in numerical and quasi-numerical terms, accuracy and validity, importance, scope, size, clarity, exceptionalness, intensity, likelihood, certainty, and extremity (i.e., emphasizing slowness rather than speed, infrequency rather than frequency; Dunphy et al., 1989).

63. This kind of primitive disambiguation is only a modest step. Chief among its practical advantages is that it relies on inexpensive technology. Computers can process large amounts of text quickly at nominal cost.

64. The results of the computer-aided classification and statistical procedures suggested both the duration and interpretation of this thematic cycle. The following excerpts span 67 years, which is close enough to the 72-year average cycle.

65. "Class conflict" is probably not appropriate here because industrial capitalism had yet to appear and the country was firmly in the grips of mercantilist theories and practices.

66. The integrative issue is itself interpreted as part of a four-phase problem-solving sequence posited by Bales (1950, 1953; Bales and Strodtbeck, 1953) and Parsons (Parsons and Bales, 1953; Parsons, Bales, and Shils, 1953; see Parsons and Smelser, 1956) the purpose of which is the pursuit of system rather than subgroup (e.g., class) goals.

REFERENCES

AGER, D. E., KNOWLES, F. E., and SMITH, J. (1979) Advances in Computer-Aided Literary and Linguistic Research. University of Aston, Birmingham, England: Department of Modern Languages.

AITKEN, A. J., BAILEY, R. W., and HAMILTON-SMITH, N. (eds.) (1973) The Computer and Literary Studies. Edinburgh: Edinburgh University Press.

ALLEN, J. (1987) Natural Language Understanding. Menlo Park, CA: Benjamin/Cummings.

ALTHAUSER, R. P. (1974) "Inferring validity from the multitrait-multimethod matrix: Another assessment," in H. L. Costner (ed.) Sociological Methodology 1973-1974. San Francisco: Jossey-Bass.

ALWIN, D. F. (1974) "Approaches to the interpretation of relationships in the multitrait-multimethod matrix," in H. L. Costner (ed.) Sociological Methodology 1973-1974. San Francisco: Jossey-Bass.

ANDERSON, A. B. (1970) "Structure of semantic space," in E. F. Borgatta (ed.) Sociological Methodology 1970. San Francisco: Jossey-Bass.

ARIES, E. (1973) Interaction Patterns and Themes of Male, Female, and Mixed Groups. Unpublished Ph.D. dissertation, Harvard University.

ARIES, E. (1977) "Male-female interpersonal styles in all male, all female, and mixed groups," in A. G. Sargent (ed.) Beyond Sex Roles. St. Paul: West.

ARMOR, D. J. (1974) "Theta reliability and factor scaling," in H. L. Costner (ed.) Sociological Methodology 1973-1974. San Francisco: Jossey-Bass.

AXELROD, R. (ed.) (1976) Structure of Decision: The Cognitive Maps of Political Elites. Princeton: Princeton University Press.

Ayer Directory of Publications. (1983) Philadelphia: Ayer.

BALES, R. F. (1950) Interaction Process Analysis: A Method for the Study of Small Groups. Reading, MA: Addison-Wesley.

BALES, R. F. (1953) "The equilibrium problem in small groups," pp. 111-161 in T. Parsons, R. F. Bales, and E. Shils (eds.) Working Papers in the Theory of Action. New York: Free Press.

BALES, R. F. and STRODTBECK, F. L. (1953) "Phases in group problem solving." Journal of Abnormal and Social Psychology 46: 485-495.

BERELSON, B. (1952) Content Analysis in Communications Research. New York: Free Press.

BERRY-ROGGHE, G. L. M. (1973) "Computation of collocations in lexical studies," in A. J. Aitken, R. W. Bailey, and N. Hamilton-Smith (eds.) The Computer and Literary Studies. Edinburgh: Edinburgh University Press.

BLALOCK, H. M. (ed.) (1974) Measurement in the Social Sciences. Chicago: Aldine.

BODEN, M. (1987) Artificial Intelligence and Natural Man (2nd ed.). New York: Basic Books.

BODEN, M. (1988) Computer Models of Mind. Cambridge: Cambridge University Press.

BRADY, M. and BERWICK, R. C. (eds.) (1983) Computational Models of Discourse. Cambridge: MIT Press.

BRENT, E. (1984) "Qualitative computing: Approaches and issues." Qualitative Sociology 7(1/2).

BRINBERG, D. and KIDDER, L. H. (eds.) (1982) Forms of Validity in Research. San Francisco: Jossey-Bass.

332

BRINBERG, D. and MCGRATH, J. E. (1982) "A network of validity concepts within the research process," in D. Brinberg and L. H. Kidder (eds.) Forms of Validity in Research. San Francisco: Jossey-Bass.

BRINBERG, D. and MCGRATH, J. E. (1985) Validity and the Research Process. Beverly Hills, CA: Sage.

BRUNNER, R. D. (1983) Forecasting Growth Ideologies. Discussion paper no. 7. Boulder: University of Colorado Center for Public Policy Research.

BRUNNER, R. D. (1984) The President's Annual Message. Discussion paper no. 8. Boulder: University of Colorado Center for Public Policy Research.

BRUNNER, R. D. and LIVORNESE, K. (1982) Subjective Political Change: A Prospectus. Discussion paper no. 5. Boulder: University of Colorado Center for Public Policy Research.

BUDGE, I., ROBERTSON, D., and HEARL, D. (eds.) (1987) Ideology, Strategy and Party Change: Spatial Analyses of Post-War Election Programmes in 19 Democracies. Cambridge: Cambridge University Press.

BURNHAM, W. D. (1970) Critical Elections and the Mainsprings of American Politics. New York: Norton.

BURTON, D. M. (1981) "Automated concordances and word indexes: The process, the programs, and the products." Computers and the Humanities 15: 139-154.

BURTON, D. M. (1982) "Automated concordances and word-indexes: Machine decisions and editorial revisions." Computers and the Humanities 16: 195-218.

CAMPBELL, D. T. and FISKE, D. W. (1959) "Convergent and discriminant validation by the multitrait-multimethod matrix." Psychological Bulletin 56: 81-105.

CAMPBELL, D. T. and O'CONNELL, E. J. (1982) "Methods as diluting trait relationships rather than adding irrelevant systematic variance," in D. Brinberg and L. H. Kidder (eds.) Forms of Validity in Research. San Francisco: Jossey-Bass.

CAMPBELL, D. T. and STANLEY, J. C. (1963) Experimental and Quasi-Experimental Designs for Research. Chicago: Rand McNally.

CARBONELL, J. G. (1981) Subjective Understanding: Computer Models of Belief Systems. Ann Arbor: UMI Research Press.

CARMINES, E. G. and ZELLER, R. A. (1982) Reliability and Validity Assessment. Beverly Hills, CA: Sage.

CLEVELAND, C., MCTAVISH, D., and PIRRO, E. (1974) Quester-Contextual Content Analysis Methodology. Paper presented at 1974 Pisa Conference on Content Analysis.

COOK, T. D. and CAMPBELL, D. T. (1979) Quasi-Experimentation: Design & Analysis for Field Settings. Chicago: Rand McNally.

CRONBACH, L. J. and MEEHL, P. E. (1955) "Construct validity in psychological tests." Psychological Bulletin 52: 281-302.

DEWEESE, L. C., III. (1976) "Computer content analysis of printed media: A limited feasibility study." Public Opinion Quarterly 40: 92-100.

DEWEESE, L. C., III. (1977) "Computer content analysis of 'day-old' newspapers: A feasibility study." Public Opinion Quarterly 41: 91-94.

DUNPHY, D. C., BULLARD, C. G., and CROSSING, E. E. M. (1974) "Validation of the General Inquirer Harvard IV Dictionary." Paper presented at the 1974 Pisa Conference on Content Analysis.

DUNPHY, D. C., BULLARD, C. G., and CROSSING, E. E. M. (1989) "Validation of the General Inquirer Harvard IV Dictionary," in C. Zuell, R. P. Weber, and P. Mohler,

Computer-assisted Text Analysis for the Social Sciences: The General Inquirer III. Mannheim, FRG: Center for Surveys, Methods, and Analysis (ZUMA).

DYER, M. G. (1983) In-Depth Understanding: A Computer Model of Integrated Processing of Narrative Comprehension. Cambridge: MIT Press.

FIRTH, J. R. (1957) "Modes of meaning," in Papers in Linguistics 1934-51. London: Oxford University Press.

FISKE, D. W. (1982) "Convergent-discriminant validation in measurements and research strategies," pp. 72-92 in D. Brinberg and L. H. Kidder (eds.) Forms of Validation in Research. San Francisco: Jossey-Bass.

FREEMAN, M. F. and TUKEY, J. W. (1950) "Transformation related to the angular and the square root." Annals of Mathematical Statistics 21: 607-611.

GEFFROY, A., LAFON, P., SEIDEL, G., and TOURNIER, M. (1973) "Lexicometric analysis of co-occurrences," in A. J. Aitken, R. W. Bailey, and N. Hamilton-Smith (eds.) The Computer and Literary Studies. Edinburgh: Edinburgh University Press.

GEORGE, A. L. (1959a) Propaganda Analysis. Evanston: Row, Peterson.

GEORGE, A. L. (1959b) "Quantitative and qualitative approaches to content analysis," in I. D. S. Pool (ed.) Trends in Content Analysis. Urbana: University of Illinois Press.

GERBNER, G., HOLSTI, O. R., KRIPPENDORFF, K., PAISLEY, W., and STONE, P. J. (eds.) (1969) The Analysis of Communication Content. New York: John Wiley.

GOTTSCHALK, L. A. (1979) The Content Analysis of Verbal Behavior: Further Studies. New York: SP Medical & Scientific Books.

GOTTSCHALK, L. A., LOLAS, F., and VINEX, L. L. (eds.) (1986) Content Analysis of Verbal Behavior. New York/Berlin: Springer-Verlag.

GREY, A., KAPLAN, D., and LASSWELL, H. D. (1965) "Recording and context units—four ways of coding editorial content," in H. D. Lasswell, N. Leites, and Associates (eds.) Language of Politics. Cambridge: MIT Press.

HASKEL, P. J. (1971) "Collocations as a measure of stylistic variety," in R. A. Wisbey (ed.) The Computer in Literary and Linguistic Research. Cambridge: Cambridge University Press.

HERZOG, A. (1973) The BS Factor. New York: Simon & Schuster.

HOCKEY, S. and MARRIOTT, I. (1982) Oxford Concordance Program Version 1.0 Users' Manual. Oxford: Oxford University Computing Service.

HOCKEY, S. and MARTIN, J. (1987) "The Oxford Concordance program version 2." Literary and Linguistic Computing 2: 125-131.

HOLSTI, O. R. (1963) "Computer content analysis," in R. C. North, O. R. Holsti, M. G. Zaninovich, and D. A. Zinnes, Content Analysis: A Handbook with Applications for the Study of International Crises. Evanston: Northwestern University Press.

HOLSTI, O. R. (1966) "External conflict and internal consensus: The Sino-Soviet case," in P. J. Stone et al., The General Inquirer: A Computer Approach to Content Analysis. Cambridge: MIT Press.

HOLSTI, O. R. (1969) Content Analysis for the Social Sciences and Humanities. Reading, MA: Addison-Wesley.

IKER, H. P. (1965) "A computer approach toward the analysis of content." Behavioral Science 10: 173-183.

IKER, H. P. (1974) "An historical note on the use of word-frequency contiguities in content analysis." Computers and the Humanities 8: 93-98.

IKER, H. P. and HARWAY, N. I. (1969) "A computer systems approach to the recognition and analysis of content," in G. Gerbner et al. (eds.) The Analysis of Communication Content. New York: John Wiley.

JANIS, I. L. (1965) "The problem of validating content analysis," in H. D. Lasswell, N. Leites, and Associates (eds.) Language of Politics. Cambridge: MIT Press.

JOHNSON, D. B. (1979) National Party Platforms 1840-1976 (2 vols.). Urbana: University of Illinois Press.

JOHNSON, D. B. (1982) National Party Platforms of 1980. Urbana: University of Illinois Press.

JONES, A. and CHURCHHOUSE, R. F. (eds.) (1976) The Computer in Literary and Linguistic Studies. Cardiff: University of Wales Press.

JÖRESKOG, K. G. and SÖRBOM, D. (1979) Advances in Factor Analysis and Structural Equation Models. Cambridge, MA: Abt.

JÖRESKOG, K. G. and SÖRBOM, D. (1984) LISREL VI (Analysis of Linear Structural Relationships by the Method of Maximum Likelihood) Users Guide. Mooresville, IN: Scientific Software, Inc.

KELLY, E. F. and STONE, P. J. (1975) Computer Recognition of English Word Senses. Amsterdam: North Holland.

KIM, J. -O. and MUELLER, C. W. (1978) Factor Analysis: Statistical Methods and Practical Issues. Beverly Hills, CA: Sage.

KLINGEMANN, H. D., MOHLER, R. P., and WEBER, R. P. (1982) "Cultural indicators based on content analysis." Quality and Quantity 16: 1-18.

KRIPPENDORFF, K. (1980) Content Analysis: An Introduction to Its Methodology. Beverly Hills, CA: Sage.

LASSWELL, H. D. and KAPLAN, A. (1950) Power and Society: A Framework for Political Inquiry. New Haven: Yale University Press.

LASSWELL, H. D., LEITES, N., and Associates (eds.) (1965) Language of Politics. Cambridge: MIT Press.

LASSWELL, H. D., LERNER, D., and POOL, I. D. S. (1952) The Comparative Study of Symbols. Stanford: Stanford University Press.

LEHMAN, E. W. (1977) Political Society: A Macrosociology of Politics. New York: Columbia University Press.

LOHMOLLER, J. -B. and WOLD, H. (1984) "Introduction to PLS estimation of path models with latent variables including some recent developments on mixed scale variables," in G. Melischek, K. E. Rosengren, and J. Stappers (eds.) Cultural Indicators: An International Symposium. Vienna: Austrian Academy of Sciences.

LONG, J. S. (1983a) Confirmatory Factor Analysis: A Preface to LISREL. Beverly Hills, CA: Sage.

LONG, J. S. (1983b) Covariance Structure Models: An Introduction to LISREL. Beverly Hills, CA: Sage.

LORD, F. M. and NOVICK, M. R. (1968) The Statistical Analysis of Mental Test Scores. Reading, MA: Addison-Wesley.

MARKOFF, J., SHAPIRO, G., and WEITMAN, S. (1974) "Toward the integration of content analysis and general methodology," in D. R. Heise (ed.) Sociological Methodology, 1975. San Francisco: Jossey-Bass.

MELISCHEK, G., ROSENGREN, K. E., and STAPPERS, J. (eds.) (1984) Cultural Indicators: An International Symposium. Vienna: Austrian Academy of Sciences.

MERRIAM, J. E. and MAKOWER, J. (1988) Trend Watching: How the Media Create Trends and How to be the First to Uncover Them. New York: American Management Association.

MERRITT, R. L. (1966) Symbols of American Community 1735-1775. New Haven: Yale University Press.

MOSTELLER, F. and WALLACE, D. L. (1964) Inference and Disputed Authorship: The Federalist. Reading, MA: Addison-Wesley.

NAISBITT, J. (1982) Megatrends. New York: Warner Books.

NAMENWIRTH, J. Z. (no date) The Namenwirth Political Dictionary. Unpublished manuscript.

NAMENWIRTH, J. Z. (1969a) "Marks of distinction: A content analysis of British mass and prestige newspaper editorials." American Journal of Sociology 74: 343-360.

NAMENWIRTH, J. Z. (1969b) "Some long and short term trends in one American political value," in G. Gerbner et al., The Analysis of Communication Content. New York: John Wiley.

NAMENWIRTH, J. Z. (1970) "Prestige newspapers and the assessment of elite opinions." Journalism Quarterly 47: 318-323.

NAMENWIRTH, J. Z. (1973) "The wheels of time and the interdependence of value change." Journal of Interdisciplinary History 3: 649-683.

NAMENWIRTH, J. Z. (1984a) "Why cultural indicators?" in G. Melischek, K. E. Rosengren, and J. Stappers (eds.) Cultural Indicators. Vienna: Austrian Academy of Sciences.

NAMENWIRTH, J. Z. and BIBBEE, R. (1975) "Speech codes in the press." Journal of Communication 25: 50-63.

NAMENWIRTH, J. Z. and LASSWELL, H. D. (1970) The Changing Language of American Values: A Computer Study of Selected Party Platforms. Beverly Hills, CA: Sage.

NAMENWIRTH, J. Z. and WEBER, R. P. (1987) Dynamics of Culture. Winchester, MA: Allen & Unwin.

NORTH, R. C., HOLSTI, O. R., ZANINOVICH, M. G., and ZINNES, D. A. (1963) Content Analysis: A Handbook with Applications for the Study of International Crises. Evanston: Northwestern University Press.

OAKMAN, R. L. (1980) Computer Methods for Literary Research. Columbia: University of South Carolina Press.

OGILVIE, D. M. (1966) "Procedures for improving the interpretation of tag scores: The case of Windle," in P. J. Stone et al., The General Inquirer: A Computer Approach to Content Analysis. Cambridge: MIT Press.

OGILVIE, D. M., STONE, P. J., and KELLY, E. F. (1980) "Computer-aided content analysis," in R. B. Smith and P. K. Manning (eds.) Handbook of Social Science Research Methods. New York: Irvington.

OGILVIE, D. M., STONE, P. J., and SHNEIDMAN, E. S. (1966) "Some characteristics of genuine versus simulated suicide notes," in P. J. Stone et al., The General Inquirer: A Computer Approach to Content Analysis. Cambridge: MIT Press.

ORWELL, G. (1949) Nineteen Eighty-Four, A Novel. New York: Harcourt Brace.

OSGOOD, C. E., MAY, W. H., and MIRON, M. S. (1975) Cross-Cultural Universals of Affective Meaning. Urbana: University of Illinois Press.

OSGOOD, C. E., SUCI, G. J., and TANNENBAUM, P. H. (1957) The Measurement of Meaning. Urbana: University of Illinois Press.

336

PARSONS, T. (1969) "On the concept of political power," in T. Parsons, Politics and Social Structure. New York: Free Press.

PARSONS, T. and BALES, R. F. (1953) "The dimensions of action-space," pp. 63-109 in T. Parsons, R. F. Bales, and E. A. Shils (eds.) Working Papers in the Theory of Action. New York: Free Press.

PARSONS, T., BALES, R. F., and SHILS, E. A. (1953) "Phase movement in relation to motivation, symbol formation, and role structure," pp. 163-268 in T. Parsons, R. F. Bales, and E. A. Shils (eds.) Working Papers in the Theory of Action. New York: Free Press.

PARSONS, T. and SMELSER, N. (1956) Economy and Society. New York: Free Press.

POOL, I. D. S. (1951) Symbols of Internationalism. Stanford: Stanford University Press.

POOL, I. D. S. (1952a) The "Prestige Papers": A Survey of Their Editorials. Stanford: Stanford University Press.

POOL, I. D. S. (1952b) Symbols of Democracy. Stanford: Stanford University Press.

POOL, I. D. S. (ed.) (1959) Trends in Content Analysis. Urbana: University of Illinois Press.

PRESTON, M. J. and COLEMAN, S. S. (1978) "Some considerations concerning encoding and concording texts." Computers and the Humanities 12: 3-12.

ROSENGREN, K. E. (ed.) (1981) Advances in Content Analysis. Beverly Hills, CA: Sage.

ROSENTHAL, R. (1984) Meta-Analytic Procedures for Social Research. Beverly Hills, CA: Sage.

ROSENTHAL, R. and ROSNOW, R. L. (1984) Essentials of Behavioral Research: Methods and Data Analysis. New York: McGraw-Hill.

RUMMEL, R. J. (1970) Applied Factor Analysis. Evanston: Northwestern University Press.

SALTON, G. (1989) Automatic Test Processing. Reading, MA: Addison-Wesley.

SARIS-GALLHOFER, I. N., SARIS, W. E., and MORTON, E. L. (1978) "A validation study of Holsti's content analysis procedure." Quality and Quantity 12: 131-145.

SCHANK, R. C. and ABELSON, R. P. (1977) Scripts, Plans, Goals, and Understanding. Hillsdale, NJ: Lawrence Erlbaum.

SCHUESSLER, K. (1970) Analyzing Social Data: A Statistical Orientation. Boston: Houghton Mifflin.

SLATER, P. (1966) Microcosm. New York: John Wiley.

SMITH, R. G. (1978) The Message Measurement Inventory: A Profile for Communication Analysis. Bloomington: Indiana University Press.

SNIDER, J. G. and OSGOOD, C. E. (eds.) (1969) Semantic Differential Technique: A Sourcebook. Chicago: Aldine.

STEFFLRE, V. (1965) "Simulation of people's behavior toward new objects and events." American Behavioral Scientist 8: 12-15.

STEINER, G. (1975) After Babel: Aspects of Language and Translation. Oxford: Oxford University Press.

STONE, P. J., DUNPHY, D. C., SMITH, M. S., and OGILVIE, D. M. (1966) The General Inquirer: A Computer Approach to Content Analysis. Cambridge: MIT Press.

TUFTE, E. R. (1978) Political Control of the Economy. Princeton: Princeton University Press.

WALKER, A. W. (1975) The Empirical Delineation of Two Musical Taste Cultures: A Content Analysis of Best-Selling Soul and Popular Recordings from 1962-1973. Unpublished Ph.D. dissertation, New School for Social Research.

WEBB, E. J., CAMPBELL, D. T., SCHWARTZ, R. D., and SECHRIST, L. (1981) Nonreactive Measures in the Social Sciences. Boston: Houghton Mifflin.

WEBER, R. P. (1981) "Society and economy in the Western world system." Social Forces 59: 1130-1148.

WEBER, R. P. (1982) "The long-term problem-solving dynamics of social systems." European Journal of Political Research 10: 387-405.

WEBER, R. P. (1983) "Measurement models for content analysis." Quality and Quantity 17: 127-149.

WEBER, R. P. (1984a) "Content analytic cultural indicators," in G. Melischek, K. E. Rosengren, and J. Stappers (eds.) Cultural Indicators: An International Symposium. Vienna: Austrian Academy of Sciences.

WEBER, R. P. (1984b) "Content analysis: A short primer." Qualitative Sociology 7: 126-147.

WEBER, R. P. and NAMENWIRTH, J. Z. (in press) "Content analytic culture indicators: A self-critique," in Advances in Computing and the Humanities (vol. 3). Greenwich, CT: JAI.

WEIZENBAUM, J. (1976) Computer Power and Human Reason. San Francisco: Freeman.

WILLIAMS, R. (1985) Keywords: A Vocabulary of Culture and Society (rev. ed.). New York: Oxford University Press.

WINOGRAD, T. (1983) Language As a Cognitive Process, Volume 1. Syntax. Reading, MA: Addison-Wesley.

WINOGRAD, T. and FLORES, F. (1986) Understanding Computers and Cognition: A New Foundation for Design. Norwood, NJ: Ablex.

WISBEY, R. A. (1971) The Computer in Literary and Linguistic Research. Cambridge: Cambridge University Press.

WOLD, H. (1975) "Soft modelling by latent variables: The non-linear iterative partial least squares (NIPALS) approach," in J. Gani (ed.) Perspectives in Probability and Statistics, Papers in Honour of M. S. Bartlett. London: Academic Press.

WOLD, H. (1981) "Model construction and evaluation when theoretical knowledge is scarce: On the theory and application of partial least squares," in J. Kmenta and J. Ramsey (eds.) Evaluation of Econometric Models. New York: Academic Press.

ZELLER, R. A. and CARMINES, E. G. (1980) Measurement in the Social Sciences. Cambridge: Cambridge University Press.

ZIPF, G. K. (1932) Selected Studies of the Principle of Relative Frequency in Language. Cambridge, MA: Harvard University Press.

ZIPF, G. K. (1965) Psycho-biology of Language. Cambridge: MIT Press.

ZUELL, C., WEBER, R. P., and MOHLER, P. P. (1989) Computer-assisted Text Analysis for the Social Sciences: The General Inquirer III. Mannheim, FRG: Center for Surveys, Methods, and Analysis (ZUMA).

ACKNOWLEDGMENTS

Acknowledgments for Second Edition

Much of the material discussed in Chapter 4 will be covered in greater depth in a much longer piece coauthored with Zvi Namenwirth (Weber and Namenwirth, in press); Namenwirth's contribution, comments, and suggestions are greatly appreciated. Connie Zuell, Peter Philip Mohler, and Philip J. Stone provided continued encouragement and support, for which I am grateful. Much of the editing and rewriting was done in the *Patisserie Francaise* near Harvard Square. Many thanks to Elie and Salwa Matta and to Alexis (Gigi) Andrews for good food and hospitality.

Acknowledgments for First Edition

This research was supported in part by ZUMA, the Center for Surveys, Methods, and Analysis, Mannheim, FRG. I remain indebted to the generosity of past and present Directors and staff, especially, Hans-Dieter Klingemann, Peter Philip Mohler, Karl Ulrich Mayer, Max Kaase, and Manfred Keuchler. Additional support was provided by Kurzweil Computer products, Inc., a subsidiary of Xerox Corp. Sue Williamson of Kurzweil played a key role, and her generosity and help is gratefully acknowledged. Randi Lynn Miller assisted with data entry at an earlier phase of the research. Thanks to Nancy Marshall, J. Zvi Namenwirth, Barbara Norman, Philip J. Stone, Kathrine Tenerowicz, and two anonymous reviewers for detailed comments on earlier drafts. Thanks also to the Harvard University Computing Center for computer resources.

Thanks to Zvi Namenwirth for permission to quote extensively from Namenwirth and Bibbee (1975); to Dexter Dunphy for permission to reproduce a figure from Dunphy, Bullard, and Crossing (1974); to Human Sciences Press for permission to adapt or reprint some material from Weber (1984b); to Elsevier Publishing Company for permission to adapt or reprint some material from Weber (1983); and to the Austrian Academy of Sciences for permission to adapt or reprint some material that appeared in Weber (1984a).

USING   PART V
PUBLISHED DATA
Errors and Remedies

HERBERT JACOB

INTRODUCTION

Libraries and computerized data archives are bursting with data ready to be analyzed. They hold thousands of statistical reports published by U.S. government agencies in addition to the reports from United Nations agencies and foreign governments. Moreover, private data collections are often readily available either in published form or by connecting to a computerized data bank.

These data are like the apple in the Garden of Eden: tempting but full of danger. Although the data are often published in formats that suggest that they are authoritative and trustworthy, they are almost always riddled with errors of one sort or another. This essay seeks to alert the unwary researcher of some of the pitfalls in using them. I shall set out both the problems and some remedies. Readers should not be discouraged. For almost every problem there is a solution or at worst an acceptable compromise. It will sometimes seem that the dangers outrun the remedies; that should give us pause as we undertake research based on these data or rely on analyses that use such sources. But it need not paralyze our research.

1. SAMPLES, CENSUSES, AND SAMPLING ERROR

The data one finds in publications are counts of one sort or another, which for many reasons may be incorrect. They may come from com-

AUTHOR'S NOTE: *This paper is the outgrowth of many discussions with Robert L. Lineberry and the substantial assistance of Michael J. Rich. I also benefited greatly from suggestions on an earlier draft by several anonymous referees; by John Sullivan; and by my colleagues, Tom Cook, Andrew Gordon, Alex Hicks, Kenneth Janda, and Wesley Skogan. None of them, however, bears any responsibility for its contents.*

plete counts or from partial counts. The U.S. Decennial Census is the best example of a data source that claims to be a complete count. It purports to be a total count of all persons living in the United States at a particular time. Vote counts are another example; they purport to be a count of all ballots in an election. Partial counts claim to represent a larger population or universe. The best such partial count is a random, probability sample. A simple random sample is a partial count in which each element of the whole population has an equal chance of being included and every combination of elements in the population has an equal chance. Those elements chosen are selected randomly (Kish, 1965; Warwick and Lininger, 1975; Selltiz et al., 1976: 522). Many variations of the random, probability sample exist. Some seek to stratify the sample according to known characteristics of the population; others seek to cluster the points from which the data will be collected. Many samples, however, are not based on the principles of random selection. Quota samples, for instance, choose data to fill a quota that reflects known traits of the population. Other collections are simply based on convenience. Observations are included because they happened to be available when the researchers went looking for their data.

The distinction between random samples and other collections of data is crucial because of the errors that all data collections contain. Sometimes these errors flow from the ways in which samples are selected; we call that sampling error. In other cases, the errors result from inadequacies in the measurement process; we call those measurement errors. Most of this essay deals with various kinds of measurement errors. However, we should first confront the possibility of sampling error and the steps we may take to overcome it.

Sampling error can be easily estimated *only* when one is working with data collected through a random sample. Two statistical theorems provide us with the tools for such an estimate. The *law of large numbers* states that with a large number of samples, the mean of the sample means will equal the mean of the population. The *central limit theorem* states that if we draw numerous large samples, the means of those samples will approximate the bell-shaped curve of the normal distribution (Palumbo, 1977: 276). These two theorems permit us to estimate both the mean and a point of a distribution with the formula:

$$u = \bar{X} + Z \; \frac{s}{\sqrt{n}}$$

where

- Z is the point under the normal curve of a standardized distribution corresponding to a selected confidence interval. It takes on the values of + or – 1.96 for a 95% confidence interval and a value of + or – 2.58 for a 99% confidence interval;
- s is the sample variance;
- n is the number of cases in the sample.

Let us suppose that we wish to estimate the mean age of unemployed persons in some city for a given year. If we obtain the information from a random sample of 500 persons and find from it that the sample mean is 35 and the sample variance is 2.5, our estimate of the reliability of the mean age of 35 with a 95% confidence is

$$35 + \text{or} - 1.96(2.5/\text{sqrt}500) \text{ or}$$

$$35 + \text{or} - 1.96(2.5/22.4) \text{ or}$$

$$35 + \text{or} - .22$$

A 99% confidence interval in this instance would be

$$35 + \text{or} - .29$$

Note that these estimates provide a margin of error. The more certain we wish to be of our estimate, the larger the confidence interval will be. For example, were we to estimate the number of smokers in a population from a random sample with a confidence of being correct 99% of the time, we would have a larger error range than if we were satisfied with a 95% chance of being correct. In some instances, the confidence interval allows us to conclude that the estimate we have obtained is insignificant because the estimated error is much larger than the estimate itself. In other cases, the confidence interval is so large that the estimate is useless. For instance, in the 1983 Chicago mayoral campaign, a last minute public opinion poll showed one candidate leading by 52% of the vote against his opponent's 48%, but the margin of error was estimated as + or – 6 percent. Such an inexact estimate is of little help in predicting the outcome (WMFT, April 11, 1983 newscast; same poll reported without error estimate in Chicago Tribune [1983]).

The ability to estimate error is a very important characteristic of random samples. One never knows whether or not a particular estimate is correct, but using a random sample allows one to estimate the probability that the estimate is wrong. Confidence in sample data is, therefore, always modified by a concrete estimate of the chance that the data are incorrect. Consequently, almost every publication of data based on samples should carry with it a discussion of the error estimate. Many reports based on samples now do so.

By contrast, when data are collected by some nonrandom procedure, no such statistical estimates of sampling error are possible. One can be certain that errors exist, but one does not know how large they might be or what the probability is for a given error range. In addition, because the data collection did not use random selection procedures, the errors may not be symmetrically arranged around the mean. They may all be clustered at one end of the distribution or another, and one can never know what direction the errors will take. For instance, the error may be larger in rural than urban areas or the reverse may be true; minorities may be overcounted or undercounted; too many or too few voters may appear in the data base. There is no way of accurately estimating such biases in nonrandom samples.

Our inability to specify sampling error occurs with both nonrandom samples like a television call-in poll and full counts like the census. They are full of selection errors, the extent of which we cannot estimate with any statistical reliability. Only when one is counting a very small group that is directly under close observation, can one have confidence in the results. For instance, I can know with considerable confidence how many students are enrolled in a small seminar. Those not present on any given day can be easily traced; I am made aware of those who drop. That is not true for my large lecture classes. When I teach more than 200 students, I never know how many are actually enrolled in the course. Some are absent every day because of illness; some miss tests. Some will drop without telling me, and others will enter the course. Even the listing that the registrar provides will often be inaccurate. At the very end of the semester, I can report the number of students for whom I have complete grades, but often one or two students will announce themselves as having been present for part of the course and eligible for a final grade.

Such difficulties are multiplied a thousandfold for a national census. It is well known that many persons are missed by such a census—

because they failed to fill out a form, were never contacted by a census worker, lived in an area considered too dangerous for census workers to go to, or were in transit. Middle-class white Americans who live stable lives are most easily counted by the census. They can be reached at a known address, are able to read the census form, and feel an obligation to return it. That is not equally true for members of many minority groups. Blacks have been consistently undercounted both because many are more suspicious of government agents and because they are more difficult to reach than white middle-class Americans. Hispanics present a still different problem because some of them are illegal aliens who fear that being counted by the census might endanger their continued residence in the United States (even though census records are not available to immigration or other law enforcement agencies). Still other persons are confused by census questions about their ethnicity. In states where few Hispanics are reported to live, sizable numbers of people misidentified themselves as Hispanic in the 1980 census. In the words of a census official, "Apparently many people did not know what a Mexican-American was, spotted the 'Amer.' on the form and marked it, even though we had American abbreviated and squeezed in between Mexican and Chicano" (New York Times, 1983).

Because of such problems, population counts are always somewhat incorrect. They contain greater errors for some groups (e.g., blacks and Hispanics) than for others (U.S. Congress, Subcommittee on Census, 1977, 1980a). Custom and legal precedent lead government publications to display figures down to the last whole number. In fact, the numbers have a margin of error that may be as high as 5 percent. The result is that "complete" counts may be less reliable than random samples! Both are certain to have errors, but the sampling error in random samples can be estimated with a high degree of accuracy, whereas the selection error in full counts can only be guessed at.

These problems, however, do not present insuperable barriers to the productive use of published statistics, even when we are not told the margin of error or when the data are supposed to be complete counts. Where the data come from random samples, one must often search further for information about sampling error. The data one finds in published sources such as the *Statistical Abstract of the United States* (U.S. Bureau of the Census, 1981, 1982-83) are often extracted from exhaustive studies that include much information about sampling error.

Consequently, one needs to go to the original source that is cited in the *Statistical Abstract*; sometimes that source will send the reader to other technical publications that provide estimates of sampling error. It is a trip worth taking.

Data that are not collected by a random probability sample cannot be evaluated in the same way. In the case of the U.S. Census, detailed technical studies exist that examine undercounts and overcounts; these are based on an analysis of the internal consistency of responses to census questions, on comparisons with recounts, and on comparisons with random sample data for the same populations. Such studies provide careful researchers with considerable information about the likely scope of counting error. For most other counts, however, no such studies exist. Nevertheless, there is another remedy. Many data based on a full count are reported down to the last digit. For instance, the 1970 population of Sacramento, California is reported to have been 257,105 (U.S. Bureau of the Census, 1977: 624). We can be reasonably certain that the population in fact was around 250,000, but we have no idea whether it was 259,872 or 252,307. For most uses, it makes little difference, although if Sacramento qualified as a first-class city under state law when it surpassed a quarter-million population, the addition or subtraction of a few inhabitants could have serious consequences.

The problem is more complicated when one uses population counts in cross-national analyses. Some nations schedule census counts as regularly as the United States and have counting procedures that are as good as or better than those in the United States. In many nations, however, census counts are occasional events; such countries lack the bureaucratic machinery to organize accurate counts. In more than a few instances, population statistics are politically sensitive, and regimes have a stake in overestimating or underestimating particular ethnic groups or other components of the population. Population counts and estimates may be found in the official publications of individual nations, in UNESCO reports, and in the *World Handbook of Political and Social Indicators* (Russet et al., 1964; Taylor and Hudson, 1972). The World Handbook provides some information about potential sources of error. Moreover, it estimates the size of the error margin for each country. For instance, for the United States, it reports an error margin for the 1965 population estimate of 2%; by contrast, the error margin for

Saudi Arabia is 30.8% (Taylor and Hudson, 1972: 295, 296). Understanding the significance of these numbers, however, requires careful reading of the text and the notes that accompany the table; indeed, the table itself does not even indicate the year for which the population is given. Careful reading is always a prerequisite for use of published statistics.

The error estimates provided by the *World Handbook* are an example of a rule of thumb that may be used to mitigate excessive specificity in full counts. Where specific error estimates do not exist, we must turn to other stopgap measures. One such expedient is to take advantage of the fact that many government publications round population counts to the nearest 1000. That does not merely save space on the printed page but also reflects skepticism about the last digit accuracy of the numbers. It calls the reader's attention to the likelihood that the numbers are not fully accurate. The consequence of such a precaution is to minimize small differences that may well be the result of error rather than reflecting a difference in the true occurrence of whatever it is we are studying. The precise degree of rounding will depend on the character of the data. With very large numbers and the likelihood of substantial error, it may be prudent to round to the nearest million rather than to the nearest thousand. Researchers must make that decision for themselves for every data set they use. Awareness of sampling or selection error is more important than the precise size of the correction because it alerts readers to the presence of possible unspecified error. (For a more detailed discussion of sampling designs and sampling error, see Kalton [1983].)

2. MEASUREMENT ERRORS AND INVALIDITY

Sampling and selection errors are only one source of inaccuracy in published data; in many instances, they are not the most significant source of error. A second deficiency that generally affects published data is measurement error. Measurement error takes many forms. Some errors arise from mistakes in conceptualization; others flow from structural characteristics of the data collection process. Let us first turn to errors stemming from conceptual problems. These may be particularly acute for users of published data because they have little control over the ways in which concepts have been operationalized. Users of published data are prisoners of decisions about conceptualization made by those who originally collected the data.

Conceptualization Errors and Construct Validity

Differences in meaning between concepts and indicators are the cause of many errors in interpreting analyses using published data. All empirical research moves from abstract concepts to concrete measures. Researchers must concern themselves both with a careful specification of their concepts and a faithful operationalization of those concepts in concrete terms.

Concepts themselves posit some "true" value for a variable. For instance, the concept of "cost of living" presumes that one can imagine some number that truly represents how much it costs to live in a middle-class style or some other style in the United States. "Literacy" posits a measurement of the ability to read and write at a specified level. "Budget deficit" infers an excess of spending over revenues. Every question that a social scientist wishes to research is defined by such a set of concepts. A political scientist may wish to examine the ways in which "politics" affects the "outputs" of "government." A criminologist may concern herself with the "sources" of "criminal behavior." A sociologist may focus on "family structure." An economist may wish to analyze the concomitants of "unemployment." Each of these concepts has many commonplace meanings. Social scientists, however, usually wish to attach a very particular definition to concepts that, through a series of operations, permit them to measure their occurrence. That way of defining concepts is called operationalization.

In operationalizing concepts, one always must substitute concrete indicators for the abstract, true value of the concept. Those indicators may miss the mark because they lack validity or they may be faulty because of unreliability. In this section we concern ourselves only with validity.

An indicator is said to be valid when the fit between it and the underlying concept is close. Although this is an elementary rule of empirical research, it is by no means simple to observe. Concepts are abstract, while measurements of indicators are concrete. The two are rarely identical and, when not identical, the gap between them introduces error into analyses. Even with such physical concepts as "heat" the gap is considerable. Heat is measured by temperature; the temperature that must be attained to boil water or melt iron at a given altitude is well known and can be determined with minimal error. However, the associated concept, "I am hot" is far trickier. A reading of 80 degrees Fahrenheit will feel hot to one person while another will find it comfortable. For that reason weather reports often speak of such measures as a "temperature-humidity index" or a "wind chill factor." Even such measures, however, do not tap the prior experience of those who are exposed to the elements, a factor that is important because it is a commonplace observation that 40 degrees in February feels much warmer than 40 degrees in June; likewise, a 40 degree day in February in Miami is "freezing cold" while the same day in Chicago is unseasonably warm. Thus a gap remains between concept and indicator. When the concept being considered is as complex as the subjective perception of "hot" or "cold", numbers on a gauge provide only a guide; considerable error remains in applying those numbers to the concept in question. Most readers probably think that "hot" and "cold" are simple concepts. Social concepts are often considerably more complex.

A partial remedy for these problems is to follow the example of weather forecasters and utilize several measures for a concept, all the while recognizing that the fit between measure and concept will not be perfect. Take for instance the concept of "deficits" as applied to governmental finances. In everyday language, "deficit" means an excess of expenditure over revenue. Governments, however, have much more complex financial arrangements than individuals or small businesses. They have many accounts, some of which may be overdrawn while others are solvent. With the federal government, the size of the deficit is quite different if one includes all social security revenues and payments or if one treats them separately. In addition, there is a considerable difference between the amount actually paid out during any given time span and the amounts obligated but not yet paid.

Procedures for determining whether a measure is valid or not have been most fully developed by psychologists dealing with nonexperimental data (Campbell and Fisk, 1959; Campbell and Stanley, 1966; Cook and Campbell, 1979; see also Carmines and Zeller, 1979; Sullivan and Feldman, 1979). They suggest that we examine convergent and discriminant validity. A measure is valid when it converges with expectations derived from other knowledge about the subject matter or when it discriminates between different concepts. With respect to the ways in which official publications define deficits, one may ask whether those governmental units that report deficits also report borrowing funds; moreover, if they are legally prohibited from having deficits (as many state and local goverments in the United States are), we should find some indication of fiscal stress when deficits occur. If neither borrowing nor indicators of stress exist, the operationalization of the concept of "deficit" that we find in official sources needs to be questioned.

Another example of convergent validity is the measure of "communications development" in various nations. Clearly it is important for many analyses that seek to compare political processes across nations to have a rough measure of the capacity of governments and the populace to communicate with one another. Measures of newspaper circulation, of the number of radio and television sets, of mail use, and the number of telephones each represent only a portion of the concept and each are full of potential errors. However, if these measures correlate closely with one another, they can be combined into an index of communications development (cf. Taylor and Hudson, 1972: 208-209). We may have more confidence in such a combined index of convergent measures than in a single indicator.

Discriminant validity is useful in considering ways in which we might infer family size from census data. Suppose one wishes to compare the income of nuclear families with that of extended families. Unfortunately, the census counts households rather than families. The nuclear family, as used by sociologists, usually refers to a unit with a husband and/or wife with their minor children. Extended families also include stepchildren, grandparents, adult children, cousins or others who do not necessarily live together (Barber, 1953: 3-4; Cherlin, 1981: 30-31). Households, as defined by the census, include not only related persons but also people who are not related by blood or marriage but who are living together. Note that even a measure that counts people living together is not entirely clear, because some people sleep in the same place without regularly taking meals together while others regularly take meals together without sharing sleeping space. For the social scientist who wishes to use census data on households for studies in which the concept, "nuclear" or "extended" family is important, the problem is that census indicators of "households" do not discriminate among different kinds of families. Failing to make such a discrimination should alert us to a potentially invalid measurement.

Control over the validity of indicators varies with the degree to which researchers are involved in collecting their data. Where researchers can design the measures they use, they usually have considerable control over their validity. Even in such circumstances, validity remains problematic, but the researcher can devise alternative measures if her first attempt fails the test of convergent or discriminant validity. When she uses published data, however, she has almost no control over the measurements. In such a case, she must examine closely the construction of the indicators in the source she is consulting and evaluate their validity for her use.

The dilemma as well as a potential solution is illustrated by the problems confronting the political scientist wishing to examine the impact of inflation on political stability. Let us suppose that her model is one that leads her to think that perceptions of inflation will lead to political unrest. Moreover, she may have substantial reason to believe that price rises will have variable effects on different elements of the population. She might reach for the *Statistical Abstract* to examine the Consumer Price Index (CPI) as her measure of inflation. That would clearly be an error. She needs data on *perceptions* of inflation or on its incidence on different strata of the population. The CPI provides neither. However, examination of Gallup or Harris public opinion polls as well as polling data available in computer readable form from the Interuniversity Consortium for Political and Social Research at the University of Michigan might provide the perceptual data desired. The CPI, however, is inappropriate because it does not discriminate between the incidence of inflation and perceptions of inflation. Even if it shows a rise, many people may not be aware of increased prices; when it falls, other people will persist in believing that inflation is still rampant. In these situations, analysts may have no influence over the collection of the data or the construction of the measure. But they retain control over their choice of alternative data sets and continue to be free to formulate their research in a different way. However, to exercise their choices wisely, researchers must understand the ways in which the misfit between concept and measure may introduce error into their analyses.

An example of a very high degree of care in operationalizing valid indicators of important concepts in political research may be found in Kenneth Janda's *Political Parties: A Cross National Survey* (1980). Unless one defines "party" with great precision, quite different kinds of groups might be included in countries that have varying political traditions. Janda devotes many pages to specifying the several dimensions of party organization that he considers. Moreover, he provides a detailed discussion of the ways in which he utilized a wide variety of original sources in order to validate his measures. Many of his numerical indices are accompanied by an adequacy-confidence code that conveys his evaluation of the quality of the data. Users of Janda's data and others like it are in almost as good a position as the researcher who collects his data himself. The user of such data has the information needed to determine if the fit between concept and measure is a good one.

A similar set of procedures for testing validity must be used when researchers find several indicators that appear to be measuring the same concept but that have not been combined into a single index. A good example is to be found in two widely used data sets about one of American society's most puzzling problems: crime. Crime data, like most gathered by government agencies, are not collected with a specific research problem in mind. In the United States, the concepts underlying crime reports reflect the orientations of two separate collecting agencies that use two quite different operationalizations of crime. One data set is the National Crime Survey, an ongoing national survey of "victimizations" in which people are asked by the Census Bureau about incidents in which they were criminally victimized. The second comes from police reports and is published by the Federal Bureau of Investigation as the *Uniform Crime Reports.*

The National Crime Survey asks a random sample of respondents if they have been victims of a crime within the preceding six months. Like all sample surveys, it is subject to sampling error and the publications of the survey provide information for estimating the size of the error. The major problems with these crime statistics concern the ways in which the concept of crime has been operationalized (Penick and Owens, 1976; Skogan, 1981). Since several persons may be victimized in the same incident, the number of victimizations is not equivalent to the number of crimes. Moreover, collecting information from victims produces a number of peculiarities. The first is that one can measure only those crimes for which victims can be found. No murders are reported in victimization surveys, since murder victims can scarcely be interviewed. Nor does the survey report drug, prostitution, or gambling offenses, since these are typically "victimless" crimes in the sense that the "victims" are also the offenders, and they are not likely to report on themselves to a census interviewer. Another limitation is that only those victimizations that occur to persons over the age of 12 are included; no child abuse or elementary school-yard crimes are included. These and many other considerations drive a large wedge between the concept of "crime" and the measure of criminality as reflected in victimizations.

The second set of data have different but equally severe problems (Biderman and Reiss, 1967; Skogan, 1975). These data are composed of offenses known to the police (Federal Bureau of Investigation); it is not a sample but a count. This set is available annually for most cities with more than 25,000 inhabitants since the mid-1930s. Over the years, however, the components of the data set have changed, and the data have been collected with increasing accuracy. In this data set, crime has been operationalized as those offenses that the police know about and that they record as crimes. The police may reduce this measure of crime by "unfounding" reports (that is, reclassifying them as noncrimes), by failing to record incidents, or by not responding to citizen calls about crimes. Moreover, the measure is sensitive to the willingness of citizens to call the police in the first place. If people decide that it is not worth their time to call the police after having been victimized, the incident will never be recorded as a crime. Thus this second data set is quite sensitive to variations in citizen reporting and bureaucratic recording.

Neither measure is a valid indicator of the sum total of all criminal activity in the United States. Just as several important categories of crimes remain unreported in victimization surveys, many crimes are not reported to the police, and others are sometimes not recorded by them. Both data sets fail to measure incivility like graffiti on subways, petty disorders, and unruliness that make people fearful and that many would consider crimes.

Moreover, the two measures do not converge; they do not measure the same thing. During the 1970s, the National Crime Survey (U.S. Department of Justice, 1979) reported that victimizations were essentially constant, while the *Uniform Crime Reports* indicated that they were rising (U.S. Bureau of the Census, 1981: 170). Each records quite different levels of crime, with the National Crime Survey measuring a much higher level of crime (i.e., victimizations) than does the Offenses Known to the Police indicator. Finally, the two measures have been found to be related in different ways to independent variables such as population density, unemployment, and the proportion of the population that is black (Booth et al., 1977).

We can be sure that the published data do in fact reflect some proportion of what an analyst means by "crime," but it will always be a variable proportion. Therefore, someone who wishes to study crime with these data must make two crucial decisions. The first concerns the manner in which crime is to be defined. If the focus is on the police and their interaction with offenders, the Offenses Known to the Police indicator may be the most appropriate one. If the focus is closer to victims and their involvement in crimes, the National Crime Survey data are likely to be preferred. If one wishes to include incivility in the measure of crime, neither indicator will be adequate. The second decision concerns the errors embedded in each set. One must decide whether the measurement error of the indicator can be tolerated.

The decision to accept or reject such measurement errors hinges on several factors. One is the availability of alternative data that might be superior to those at hand. Where such alternative exist, they should be used if resources can be mustered to obtain them. Often, however, alternatives have unexplored measurement errors and are costly in both money and time. A second criterion is the size of differences that are likely to be found in comparing sets of data. If the differences are very large, small validity errors may not be important. A third criterion is the purpose of the analysis. An exploratory study may tolerate larger measurement errors than one that seeks to confirm or disconfirm a set of hypotheses. A study on which important public policy consequences hinge requires more caution than one that will be limited to the classroom.

Occasions will arise when it may be wiser to abandon an analysis than to conduct it with the flawed data that have been published unless one can make the necessary corrections in them. One instance for such caution is the analysis of crime across nations. The researcher not only confronts the difficulties described for American data, but he also encounters substantial variations in what is considered and counted as criminal behavior. The problem is most evident in dealing with crime in the Soviet Union. Ordinary crimes were for many years considered to be a relic of bourgeois culture that presumably had been eradicated under Bolshevik rule. Especially during the later Stalinist years, crime was considered to be an evidence of regime failure to a much larger degree than in the United States, and crime counts were considered politically sensitive. It is generally agreed among Soviet specialists that such counts were very difficult to obtain and when obtained are likely to be quite unreliable (Shelley, 1979).

Ineptitude and organizational confusion may contaminate data in the same way as ideology. Court data about the processing of criminals in the United States provides such an example. The Department of Justice has published occasional state-by-state counts and estimates of civil and criminal cases initiated in courts (e.g., U.S. Bureau of the Census, 1982-83: 189). Those data remain fragmentary despite the agency's best efforts to standardize data categories and to collect comprehensive information. The data include the unlikely report that Illinois filed 519,000 criminal cases in 1977 while in the same year California (with more than twice the population filed only 57,000 cases (U.S. Bureau of the Census, 1981: 187). Tracing those statistics back, one discovers that they refer only to the state's highest criminal court. In Illinois, all criminal cases—both felonies and misdemeanors— go to the circuit courts, although the vast majority of cases are misdemeanors. In California, the courts that reported these statistics handle only felonies. These two different ways of operationalizing "criminal cases filed" would lead the unwary observer to the mistaken conclusion that Illinois is much more active in filing criminal cases than is California. These court statistics are so blemished that it would probably be better not to use them at all unless one can certify them through independent investigations.

Measurement mistakes flowing from the invalidity of the operationalization of abstract concepts are widespread in using published data. One may be trapped not only by one's own mistakes in operationalizing indicators, but one may also be trapped by the peculiarities of the operationalizations guiding collectors of the data. One needs to be particularly sensitive to indications that measures are convergent with concepts and that they discriminate between alternative concepts. One may need to look for additional measures of what one seeks to study, or one may have to choose between alternative data sets that are readily available. In a few cases, one may need to consider collecting one's own data or to abandon the project because the measurement problems are insuperable.

Errors Produced by Changing Circumstances

Somewhat different problems arise with concepts that have changed meaning over time. A prime example of such a concept is the standard (or cost) of living. Living styles change as new goods and technologies become available. They may change in different ways for people who live in urban rather than rural areas, for farmers and for clerks. These variations require that our measures of the cost of living must have different components for different circumstances, whether they be different countries and cultures or different time periods.

One instance of such a measure in the United States is the Consumer Price Index, which is often interpreted as an indicator of inflation or the cost of living. The CPI continually suffers from the inability of a statistical measure to keep up with changes in the social and economic environment. Although designed to measure the pace of inflation, it was itself a victim of inflation during the 1970s because of the way it was for many years calculated (Blinder, 1980; Gordon, 1981; Wahl, 1982). A major component of consumer prices or cost of living is the cost of housing. For many years this element of the index reflected the most recent real estate transactions and mortgage rates, even though the housing cost of most persons who were buying their homes was frozen at the time they made their purchase. Thus, by the early 1980s when current costs soared and the mortgage rate exceeded 15%, the CPI reflected very high housing costs, although only a small portion of home owners paid those amounts, and most paid much smaller sums because they had purchased their homes at a time when prices and interest rates were lower. Housing costs (other than taxes and utilities, which were measured separately) actually remained constant for most of the population, but the cost of living index supposed and reported the opposite. Consequently, the actual rise in the cost of living experienced by many Americans during the early 1980s was lower than what was reported by the Consumer Price Index.

Other changes in life-styles also have affected the CPI, with the result that it usually fails to reflect changing consumer preferences until many years after the fact. Thus, in 1977 the CPI was based on data reflecting consumer preferences sixteen years earlier; a revision of the index in that year used data that were already more than five years old (Gordon, 1981: 117). Keeping the index up to date involves problems of staggering detail. Gordon reports on it as follows:

> From 1918 to 1940, the CPI index that covered shaving was the price of a barber shave, and then switched in 1940 to the safety-razor blade, despite the fact that safety razors had largely replaced barber shaves in the 1920's. From 1940 to 1952 the index item was the blade, joined from 1952 to 1964 by shaving cream, followed from 1964 to 1977 by the shaving cream alone, followed since 1977 by a combination of dental and shaving toiletry products. Since 1964 there has been no blade in the CPI, and thus no consideration of the new world opened up for most men by the invention of the double-edged blade in the 1970's.

> Other products have come and gone as well. In 1940 the index dropped not only barbershop shaves, but also high button shoes, men's nightshirts, and girls' cotton bloomers. The 1953 revision eliminated salt pork and laundry soap but added televisions, frozen foods, Coca-Cola, and whiskey. Pajamas, which had replaced nightshirts in 1940, themselves disappeared in 1964, leaving only sheets and blankets to cover the sleeping American male. Appendectomies also disappeared in 1964, the year funeral services were added. Among the new product categories introduced in the 1978 revision were pet supplies and expenses, indoor sports equipment, tranquilizers, and electronic pocket calculators [Gordon, 1981: 128].

Gordon's account illustrates the difficulty of keeping up with changing life-styles. Moreover, even standardized items come in a bewildering assortment of brands and prices. No index can take that variety into account and keep pace with changing products and consumer preferences to yield a timely and affordable indicator. For some purposes, these errors may make no difference; for others they may be critical. For the political scientist who wishes to examine the effect of inflation on voters' perceptions of what issues are important in national politics, it is essential that the inflation measure reflect real rather than artifactual changes in price levels. For such an analysis, an equal measure of vigilance must be exercised with the indicator of voter perceptions. Without these precautions, the findings may simply be a product of invalid measures.

A similar difficulty accompanies cross-national comparisons of monetary sums such as governmental expenditures or consumer income. There are many problems with such comparisons, but the most obvious is the need to find a common indicator. One cannot compare dollars to marks or yen. If one converts other currencies into U.S. dollars, one must understand the distortions that are introduced by official (or unofficial) exchange rates (Taylor and Hudson, 1972: 288).

While all indices suffer from such problems to some degree, researchers who design their own index maintain some control over the dimensions of the problem. They may choose to tolerate errors of one kind while attempting to eliminate others. For instance, they might invest greater resources to make their index more accurate for urbanites while neglecting the unique problems of rural residents. Alternatively, if one were particularly concerned about the effects of unemployment on urban black youth, one would design an index that would pick up not only those youth actively looking for work (as the present unemployment indicators do) but also those discouraged from job seeking, who are excluded from the published unemployment statistics. If one were studying the effects of middle-class unemployment, one would want an index that also considered the effects of underemployment (both in time and in skills), but this is not important for studying unemployment among teenagers with few skills. Researchers using published data rarely enjoy such options. They must take indicators as they are published, even when they are inadequate for their purposes.

A related set of problems arises from shifts in the definition of indicators. Such shifts occur in a number of ways. One common problem for political scientists is that the boundaries of their units of analysis change. Students of national politics must accommodate themselves to changes in national boundaries just as researchers of city politics must deal with cities that grow by annexation. For instance, the Phoenix of 1978 bears faint resemblance to the Phoenix of 1948. During that 30-year period, the city added 265 square miles, an area larger than the city of Chicago. The population of Phoenix increased almost sevenfold from 100,000 to 690,000. By almost every measure, the unit that the analyst is studying may be different in one time period than in the other. Every measure associated with the city has a different meaning in 1978 than it had in 1948, yet it is often considered as if it were unchanged. Scholars using national boundaries face the same problem. These boundaries rarely remain the same for all countries even during as short a period as a decade.

Other units of measurement also change. One example of such a change is reported by Morgenstern, who quotes Oskar Anderson with respect to a change in the calendar:

> According to the census of January 1, 1910, Bulgaria had a total of 527,311 pigs; 10 years later, according to the census of January 1, 1920, their number was already 1,089,699, more than double. But, he who would conclude that there had been a rapid development in the raising of pigs in Bulgaria (a conclusion that has indeed been drawn) would be greatly mistaken. The explanation is quite simply that in Bulgaria, almost half the number of pigs is slaughtered before Christmas. But after the war, the country adopted the "new" Gregorian calendar, abandoning the "old" Julian calendar, but it celebrates the religious holidays still according to the "old" manner, i.e. with a delay of 13 days. Hence January 1, 1910 fell after Christmas when the pigs were already slaughtered and January 1, 1920, before Christmas when the animals, already condemned to death, were still alive and therefore counted. A difference of 13 days was enough to invalidate completely the exhaustive figures [Morgenstern, 1963: 46-47].

Yet another source of this problem is a change in the application of some otherwise apparently constant rules. For instance, the concept of legal majority, when persons are held responsible for their own acts, seems on the surface to have remained relatively constant in recent times. However, the age at which young people assume the legal responsibility of adults has been changed in most places in the United States from 21 to 18 during the last 15 years, thus changing the meaning of many age categorizations. Likewise, the official definition of poverty in the United States changes with each administration; the definition of metropolitan area shifts every second or third decade.

Survey data also often present troubling challenges to researchers. Where the researcher wishes to analyze changes of public attitudes or perceptions over time, she must rely on questions in a series of surveys. In some instances, the questions will have been altered in minor or major ways from one survey to the next. Such changes make it difficult to decide whether findings are the result of real changes in attitudes or whether they are the artifact of the changes in the questions. The debate over that question is articulated well in an exchange between three sets of scholars in the *American Journal of Political Science*. Two groups (Sullivan et al., 1978; Bishop et al., 1979) asserted that the finding of greater conservatism and policy consistency among voters in the 1970s as compared with earlier voters might be the product of changes in the wording of the surveys. The third group, (Nie and Rabjohn, 1979) responded by showing that the findings were consistent with results in surveys where the questions were not changed. The exchange illustrates the care that must be exercised when using data from a series of surveys.

The problem does not always disappear when survey questions remain constant. That alone does not guarantee their validity. Social reality and popular understandings change over time; in order to capture such changed meanings, it may be necessary to alter question-naire items. Such changes confront the social researcher with a dilemma. If researchers retain constant items, their measures will increasingly depart from the social reality they are attempting to capture because that reality is continually changing. But if they alter the measure to keep up with the changing reality, they lose continuity with earlier measures. The problem has no entirely satisfactory solution. Some agencies attempt to straddle the dilemma by using both an "old" and a "new" index and devising conversion factors by which one may find equivalent values for the "old" concept using the new measure. Such conversion factors, while often the best available solution, are of dubious validity because the old indicator did not tap the phenomena measured by the new index, the reason being that these phenomena did not yet exist. Unless, by chance, one possesses measures of some underlying social phenomenon that has remained constant, one cannot validly measure social change using indicators whose definitions shift. The most promising solution is to conduct separate analyses for each portion of the time period during which the indicator remained constant. The weakness of this solution is that when one breaks a data set into several segments, one often does not have sufficient data points in each portion to conduct the type of analysis that is desired (Cook et al., 1980: 128-129).

One example of a partially successful way to address this kind of problem concerns the changing value of money. It changes in response to inflation or recession and (what Americans rarely have experienced) revaluation. Although most people think in terms of current dollars— that is, the actual number they have on their paycheck or in their bank account at any one time—economists have long converted those amounts into so-called constant dollars. Constant dollars are obtained by using a price deflator and multiplying current dollars with it. The difficulty with that procedure is that, as we have already seen with our discussion of the Consumer Price Index, such deflators themselves contain considerable error. If one wants to know how much better off one was in 1982 than in 1972, use of constant dollars is undoubtedly better than use of current dollars. However, one must be careful not to use such indicators inappropriately or to take them too literally. It may, for instance, be more valid to use current dollars when inflation is steady but slow and one wishes to make inferences about how wealthy or poor people *feel* because it is current dollars that people deal with.

Errors Arising from Inappropriate Transformations

The problem presented by the changing value of money occurs more generally. Many of the data that appear in published sources are not presented in raw form. Rather, they have been standardized by some other statistic. Just as fiscal data are often presented in constant rather than current dollars, many social statistics are the product of a transformation that involves use of another indicator. The most frequently used standard is population. Innumerable statistics are given on a per capita basis. Several errors may occur through such standardizations. Some of them arise from the use of inappropriate measures; others arise from the errors in the statistic used to make the transformation.

Mistakes are often made in choosing an appropriate measure to standardize an indicator. If one merely wishes to provide "more meaningful" comparisons, standardizing by the population is often helpful because it avoids confusing large and small effects that are simply the consequence of population size. Often, however, it is blatantly wrong to use population as a standardizer. For instance, it makes little sense to report rapes per capita when rapes are committed almost entirely against women. Yet in most of its statistical tables, the *Uniform Crime Reports* show the rape rate per 100,000 inhabitants. Moreover, it makes little sense to include young girls in the base because very few pre-adolescent girls are the victims of reported rapes. The consequence of using the inappropriate base in this instance is that rapes appear to be a much less common event than they in fact are. Education expenditures per capita also make little sense. If they are intended to show how much money was addressed to a problem, the correct measure of the "problem" is the number of school-age children, not the entire population. On the other hand, if the indicator is intended to show the resource base for such expenditures, the number of adults (excluding children) is more appropriate.

Once one becomes sensitive to this issue, one finds that a large number of indicators are calculated on the incorrect base. The correct choice is not mandated by some general rule. Rather, the base must be chosen so that it validly reflects the concept that the indicator is to measure. Inappropriate choices are sometimes made because a more appropriate base figure is unavailable or difficult to obtain. More often, standardized data are simply copied from the published source without consideration for potential misinterpretations and the availability of alternatives. Nevertheless, there may be occasions when one cannot avoid using a base that is less than optimal. When one does so, however, one should be quite conscious that the results are contaminated with the error inherent in such a choice.

In addition to the danger of choosing an inappropriate standardizer, we need to recognize the possibility that the measures used for standardization may be errorful. We have already seen how the Consumer Price Index is subject to error from many sources. We have also seen that many of the same errors and some additional ones are embedded in the population statistics from the U.S. Census (U.S. Congress, Subcommittee on Census and Population). Use of more errorful population estimates creates even more dubious statistics. Take, for example, cross-national per capita estimates. The *World Handbook* (Taylor and Hudson, 1972) reports many such statistics. For instance, it reports the number of students per one million population. For Saudi Arabia, the number is given as 240 in 1964 with no warning that this might be a biased estimate (p. 231); however, as we have seen, the editors indicate on another page (296) that the population estimate for Saudi Arabia has a 30.8% error margin. Regardless of the accuracy of the count of students (or anything else), when standardized by an errorful population estimate, the per capita statistic itself becomes contaminated with error. Whenever a measure is standardized by some other indicator, the careful researcher needs to investigate the validity and reliability of the standardizing measure. One cannot take for granted the accuracy of population statistics, monetary indices, or any of the other social indicators that are used to standardize statistics.[1]

Still another source of error in population counts and other standardizing statistics is their unavailability for the time period the researcher needs. Suppose one wishes to calculate crime rates or per capita divorce rates for cities on an annual basis. The required population statistics exist only for years in which the census was taken— for instance, 1960, 1970, and 1980 in the United States. To produce annual crime or divorce rates one needs to estimate population for each of the intervening years. That is most appropriately done when one knows the population count both for the beginning and the end of the period one is concerned with. Then one may estimate the intervening years by apportioning the change (growth or decline) to each of the nine years between censuses (Smith and Zopf, 1976; 574-579). Usually that ought not to be done by simply dividing the difference by nine; such an estimate assumes an equal growth or decline for each of the nine years, something that is quite unlikely. Rather, demographers tend to use a log-linear estimate, which has the effect of adding last year's change to the base before calculating the next data point. It assigns the largest proportion of the change to later years. Even that solution, however, still depends on uncomfortable assumptions. Without further information, one does not know whether growth occurred only during some years while during others there was a decline. One also does not know whether the growth occurred in relatively regular amounts or whether there were spurts during some years (for instance, during years of substantial economic growth) while it tapered off during other years.

Consequently, one may seek additional information about population change from such sources as utility hook-ups, health department records, or building permits. In most cases, however, few of those sources are readily available, and all are subject to their own errors. Therefore, researchers face the unenviable choice of selecting an inappropriate measure (for instance, one that is badly outdated) or using one that is full of unknown errors. It is a decision that is routinely made, but often the choice is exercised without an awareness of the possible extent to which an analysis may be damaged by it. In order to avoid misleading readers by inappropriate confidence in one's data, researchers are obligated to report their awareness of validity problems with their data and to indicate the consequences those problems pose for the researcher's conclusions.

Another danger lurks in the use of errorful standardizers (Schuessler, 1974; Fuguitt and Lieberson, 1974; Uslaner, 1976; Long, 1980). When one uses standardized indicators in multivariate analyses, the errors in the standardizer will obviously introduce unknown error into the analysis. That error cannot be estimated by referring to standard estimates of error that such analyses routinely produce, because those estimates of error refer to simple sampling error in the variables and not to the compounded error produced when two indicators are multiplied or divided by one another. In addition, one needs to take care not to include the same variable on both sides of the equation as the result of standardizing variables in terms of rates; that produces some degree of spuriousness in the analysis. For instance, one should not rely on the correlation coefficients between crime rate and per capita income because some of the relationship is produced by the population element that is common to both indicators. The recommended solution is to leave the dependent variable (the crime count in the example above) in its raw form and use the standardizing variable (for example, population) as one of the independent variables. Such procedures avoid the error of spurious correlation although they do nothing to reduce the errors that are inherent in the standardizing indicators.

Summary

Challenges to validity of measures are a fundamental problem that researchers using published data must address. Concepts that interest the researcher are often not those motivating those who collect data or who devise measures for public agencies. Challenges to validity arise from the inability of researchers who use published data to design their own indicators and the consequent gap between concept and indicator. Other problems arise from changes in concepts that may be inadequately reflected by published indicators. Still other problems come from the use of inappropriate indicators for standardizing measures. Sensitivity to these problems is the first requirement for sensible use of such data. Such sensitivity alerts the researcher to look for analysis errors that are the consequence of a mismatch between concepts and data. When compromises must be made, as is often the case, they should also be reported.

3. RELIABILITY

Reliability is the third major concern of empirical researchers. Reliability refers to the ability to obtain consistent results in successive Reliability refers to the ability to obtain consistent results in successive measurements of the same phenomenon. A scale is considered reliable if it records the same number each time a five-pound weight is placed on it. A count of the number of schools is reliable if successive counts (for the same date) produce identical results.

Reliability does not come cheaply. Consider, for instance, forecasting the size of the Florida orange crop. A reliable forecast depends on many factors; fundamental to all is knowledge of the condition of the crop. According to the *Wall Street Journal* [September 14, 1983: 1], sixty men were employed in 1983 to climb 4500 trees. Their job was to count the number of oranges on the tree limbs. Tree limbs were selected randomly, and the men climbed up them to count the oranges. The oranges on each limb were counted by two different men; if their count was not the same, they were told to recount. If they still did not agree, the supervisor climbed up and his count became the official one. One wonders, of course, what happens when no reporter is watching. Sometimes counts are faked in such operations. If every published statistic were collected with the care exhibited by the orange counters, reliability would be a smaller problem.

The user of published data cannot take it for granted that care has been exercised in the collection and reporting of information. A colleague tells a story of how a count of date trees was conducted in a village of a Third World country. An official from the central agriculture ministry arrived at the village and asked the village elder how many date trees were in the village. The elder replied, "Who knows?" After several exchanges of this sort, the elder finally exploded with impatience and told the official to write down "sixty." And sixty it became in the official statistics. Such problems, however, are not limited to Third World data. Suppose, for instance, that you were interested in analyzing gender gap in voter turnout in the United States. A number of different studies report voter turnout by sex. Table 1 shows the data from four studies for the year 1968. All four claim to be relying on the same data source—the sample surveys of the Survey Research Center at the University of Michigan—yet none of the four studies agrees with any of the others. For other years, the estimates are sometimes closer and sometimes farther apart. The analyst's conclusions appear to hinge on whether the data were taken from an earlier or later data tape, or from a published report of the data. Such mutations of data from an apparent common source often result from successive handling by archival employees and analysts.[2]

Reliability is very much a function of the characteristics of the organizations that produce and publish the data. All data are collected by organizations, large or small. Even the individual researcher often relies on assistants to photocopy or hand copy data from published sources. Such assistants are likely to make mistakes as the orange counters do, and the researcher must take the same precautions to check his assistant's accuracy. The problems increase exponentially when one depends on other organizations for one's data collection, because the

TABLE 1
Voting Turnout by Sex in 1968 in the United States (percentages)

Source	Men	Women
Lansing (1974: 8)	76	73
Lynn (1979: 406)	69	66
Poole and Zeigler (1982: Table 2)	77	72.4
Miller et al. (1980: 317)	78.1	74.1

researcher has no influence on the organizational procedures that produce his data. The more one relies on published data, the more one needs to know the organizational quirks that governed the collection and archiving of the materials.

Clerical Errors

Simple clerical errors are the bane of every research endeavor. Every research organization must make some attempt to identify their source and to minimize their effect. The usual measures include screening personnel so that the careless are given other work or are not hired at all. Those assigned to work with data must be trained so that they carry out their tasks correctly. Someone must check the data for accuracy. This may include repunching the data (using a verifier) and comparing the collected data with some other set. Incentives must exist for accurate work. No data that have not been subjected to such checks warrant our trust.

Yet some important data sets are routinely used even though they have not been subject to such precautions. The most prominent of these are election returns. Ballots are counted in tens of thousands of precincts across the country. Some of them are printed ballots on which voters indicated their choice with pen or pencil; these need to be counted manually. Others are cast on machines that automatically tally the results; still others are cast on punch cards which must be run through a counting machine. After the count has been determined, it must be recorded, telephoned to a central office where the results again must be copied, tallied, and recorded.

The employees who perform these tasks in the United States are barely trained part-timers. They are recruited by party organizations mostly for individual elections. They work a single long day from early in the morning when the polls open until the ballots have been counted in the evening. At best, most receive a few hours of training before election day, but many are doing it for the first (and last) time because counting ballots is not a task that is routinely and repetitively performed. Thus it is little wonder that results are not accurate to the last ballot even in honest elections, and we know that not all elections in our past have been honest. In most elections, counting errors make no difference in the outcome since the margin of victory is more than five percentage points and the error is probably less. But when a race is especially close, the winner is probably determined by error. For instance, in the 1982 Illinois gubernatorial contest, the margin between the incumbent James Thompson and his Democratic challenger, Adlai Stevenson III, was only 5,000 votes out of 3,6000,000 ballots. Because this is a population count rather than a random sample, we cannot precisely estimate the margin of error, but it seems likely that the official margin, which was less than two-tenths of one percent, was well within the boundaries of such an error. Assume no systematic error (such as ballot theft) in the original count; if 100 recounts were taken, one would expect Thompson to win about 50 and Stevenson to win the other 50. In such close elections, one cannot determine the winner with any confidence; one can only surmise that the race was a virtual tie.

How should researchers treat election results and similar counts when doing research? Some caution is certainly in order. When using raw totals for large jurisdictions, it is absurd to believe that the count is accurate to more than the closest thousand. In other words, one would be well advised to disregard the last three (or perhaps even four) digits of the official count. In elections and in many other instances, the official count is required by law to report the returns down to the last item. To do otherwise in elections would imply that individual votes didn't matter because they were not counted; moreover, a winner has to be designated. Consequently, voting statistics are often published, as in *America Votes* (Scammon et al., annual), with excessive pseudo-accuracy. Researchers, knowing that errors are inevitable in the counting process, should treat the count in rounded-off thousands or ten thousands.

Searching for such counting errors and the other reliability problems we will discuss below must have a high priority for all users of published statistics. Several procedures are available. Whether one has cross-sectional data (many observations at one point in time) or longitudinal data, one needs to display them in a scatter plot. Such a plot will reveal whether any cases are so deviant from the mean or the regression line that they require further investigation. Moreover, one can compare the display of one set of data with other sets that, according to one's knowledge of the phenomena, should look similar. If they do not, they bear further investigation. For instance, the data on per capita newspaper circulation in the *World Handbooks* appear suspect when one compares the numbers from the first two editions. For the United States, the per capita figures for 1960 are 326 and for 1965, 310 (Russett et al., 1964: 108; Taylor and Hudson, 1972: 242). The drop in per capita newspaper circulation seems correct if one compares it with the rise in television sets and assumes that people are substituting television for newspapers. However, if one then looks at Sweden, one finds the reported per capita newspaper circulation rose between 1960 and 1965, while the number of television sets increased even more than in the United States. Either the Swedes did not substitute television for newspapers or the data for the United States or Sweden are incorrect. On the surface, at least, such a comparison casts doubts on the reliability of the reported data. Without comparing the data from several years, one is likely to accept the numbers from one volume or the other uncritically because the tables themselves give the reader no reason to exercise exceptional caution. The comparison forces the researcher to examine the data more closely.

Changes in Collection Procedures

Official statistics often change in subtle ways that reflect changes in the organizations that collect them. The headings in official tables remain the same even though the numbers mean something slightly different because of the way in which they were collected. One needs to search for such organizational changes and take them into accont when using the data that organizations produce. Again, we may use voting statistics as an example. Registration statistics may reflect not only changes in the number of persons registering but also changes in registration requirements such as the decline in use of literacy tests and the reduction in the voting age. Other changes may be more subtle, such as alterations in the ballot-counting process that took place in the 1960s and 1970s. Paper ballots were disappearing while some form of machine readable ballot or voting machine came into increasing use. Consequently, the error discount that we attach to the vote count ought probably to be higher for election results preceding 1960 than for more recent ones. One must exercise similar caution in interpreting statistics on the incidence of particular diseases, because they reflect not only the actual incidence of those illnesses but also variations in the health agency's ability to detect them. As medical knowledge and instrumentation improve, more illnesses can be identified and reported.

Corrections Made by Collection Agency

Data are sometimes inconsistent from one report to the next because they have been subjected to an internal review and correction process. Thus, the numbers reported for a given year change from one volume to another of a statistical report. These changes reflect corrections for errors of which the agency has become aware. Sometime these corrections are simply for printing errors. Often, however, the alterations reflect an ongoing or periodical cleansing process. Some agencies inspect their data and issue corrections when they feel it is necessary. Researchers need to be aware of this correction process for several reasons. First, if they wish to use data with the least number of clerical errors, they need to know what cleansing process the organization used and the publication schedule for the corrected information. Second, if researchers are constructing a time series, they need to be aware that the earliest points of their series may be composed of corrected data while more recent points in their series may be uncorrected or partially corrected. Greater errors may be contained in the latter than in the former.

Many of the most frequently used economic indicators are treated in this way, and the differences between early estimates and "final" statistics may be quite substantial. An example is the gross national product (GNP), one of the most frequently used economic indicators.

TABLE 2

The 1976 Gross National Product as Reported in Five Successive Volume of *Statistical Abstract of the United States*

Year	Billions of Dollars
1977	1691.6
1978	1706.5
1979	1700.1
1980	1702.2
1981	1718.0

SOURCES: U.S. Bureau of the Census, Statistical Abstract of the United States (1977: 428; 1978: 440; 1979: 435; 1980: 437; 1981: 420).

Table 2 shows the United States' GNP for 1976 from five recent *Statistical Abstracts.* The difference between the 1977 and 1981 reports is $26.4 billion or 1.5%. It is particularly large between 1980 and 1981 because in 1981 a substantial correction was made that affected many of the previous years. Such large corrections are more often made during the first one or two years after a statistic is published than later. In the GNP series, the correction between first publication and the second year often exceeds $2 billion.

The propensity of agencies to correct their data poses special problems for the researchers who collect their data at one time and then use it several years later. Unless they update their data in the same way as the agency does, their published findings may be at variance with other analyses that use the newer versions of the data.

As with the vote count, there is a tendency to publish economic statistics with exaggerated accuracy even when no legal or ritualistic reason exists (as it does with the vote count) to justify it. Notice that the data in Table 2 are published to the nearest $100 million. Both public and private organizations often publish data to the nearest one or two decimal places, although the error inherent in those data are 10 or 100 times greater than that. In the case of GNP data, little would be lost if we rounded to the nearest billion or even nearest 10 billion. Such rounding signals the user that the data are not accurate to the last integer, not to speak of the last decimal place. It prevents the analyst and reader from assuming greater precision than in fact exists.

Manipulation of Data

Another set of problems arises from the contamination of data by ideological or organizational values. The data that organizations collect can have favorable or unfavorable consequences for them; sometimes organizations try to tilt the data collection process in their favor. An illuminating although fictional example was given by Alexander Solzhenitsyn in his novel, *Cancer Ward* (1969). The hospital in which much of the action takes place managed to keep its mortality rate low by discharging terminally ill patients several days before their death. When the patients died, they died at home and were not counted among those dying while under the hospital's care.

It is difficult to know how widespread such practices are, but we can be certain that they occur. In an American state mental institution, for instance, a worker reported two major changes in its apparent workload that reflected budgetary constraints rather than changes in either the population the hospital served or in the characteristics of its patients. The first change was that between 1981 and 1982 the number of violent juveniles sent to it plummeted. However, that did not reflect a decline in youthful violence. Rather, whereas in 1981 violent youths were sent to the mental hospital, in 1982 they were handled by the criminal justice system and sent to jail.

The second change was the number of patients with suicidal tendencies declined according to official records. This decline, however, did not reflect a drop in patients with suicidal tendencies, but rather resulted from a change in record keeping. Because the institution's budget had been cut and it was short-staffed, its doctors were loathe to categorize patients as suicidal since that would require the hospital to provide closer supervision for them. The hospital no longer had the staff to provide such care. Yet, if such supervision were not given to patients recorded as suicidal, the institution might be sued for medical malpractice. Hence the solution was to alter the records and report fewer patients with suicidal tendencies.[3]

Another example is the well-known tendency for schools to prep their pupils just before giving them standardized tests on which their success in educating children will be judged. The test scores may therefore not tap general knowledge of a subject but only reflect the degree to which pupils remembered answers to particular questions that they had been given earlier. Parents are also familiar with the juggling that accompanies the number of days that children are officially in school. Children are sometimes kept in school in the morning just long enough for the day to count before being sent home either because of a snow storm or because in-service training or conferences are to take place. It is important to the school to have the day recorded as a school day in the official attendance count because the size of the school's state grant often depends on the number of days it is officially in session.

Legislative roll calls produce false statistics for still another reason. Adoption of legislation involves many votes. Some are on procedural issues; others are on amendments; finally, the bill as completed must be voted upon. These votes have varying significance. Sometimes the crucial vote comes on a procedural issue; at other times one or another amendment would have the effect of gutting the bill or changing it substantially, and the vote on that amendment is the crucial one. The final vote often, but not always, has the least significance. The *Congressional Record* and the journals of many other legislative bodies record roll call votes without weighting their significance. Consequently, all serious students of legislative roll calls must make their own assessment of the votes and weight them accordingly. Simple indices based on all votes or on all final votes will necessarily be quite misleading because the votes do not mean what they appear to mean.

Data do not only mirror internal characteristics of the organizations collecting them; they also reflect the organization's ability to withstand external pressures. Even such a well-respected agency as the Bureau of Labor Statistics is subjected to enormous pressure to juggle its statistics. Our earlier discussion of the Consumer Price Index may have led an unwary reader to think that treating housing costs was simply a technical matter. In fact, it was a very political one, because the outcome had important consequences for all those people whose wages and pensions were linked to the index. The current housing cost exaggerated inflation, and many persons favored retaining it as a component of the index because it kept their payments ahead of real inflation. Moreover, many government agencies simply do not publish data that might be damaging to them (Gordon and Heinz, 1973). While "freedom of information" requests may pry such data from agencies, it is a difficult and time-consuming process that is beyond the financial reach of many researchers. Often government data are even beyond the reach of freedom of information requests, or the very nature of the activity may lead to the generation of false statistics. One example is the expenditure level for government intelligence activities. Such activities are usually disguised in a variety of ways. The published budget of the Central Intelligence Agency in the United States and parallel agencies elsewhere includes only a portion of the funds used for intelligence gathering. Other intelligence activities are scattered among the budgets of many other agencies. An analyst cannot discover how much money is spent on intelligence activities either for the United States or for any other country.

There are many other occasions for dissembling, and they affect sample surveys as well as data collected by other methods. For instance, it is well known that respondents in sample surveys may be reluctant to reveal information that they consider sensitive (Bradburn et al., 1979: 64-106). In some contexts that involves revealing their age; in others, it means that they will not provide accurate income data; they often will not give information about activities that are considered illicit. Thus, income data that come from sample surveys may be inaccurate; age distributions may be distorted; and information about drug use and handgun ownership may be quite misleading. Those conducting sample surveys are generally sensitive to these problems because they specialize in survey design. Secondary users who see the results of the surveys in some publication are much less likely to be aware of their limitations.

Government statistics are not the only ones subject to manipulation and misinterpretation. For instance, one cannot take at face value many of the balance sheets of private corporations, because they treat some important assets and liabilities in quite variable and arbitrary ways. Procter and Gamble, for instance, routinely has included "goodwill" among its current assets; in 1982 its annual report listed "goodwill and other assets" as being worth $440 million. Lockheed Corporation, on the other hand, did not list one penny for goodwill. Clearly such entries on the balance sheets are arbitrary estimates of assets that are extremely difficult to evaluate. Their presence on some balance sheets and absence on others represents quite different ways of handling important financial information. Similarly, seemingly technical accounting decisions to use LIFO (last-in, first-out) instead of FIFO (first-in, first-out) to determine the cost of inventory can dramatically change a corporation's balance sheet. Occasionally, one even reads of corporate officers pushing one quarter's sales back into a previous quarter in order to improve their record and enhance their chances for promotion or to increase their bonus.

Instrumentation

All data are the consequence of one person asking questions of someone else. There is a large body of literature on the art of asking questions productively in the context of a sample survey (Cannell and Kahn, 1968; Bradburn et al., 1979). Every manual will tell the neophyte that questions must be worded clearly, that they must ask for only one bit of information at a time, and that they should avoid a format that might lead to an acquiescence response set or one that might lead to respondent fatigue. To determine whether such problems existed for a particular data set, investigators should ferret out the particular questions used to elicit the information being analyzed. Sometimes it is possible to obtain copies of the entire survey instrument. That information is essential to the secondary users' ability to evaluate the reliability of the information they wished to use.

Although it is rarely acknowledged, the same strictures apply to other forms of information that are found in published sources. They are also the result of someone's asking questions. The way in which those questions are posed affects the reliability of the responses. Much statistical information is collected by forms that are routinely filled out by those in possession of the information. The categories in which the information is to be recorded must be meaningful to the persons filling out the data form. The respondents must be completely clear about the meaning of such terms as "operating" expenditures as opposed to "capital" expenditures, or cases "filed" as against cases "closed." If the forms are confusing or tiresome, the information that is recorded will be full of indeterminate errors. Some agencies are reputed to be quite careful about such matters. The U.S. Census Bureau in collecting expenditure information from local governments, for instance, sometimes sends its own workers into the field to check the accuracy of the recorded information or will make telephone calls to clarify apparent inconsistencies or ambiguities in responses. It behooves researchers using such data to examine the data collection sheets and to learn what checking procedures the collecting agency performed before embarking on their own analysis of data. Often such inquiries require a telephone call or letter to the collecting agency. Without such checking, researchers run the danger of anchoring their conclusions on differences in the data that reflect reliability errors rather than true differences in the phenomena that they are examining.

Categorization

All data must be classified in some manner. It is impossible to publish everyone's income in the census or to reproduce the full detail of every government agency's budget. The categories that are chosen, however, often introduce errors quite apart from the approximations that they represent because they may not be consistent from one year to the next or may differ in various data sources. Take, for instance, expenditures for police services. In some places in the United States, all urban police services are provided by the city police department. Its expenditures are synonymous with police expenditures. Other places, however, have police forces that operate outside the jurisdiction of the police department. The transit system may have its own police force and so may the housing authority. The parks may have another police force. However, these police expenditures are likely to be buried in the operating budgets of the transit, housing, and park agencies. Whereas in one city police expenditures include 99% of all policing activities, in another they may include only two-thirds.

That difficulty exists with many data categories. Money income by household status reported from census sample surveys depends on the surveyors' correctly categorizing the household from which they are obtaining information; it also depends on the respondents' correctly understanding the categories they are being asked about. Whether a household is composed of related or unrelated individuals is not easily, quickly, or consistently discernible. One finds the same kind of problem with obtaining information about the number of motor vehicle accidents. For instance, the U.S. Census Bureau (1982-83: 615-616) reports different data for the number of deaths from motor vehicle accidents in two adjacent tables. In one table the data are categorized by the date of the accident; in the other, they are categorized by the year of the death. Moreover, the deaths are classified by the state in which they occurred rather than the state in which the victim lived. Those classification decisions may make no difference for some analyses, but for others they will be crucial.

Summary

I have pointed to five factors that require particular attention. The first is the amount of training and supervision provided those who collect the data. The less it is, the greater the error that will have to be discounted. The second element that needs to be discovered is the internal purposes served by the data and the internal implications of statistics for an organization. Third, one needs to be concerned with potential instrumentation problems. Fourth, if researchers use data collected repeatedly over some period of time, they need to determine what changes took place in the training and supervision of the persons who collected the data they are using. The data are likely to be more accurate for some periods than for others; alternatively, the error will be in one direction during one period and in the opposite direction during another period. Fifth, researchers need to be aware of the implications of classification decisions made by the original collectors of the data.

4. CONCLUSION

The problems that accompany the use of published data are manifold, but so are the solutions. Both demand careful examination.

Perhaps the most important attribute for the user of published data is a large dose of skepticism. Whether data are found in libraries or data archives, they should not be viewed simply as providing grand opportunities for cheap analyses; they should be seen as problematic. In every case the analyst should ask, Are these data valid? In what ways might they have been contaminated so that they are unreliable? In many instances the data will pass muster. However, in many other cases the data will be revealed as flawed in some fundamental way. It is the duty of the analyst to discover the flaws and, if possible, to correct them.

Researchers must subject published data to as many tests as they can devise. They must look for convergent and discriminant validity. They must display them on scatter plots to identify suspicious deviant data points. When they find them lacking, they must devise remedial strategies. In many cases one can improve validity and reliability by joining the data with other bits of information. One can go beyond the published source to persons in the agency to learn what might be done to improve data quality. When it is not possible to improve it, one can use them with extra precautions employing such measures as avoiding exaggerated precision, alerting readers to data quality problems, and erring on the side of conservatism in interpreting one's results. In a few instances the contaminations are irremediable and the task must be abandoned.

In the preceding pages I have described many of the most common problems encountered in using published data and some of some ways of overcoming them. I summarize them in Table 3.

Most of the remedies have been sufficiently illustrated in the preceding pages; a few, however, need further elaboration. One of those is among the simplest available to the analyst: directly requesting further information about published data from the collecting agency. Two steps are required in most instances. The first is a series of telephone calls to determine who in the agency possesses the technical information that is required. This may be necessary even if the data come from a reputable archive like the Inter-University Consortium of Political and Social Research. Errors may have been introduced during the archival process; often they can be traced only by comparing the data obtained from the archive with the original data from its collector. A preliminary conversation with that person is often helpful. Such a conversation, however, must often be followed by a letter specifying the information that is needed. Correspondence is important because oral requests are often poorly formulated, misunderstood, and mislaid. In many instances, requests for technical information will receive quick and thorough attention.

TABLE 3
Summary of Data Problems and Potential Solutions

Problem	Solution
Selection Error	For random samples, specify sampling error. For counts and nonrandom samples, round off to signal error and avoid exaggerated accuracy.
Invalidity	
Construct validity: Misfit between collector's and user's conceptualization	To diagnose, look for convergence with other measures and/or ability to discriminate from other concepts. Then use multiple measures, choose most appropriate alternative measure, or abandon study if no valid measure exists.
Changing circumstances causes invalidity	Search for and use indicator underlying variable common to past and present phenomenon. Calculate "conversion" factor from old to new. Undertake separate analyses for time periods when definition remained constant.
Inappropriate transformations	Use correct variable for transforming data. Watch for errors in variable used for making the transformation. Take into account potential invalidity of transforming variable. Avoid using same transformation for both dependent and independent variables.
Unavailability of data for required data points	Interpolate using log-linear methods, supplemented by additional data.
Reliability	
Clerical errors	Look for deviant cases in scatterplot. Check amount of training given by collecting agencies. Round off.
Change in collection procedures	Make separate reliability assessments for each segment of the data.

(continued)

TABLE 3 (Continued)

Problem	Solution
Corrections made by collection agency	Look for accounts of correction procedures and the times when they were applied.
Manipulation of data	Look for media and congressional accounts of such manipulations. Talk to insiders.
Instrumentation	Search for copy of data collection instrument and examine it for instrumentation errors.
Categorization	Look for inconsistencies across place and time. Try to recombine data into more consistent categories

Scatterplots have widespread use in identifying potential trouble in a data set. They should be routinely employed during the first examination of a set of data. One should look for two warning signals. The first is deviant points that cannot be readily explained by the theory one is testing. Such deviant points do not invariably represent data errors, but often they do. One can save many hours of work and much embarrassment by searching for the errors before elaborating some new theoretical statement to account for the deviant data. One method for examining these deviant points further is to collect additional information. If the points are in a cross-sectional data set, one should look at a time series for the questionable points. For example, if Philadelphia crime statistics look suspiciously low when compared to other cities of similar size, one should examine them for a number of years before and after the original point. If the point that one originally examined does not stick out suspiciously in the time series, one can be a little more certain that the observation is not a reflection of random error. It may, of course, reflect systematically different ways of counting the data in that jurisdiction. On the other hand, if the data point is also deviant in the time series, one may find the explanation by examining the data collection methods that produced that observation. It may reflect an error or it may represent some unusual occurence.

The second test one should apply to scatter plots is whether they show much *less* variability than one would otherwise expect. A completely flat line in one time series when many others show considerable variation should lead the researcher to suspect that something may be amiss. Once more, further examination is required.

Careful examination of published data can save one from absurd results. A dramatic example comes from the work of Coale and Stephan (1962: 338) on census data that seemed to show a surprising number of teenage widowers:

> The number [of teenage widowers] listed by the Census . . . were 1,670 at age 14; 1,475 at age 15; 1,175 at 16. . . . Not until age 22 did the listed number of widowers surpass those at 14. Male divorces also decrease in number as age increases from 1,320 at age 14 to 575 at age 17.

The explanation for this curious set of numbers was that some keypunch operators moved the data one column to the right so that middle-aged males became teenagers in the census reports. In this instance Coale and Stephan simply used their prior knowledge of American culture to identify potentially incorrect data. They could not be certain that teenage widowers did not exist in the numbers originally reported by the census, but it seemed quite unlikely. Others need to follow their example. Researchers should not be afraid to apply their knowledge. As they become more familiar with their research problem, they will become more adept in identifying potential data errors.

When possible, the incorrect data should be replaced with correct information or deleted from the analysis. In some instances, however, the researcher will remain uncertain about the reliability of the data. It may look suspicious, but no definite errors can be identified. In a time series, a partial remedy may be to average observations over several time points. One may replace the original data with a rolling three- or five-year average. That has the effect of dampening the series and possibly obscuring relationships. On the other hand, if the variations reflect suspected data collection errors rather than real fluctuations, the dampening produced by the use of a rolling average is a conservative approach that avoids unwarranted findings.

Equal skepticism should be applied to cross-sectional data. Most analysts using cross-sectional indicators display little sensitivity to the effects of their choice of date at which they conduct their analysis. Many analyses use data at census years because much demographic information is available only at such time points. Other data, however, that are part of such an analysis may be drawn from continuous time series. Researchers often take those data without examining whether they are suspicious blips of a time series that indicate probable error. To do so requires some additional labor. As we have already suggested, for each suspicious cross-sectional data point, a time series of 15-20 observations should be examined to determine that the observation is not a substantially deviant case that in all likelihood reflects error rather than true variation. Only then can one proceed to the planned analysis with some confidence that the data represent relatively error-free observations.

Finally, the question of rounding data from census count or nonrandom samples will often appear troublesome because no hard rule can be recommended that will yield the exact amount of rounding to apply. Once again, researchers must depend on their knowledge of the data. If the organization that collected the data has a good reputation for collecting information carefully, a smaller rounding may be applied than when one knows that the organization is usually careless. For instance, census population counts in the United States are probably more accurate than vote counts or police crime counts. That is true because we know that census employees are trained and supervised more painstakingly than are persons who count votes or police officers who record crimes. Moreover, one has to look at the size of the statistics. Rounding three digits off numbers that are originally in the thousands is a very large correction. Reporting figures that originally are in the billions with the last three digits omitted is a much smaller correction. One must use one's best judgment in making such corrections. However, it is usually better to err in employing some degree of rounding than not to round off at all, because the rounding (whatever it is) will alert readers to data problems that might otherwise go unnoticed.

Many problems lurk among the multitude of published statistics that await researchers in their libraries. They constitute a rich lode of materials on which many substantial analyses can be performed, but these data must be refined and treated with respect. They cannot be plucked mechanically from their source and entered into an analysis. Without exception, all published statistics should be treated with suspicion. One needs to inspect them for inconsistencies and errors in reporting. One must learn about the organizations that produced them and the errors organizational preferences introduced into them. One must question the ways in which indicators were standardized. In the end, some validity and reliability problems are likely to remain unresolved, but they need never lie unaddressed in the interpretation of results.

APPENDIX: A BRIEF NOTE ON SOURCES
AND CRITIQUES OF IMPORTANT DATA SETS

A brief description of many of the most important publicly available data sets may be found in Taeuber and Rockwell (1982). The data described in that paper are all available in machine readable form; many of them are also available in published form.

The census is the richest data base on the characteristics of people in the United States. Prior to the 1980 census, most of the data were published in printed form. Much of the 1980 data are available only in microfiche or machine readable form. The Census Bureau also publishes technical reports that provide a wealth of information about particular data problems and the solutions the Census Bureau has adopted. In addition, several congressional hearings provide much information about undercounts and biases in the 1970 and 1980 censuses (see the House Subcommittee on Census and Population [U.S. Congress, 1977]; House Subcommittee on Census and Population [U.S. Congress, 1980]; Senate Committee on Governmental Affairs [U.S. Congress, 1980]).

The census is also the source of most statistics on government expenditures. Anton et al. (1980) provide a detailed and sometimes devastating critique of these numbers. Other useful critiques include Collins (1982) and Fossett and Kramer (1981).

The Consumer Price Index is a product of the Bureau of Labor Statistics. Particularly helpful critiques may be found in Blinder (1980), Gordon (1981), and Wahl (1982). Unemployment statistics are also produced by the Bureau of Labor Statistics. Some of the problems associated with these data are discussed by Shiskin (1976), Groth (1982), and statements by Norwood and Landrieu before the House Subcommitte on State, Justice and Commerce (U.S. Congress, 1976).

Economic statistics are the subject of the landmark book by Oskar Morgenstern (1963). Another more recent but more limited discussion is to be found in Parker (1982).

Crime data are cirtiqued by almost every author using them. Some of the best discussions are by Penick and Owens (1976), Skogan (1975, 1981), and Biderman and Reiss (1967).

The problems associated with vote counts have not been discussed in the literature. There are, however, some good discussions of the effects of varying registration procedures on voter turnout. For these, see Kelly et al. (1967), Kim et al. (1975), and Rosenstone and Wolfinger (1978). The counts themselves are most fully reported in Scammon et al. (annual).

The principal depository for social data is the Inter-University consortium for Political and Social Research at the University of Michigan. Its holdings include the data base for many government studies, census data, and the data files from many individual researchers and social science organizations. It also has the polling data for the Survey Research Center's election studies. Its data holdings are in machine readable form and are accompanied by considerable documentation that alerts users to potential sources of error. Other public opinion polling data are held by the National Opinion Research Center at the University of Chicago, the Roper Center at the University of Connecticut, the Institute for Research in Social Science at the University of North Carolina, and the Gallup Social Science Research Group at Princeton, New Jersey. Many smaller and specialized archives exist on other university campuses.

Cross-national data are available from a variety of United Nations publications. These are combined with data from other sources in the two editions of the *World Handbook of Political and Social Indicators*. The first (Russett et al., 1964) includes data up to 1961; the second (Taylor and Hudson, 1972) includes data through 1965. A third edition is available in machine readable form from the Inter-University Consortium for Political and Social Research and has data pertaining to the 1970s. As I indicated in the text, these data must be used with extreme caution; in many instances these volumes provide insufficient warnings about the quality of the data. A model of care for data quality is represented by Janda's *Political Parties* (1980). It provides information about political parties in 53 countries between 1950 and 1962, with further information about the history of these parties through 1978. That publication includes comprehensive information about the reliability of the reported data and the methods used to determine validity and reliability.

NOTES

1. Note, however, that when one compares two measures that are standardized with the same statistic (e.g., population size), the error introduced by that standardization is constant. In other words, one does not increase the error by using such a standardization measure.

2. I am indebted to Virginia Gray for calling my attention to these data and to the discrepancies shown in Table 1.

3. These observations were reported via personal communication with a staff member at the institution.

REFERENCES

ANTON, T. J., J. P. CAWLEY, and K. L. KRAMER (1980) Moving Money. Cambridge, MA: Oelgeschlager, Gunn & Hain.

BARBER, R. E. (1953) Marriage and Family. New York: McGraw-Hill.

BIDERMAN, A. D. and A. J. REISS, Jr. (1967) "On exploring the 'dark figure' of crime." The Annals of the American Academy of Political and Social Science (November): 1-15.

BISHOP, G. F., A. J. TUCHFARBER, and R. W. OLDENICK (1978) "Change in the structure of American political attitudes." American Journal of Political Science 22: 250-269.

———and S. E. BENNETT (1979) "Questions about question wording: a rejoinder to revisiting mass belief systems revisited." American Journal of Political Science 23: 187-192.

BLINDER, A. S. (1980) "Consumer Price Index and the measurement of recent inflation." Brookings Papers on Economic Activity no. 2: 539-573.

BOOTH, A, D. R. JOHNSON, and H. M. CHOLDIN (1977) "Correlates of city crime rates: victimization surveys versus official statistics." Social Problems 25: 187.

BRADBURN, N. M., S. SUDMAN, and Associates (1979) Improving Interview Method and Questionnaire Design. San Francisco: Jossey-Bass.

CAMPBELL, D. T. and J. C. STANLEY (1966) Experimental and Quasi-experimental Designs for Research. Chicago: Rand McNally.

CANNELL, C. F. and R. F. KAHN (1968) "Interviewing," in G. Linzey and E. Aronson (eds.) Handbook of Social Psychology, vol. 2. Reading, MA: Addison-Wesley.

CARMINES, E. G. and R. A. ZELLER (1979) Reliability and Validity Assessment. Beverly Hills, CA: Sage.

CHERLIN, A. (1981) Marriage, Divorce, Remarriage. Cambridge, MA: Harvard University Press.

Chicago Tribune (1983) April 11: 1.

COALE, A. J. and F. F. STEPHAN (1962) "The case of the Indians and the teen-age widows," Journal of the American Statistical Association 57 (June): 338-347.

COLLINS, J. N. (1982) "Uses and limitations of 1977 Census of Governments Finance Data." Review of Public Data Use 10(May): 9-22.

COOK, T. D. and D. T. CAMPBELL (1979) Quasi-experimentation: Design and Analysis Issues for Field Settings. Chicago: Rand McNally.

COOK, T. D., L. DINTZER, and M. M. MARK (1980) "The causal analysis of concomitant time series" in L. Bickman (ed.) Applied Social Psychology Annual, vol. 1. Beverly Hills, CA: Sage.

Federal Bureau of Investigation (annual) Uniform Crime Reports. Washington, DC: Government Printing Office.

FOSSETT, J. W. and K. L. KRAMER (1981) "Urban revival, federal funds and the census: an assessment of federal data on cities," Prepared for delivery at the Midwest Political Science Association meetings, Cincinnati, OH, April 1981. (mimeo)

FUGUITT, G. V. and S. LIEBERSON (1974) "Correlation of ratios or difference scores having common terms," in H. L. Costner (ed.) Sociological Methodology. San Francisco: Jossey-Bass.

GORDON, A. C. and J. P. HEINZ [eds.] (1979) Public Access to Information. New Brunswick, NJ: Transaction Books.

GORDON, R. J. (1981) "The Consumer Price Index: measuring inflation and causing it." Public Interest (Spring): 112-134.

GROTH, P. G. (1982) "Values and the measurement of unemployment." Social Science Quarterly 63(March): 154-159.

JANDA, K. (1980) Political Parties: A Cross National Survey. New York: Free Press.

KALTON, G. (1983) Introduction to Survey Sampling. Beverly Hills, CA: Sage.

KELLEY, S. Jr., R. AYERS, and W. G. BOWEN (1967) "Registration and voting: putting first things first," American Political Science Review 61: 359-377.

KIM, J. Θ. et al. (1975) "Voter turnout among the American states." American Political Science Review 69: 107-131.

KISH, L. (1965) Survey Sampling. New York: John Wiley.

LANSING, M. (1974) "American woman: voter and activist," in J. Jaquette (ed.) Women in Politics. New York: John Wiley.

LONG, S. B. (1980) "The continuing debate over the use of ratio variables: facts and fiction," in K. F. Schuessler (ed.) Sociological Methodology. San Francisco: Jossey-Bass.

LYNN, N. (1979) "Women in American politics: an overview," in J. Freeman (ed.) Women: A Feminist Perspective. Palo Alto, CA: Mayfield.

McCLEARY, R. and R. A. HAY, Jr. (1980) Applied Time Series Analysis for the Social Sciences. Beverly Hills, CA: Sage.

MILLER, W. E., A. H. MILLER, and E. J. SCHNEIDER (1980) American National Election Studies Data Sourcebook, 1952-1978. Cambridge, MA: Harvard University Press.

MORGENSTERN, O. (1963) On the Accuracy of Economic Observations. Princeton, NJ: Princeton University Press. New York Times (1983) September 7: 12.

NIE, N. H. and J. RABJOHN (1979) "Revisiting mass belief systems revisited: or, doing research is like watching a tennis match." American Journal of Politcal Science 23: 139-175.

PALUMBO, D. J. (1977) Statistics in Political and Behavioral Science. New York: Columbia University Press.

PARKER, R. P. (1982) "The quality of the U.S. national income and product accounts." Review of Public Data Use 10(May): 1-8.

PENICK, B.K.E. and M.E.B. OWENS, III [eds.] (1976) Surveying Crime. Washington, DC: National Academy of Science.

POOLE, K. and H. ZEIGLER (1982) "Gender and voting in the 1980 presidential election." Presented at the annual meeting of the American Political Science Association, Denver, CO.

ROSENSTONE, S. J. and R. E. WOLFINGER (1978) "The effect of registration laws on voter turnout." American Political Science Review 72: 22-45.

RUSSETT, B. M., H. R. ALKER, Jr., K. W. DEUTSCH, and H. D. LASSWELL (1964) World Handbook of Political and Social Indicators. New Haven, CT: Yale University Press.

SCAMMON, R. A. et al. (annual) America votes. Washington, DC: Congressional Quarterly.

SCHUESSLER, K. (1974) "Analysis of ratio variables." American Journal of Sociology 80: 379.

SELLITIZ, C., L. S. WRIGHTSMAN, and S. W. COOK (1976) Research Methods in the Social Sciences. New York: Holt, Rinehart and Winston.

SHELLEY, L. (1979) "Soviet criminology After the revolution." Journal of Criminal Law and Criminology 70: 390-396.

SHISKIN, J. (1976) "Employment and unemployment: the doughnut or the hole?" Monthly Labor Review 99(Feb): 3-10.

SIMON, J. L. (1978) Basic Research Methods in Social Sciences. New York: Random House.

SKOGAN, W. G. (1981) Issues in the Measurement of Victimization. Washington, DC: Bureau of Justice Statistics.

———(1975) "Measurement problems in official and survey rates." Journal of Criminal Justice (Spring): 17-31.

SMITH, L. T. and P. E. ZOPF, Jr. (1976) Demography: Principles and Methods. New York: Alfred.

SOLZHENITSYN, A. (1969) Cancer Ward. New York: Farrar, Strauss = Giroux.

SULLIVAN, J. L. and S. FELDMAN (1979) Multiple Indicators. Beverly Hills, CA: Sage.

SULLIVAN, J. L., J. E. PIERESON, and G. E. MARCUS (1978) "Ideological constraint in the mass public: a methodological critique and some new findings." American Journal of Political Science, 22: 233-249.

———and S. FELDMAN (1979) "The more things change, the more they remain the same: rejoinder to Nie and Rabjohn." American Journal of Political Science 23: 176-186.

TAEUBER, R. C. and R. C. ROCKWELL (1982) "National social data series: a compendium of brief descriptions," Review of Public Data Use 10: 23-111.

TAYLOR, C. S. and M. C. HUDSON (1972) World Handbook of Political and Social Indicators, second edition. New Haven, CT: Yale University Press.

U.S. Bureau of the Census (1982-83) Statistical Abstract of the United States. Washington, DC: Government Printing Office.

———(1981) Statistical Abstract of the United States. Washington, DC: Government Printing Office.

———(1977) County and City Data Book. Washington, DC: Government Printing Office.

U.S. Congress, House of Representatives, Subcommittee on Census and Population (1980a) Hearings, Com. Serial 96-63.
——(1980b) Hearings, July 30.
——(1977) Hearings, Com. Serial 95-46.
U.S. Congress, House of Representatives, Subcommittee on Commerce, Consumers and Monetary Affairs (1980) Hearings, March 18.
U. S. Congress, House of Representatives, Subcommittee on State, Justice and Commerce (1976) Hearings, July 28-30.
U.S. Congress, Senate Committee on Governmental Affairs (1980) The Decennial Census: An Analysis and Review. 96th Congress, 2d Session.
U. S. Department of Justice (1979) National Crime Survey: Criminal Victimization in the United States: 1973-79. Washington, DC: Government Printing Office.
USLANER, E. N. (1976) "The pitfalls of per capita." American Journal of Political Science 20: 125.
WALH, R. C. (1982) "Is the Consumer Price Index a fair measure of inflation?" Journal of Policy Analysis and Mangement 1(Summer): 496-511.
WARWICK, D. P. and C. A. LININGER (1975) The Sample Survey: Theory and Practice. New York: McGraw-Hill.

INDEX

Abstractions, difficulty of, 97
Accounts, literal-minded, 101-102
Accuracy, 4, 5, 259
Acquiescence responses, 120-121
Age data, 358, 372
Agree/disagree items, 95, 120, 127, 131
Alienation scores, 126
Alternative answers, 21, 97
Ambiguity:
    category definitions and, 267
    phrases and, 291
    questions and, 100-102
Analysis:
    abandoning, 352-353
    codes and, 20
    combining categories, 31
    computer-assisted data collection and,
        241-242
    data preparation for, 8, 57-58
    form design and, 17-18
    minimizing transformations during,
        20
    missing values and, 63-64
    observations and, 4
    open-ended questions and, 11, 18
    subfiles for, 78
    unit of, 356-357
Analysis of covariance, 308
Analysis of variance, 71, 265, 283, 313
Answers, 1, 112, 115
    closed-ended questions and, 14-24
    complex, 26
    creating, 22-24
    exhaustive, 14, 15-16, 26
    incomplete, 40
    internal consistency of, 344
    middle category, 118-119
    mutually exclusive, 14, 17
    nonexistent, 58-60
    range checks, 208-210
    sequence of, 182
    short open-ended, 25-26

single versus multiple, 21
study objectives related to, 30-31
summary screens and, 203-204
Arcsin square root transformation, 313
Arithmetic transformations, 66
Articles, content analysis and, 274
ASCII files, 46
Attitudes:
    behavior and, 115
    complexity of, 127-129
    data collection and, 19
    intensity of, 119-120
    latent-indicator models of, 316
    magnitude scaling of, 111-113
    measures of, 71
    questions and, 99-100, 114-115
    realistic, 105
    reporting of, 21
    structure of, 75
Audiotapes, 4
Averaging observations, 379
Averaging time use, 103-104

Background information, 143, 214-215,
    221-222
Back-translation, 320-321
Bar codes, 239
Batch processing, 44
Behavior, 7
    attitudes and, 115
    electronic equipment and, 168
    measurement of sensitive or disap-
        proved, 116
    predictors of, 115
    questions and, 99-100, 113-114
    reporting, 21
Bias, 2, 63, 130
Blacks, undercounted, 343
BMDP program, 47, 58, 60, 63, 69, 76
Books, sampling, 285
Bounded recall, 102-103, 216
Branching, 171-172, 183

ABOUT THE EDITOR

MICHAEL S. LEWIS-BECK, Professor of Political Science at the University of Iowa, received his Ph.D. from the University of Michigan. Currently, in addition to editing the Sage monograph series *Quantitative Applications in the Social Sciences (QASS)*, he is editor of the *American Journal of Political Science*. He has authored or coauthored numerous books and articles, including *Applied Regression: An Introduction, New Tools for Social Scientists: Advances and Applications in Research Methods, Economics and Elections: The Major Western Democracies,* and *Forecasting Elections.* In addition to his work at the University of Iowa, he has taught quantitative methods courses at the Inter-University Consortium for Political and Social Research (ICPSR) Summer Program at the University of Michigan and The European Consortium for Political Research (ECPR) Summer Program at the University of Essex. Also, he has held visiting appointments at the Catholic University in Lima, Peru, and the University of Paris I (Sorbonne) in France.

ABOUT THE AUTHORS

LINDA B. BOURQUE is Professor and Head of the Division of Population and Family Health, and Vice Chair of the Department of Community Health Sciences, in the School of Public Health at the University of California at Los Angeles, where she teaches courses in research design and survey methodology. Her research is in the area of intentional and unintentional injury. She is the author or coauthor of 40 scientific articles and the book *Defining Rape*. She received her Ph.D. in sociology from Duke University.

VIRGINIA A. CLARK is Professor Emeritus of Biostatistics in the School of Public Health and Biomathematics in the School of Medicine at the University of California at Los Angeles. She is an expert in multivariate analysis and has consulted in biomedical and economic studies. She is author of more than 80 scientific articles and coauthor of four textbooks: *Preparation for Basic Statistics* (with Michael E. Tarter), *Applied Statistics: Analysis of Variance and Regression* (2nd ed.) (with O. Jean Dunn), *Survival Distributions: Reliability Applications in the Biomedical Sciences* (with Alan Gross), and *Computer-Aided Multivariate Analysis* (2nd ed.) (with A. A. Afifi). She received her Ph.D. in biostatistics from the University of California at Los Angeles.

JEAN M. CONVERSE is a former director of the Detroit Area Study, University of Michigan. She is author of the book, *Survey Research in the United States: Roots and Emergence 1890-1960;* and coauthor with Howard Schuman of *Conversations at Random: Survey Research as Interviewers See It.*

HERBERT JACOB is Professor of Political Science at Northwestern University. He received his Ph.D. from Yale University and previously taught at Tulane University, Johns Hopkins University, and the University of Wisconsin, Madison. He is past president of the Law & Society Association, and has been a Fellow at the Center for Advanced Studies in the Behavioral Sciences at Stanford University and at the Centre for

Socio-Legal Research at Oxford University. He is editor of the *Law &
Politics Book Review*. He has written widely on the American legal
system. His most recent books are *Silent Revolution: The Transformation of Divorce in the United States* (1988) and *Law and Politics in the
United States* (1995).

STANLEY PRESSER, formerly director of the Detroit Area Study, is
currently director of the Sociology Program at the National Science
Foundation. He is coauthor with Howard Schuman of *Questions and
Answers in Attitude Surveys: Experiments in Question Wording, Form,
and Context,* and coeditor with Elizabeth Martin and Diana McDuffee
of the *Sourcebook of Harris National Surveys: Repeated Questions
1963-1976.*

WILLEM E. SARIS is Professor in the Department of Methods and
Techniques for Political Science at the University of Amsterdam, The
Netherlands. He received his masters in sociology at the University of
Utrecht and his Ph.D. in social science at the University of Amsterdam.
He is currently Chairman of the Sociometric Research Foundation. He
has published numerous professional articles and books. Some of his
present research interests involve: structural equation modeling, improvement of measurement in social science research, and the development of computer-assisted interviewing.

ROBERT PHILIP WEBER is currently a Principal of Northeast Consulting Resources, Inc., a Boston consulting firm. He holds a Ph.D. in
sociology, is a founding member of the Sociology of Culture section of
the American Sociological Association, and past editor of *Culture,* the
section newsletter. Dr. Weber has been a Fullbright fellow and guest
professor and lecturer in Germany, Sweden, the Netherlands, and the
UK. The author of more than a dozen papers on content analysis and on
long-term social, economic, political, and cultural change, he is also
coauthor with J. Z. Namenwirth of *Dynamics of Culture* (1987) and
coauthor with C. Zuell and P. Ph. Mohler of *Computer-Assisted Text
Analysis for the Social Sciences: The General Inquirer III* (1989). With
P. J. Stone, he is coauthor of the article on "content analysis" in the
Encyclopedia of Sociology (1992).